Mastering Public Health

ESSENTIAL SKILLS FOR EFFECTIVE PRACTICE

EDITED BY

BARRY S. LEVY

JOYCE R. GAUFIN

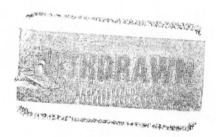

OXFORD
UNIVERSITY PRESS

OXFORD
UNIVERSITY PRESS

Oxford University Press, Inc., publishes works that further
Oxford University's objective of excellence
in research, scholarship, and education.

Oxford New York
Auckland   Cape Town   Dar es Salaam   Hong Kong   Karachi
Kuala Lumpur   Madrid   Melbourne   Mexico City   Nairobi
New Delhi   Shanghai   Taipei   Toronto

With offices in
Argentina   Austria   Brazil   Chile   Czech Republic   France   Greece
Guatemala   Hungary   Italy   Japan   Poland   Portugal   Singapore
South Korea   Switzerland   Thailand   Turkey   Ukraine   Vietnam

Copyright © 2012 by Oxford University Press, Inc.

Published by Oxford University Press, Inc.
198 Madison Avenue, New York, New York 10016
www.oup.com

Oxford is a registered trademark of Oxford University Press

Library of Congress Cataloging-in-Publication Data

Mastering public health : essential skills for effective practice / edited by Barry S. Levy, Joyce R. Gaufin.
    p. ; cm.
  Includes bibliographical references.
  ISBN 978-0-19-975397-0 (pbk. : alk. paper)
  I. Levy, Barry S. II. Gaufin, Joyce R.
  [DNLM: 1. Public Health Practice. WA 100]

  LC classification not assigned
  362.1068—dc23   2011029793

9 8 7 6 5 4 3 2 1

Printed in China
on acid-free paper

This material is not intended to be, and should not be considered, a substitute for medical or other
professional advice. Treatment for the conditions described in this material is highly dependent on the
individual circumstances. And, while this material is designed to offer accurate information with respect
to the subject matter covered and to be current as of the time it was written, research and knowledge about
medical and health issues is constantly evolving and dose schedules for medications are being revised
continually, with new side effects recognized and accounted for regularly. Readers must therefore always
check the product information and clinical procedures with the most up-to-date published product
information and data sheets provided by the manufacturers and the most recent codes of conduct and
safety regulation. The publisher and the authors make no representations or warranties to readers, express
or implied, as to the accuracy or completeness of this material. Without limiting the foregoing, the
publisher and the authors make no representations or warranties as to the accuracy or efficacy of the drug
dosages mentioned in the material. The authors and the publisher do not accept, and expressly disclaim,
any responsibility for any liability, loss or risk that may be claimed or incurred as a consequence of the use
and/or application of any of the contents of this material.

Foreword

"Where is the wisdom we have lost in knowledge?
Where is the knowledge we have lost in information?"
—T. S. Eliot

Seldom do we see a book that so clearly and persuasively presents fresh practical information as in the case in this "labor of love" compiled by two wise leaders—Barry Levy and Joyce Gaufin. As I read the chapters, I continued to say to myself, "That is exactly what public health practitioners need to know now." This book very effectively addresses the needs of public health leaders and managers who will say, "I wish I had this book years ago!" In effect, the book helps all of us to find the wisdom we have lost in the avalanche of information that daily inundates public health practitioners.

Why will *Mastering Public Health* be so useful?

First, the authors are wise and very experienced public health leaders with a wide range of expertise and decades of front-line experience at the local, state, and national level. As I read through the book, I concluded that "they know whereof they speak."

Second, they have taken the time to reflect on these experiences and distill them down into very practical guidance that busy practitioners can put to use immediately. This is a practical book for thoughtful practitioners containing many "best practices" that are succinctly presented.

Third, *Mastering Public Health* clearly stands apart from any existing book dedicated to the learning needs of public health practitioners. It is truly unique. Furthermore, it comes along at a pivotal time in the history of public health practice in the United States. Developing the skills of public health leaders and managers is needed now more than ever before.

This book will be a vital resource for the network of public health leadership and management institutes across the nation, which Joyce Gaufin and others of us have helped to create. Schools of public health and other academic institutions will now have a book that students will *love* because it will help them prepare for the work they will be doing once they enter "the real world."

The individual chapters of the book—focusing on such topics as communication, organizational development, cultural competency, systems thinking, and leadership and management practice—"cover the waterfront" of public health practice. The authors not only share a wealth of experience but also reference relevant literature. As a result, the book effectively synthesizes a wealth of practice experience with the expertise of researchers and subject-matter experts who have studied these areas of leadership and management practice.

I can hardly wait to use this book! I know many others will use the book as we teach the next generation of public health leaders. It fills a vital niche in the public health practice literature and will become a "must-have" text for those who are committed to building a stronger public health workforce that can effectively take on the challenges ahead.

Congratulations to Barry Levy, Joyce Gaufin, and all of the contributors to *Mastering Public Health* for giving us a book that we need now and will use for years to come!

Edward L. Baker, M.D., M.P.H.
Chapel Hill, North Carolina

Preface

Warning: Your reading this book will *not* make you a master of public health. It alone will *not* enable you to achieve mastery in this field. Put it back where you found it if that's what you were hoping to get out of opening the cover.

However, taken together with other education, training, and experience, this book *will* enable you to achieve greater mastery in the day-to-day practice of public health by learning from numerous experienced public health leaders about essential skills for effective public health practice—in government agencies, in non-governmental organizations, in academic institutions, in private-sector organizations, and other work settings.

Mastering Public Health is a "how-to" book focused on "nuts-and-bolts" skills in three broad areas of public health practice: Communication, Administration and Management, and Leadership. This book has three parts corresponding to these three areas. Each part consists of five chapters and additional commentaries on lessons learned from the experiences of leaders and experts in this field.

This book is designed to complement the content-oriented knowledge and skills you have acquired in your education, training, and experience thus far. It addresses many of the practical skills necessary for you to be effective in your work and to lay a foundation for your further career development.

We believe you will find *Mastering Public Health* to be a valuable guide—whether you are an epidemiologist in a state health department, a public health nutritionist or health educator in a community organization, a public health nurse for a city health agency, a faculty member in an academic institution, a public health director of a health-promotion program in the private sector, or any other public health professional—or student in the health professions.

Mastering of skills for public health practice is not a destination, but a journey that lasts for your entire career. We intend that this book will serve you well on this journey.

Barry S. Levy
Sherborn, Massachusetts

Joyce R. Gaufin
Dammeron Valley, Utah

June 2011

Acknowledgments

We greatly appreciate the assistance and support of many people in the development of *Mastering Public Health*. We thank the many contributing authors, who have shared their experience and advice.

We acknowledge Heather McStowe for her excellent work in preparing the manuscript and communicating with authors and the production team.

We are grateful for the outstanding work and support of Maura Roessner, Regan Hofmann, Rachel Mayer, and Leslie Johnson of the editorial and production departments at Oxford University Press; Viswanath Prasanna and Smitha Raj of Glyph International; and Wendy Walker, who copyedited the manuscript.

We express our deep appreciation to our spouses, Nancy Levy and Richard Gaufin, for their ongoing support.

Finally, we express our appreciation to our mentors and colleagues who, over the years, have taught us essential skills for effective practice in public health.

- B.S.L. and J.R.G.

Contents

Contributors

Carol Easley Allen, Ph.D., R.N.
Professor and Chair
Department of Nursing
Oakwood University
Huntsville, AL
callen@oakwood.edu

Myron Allukian, Jr., D.D.S., M.P.H.
Oral Health Consultant
President
American Association for Community
    Dental Programs
Boston, MA
MyAlluk@aol.com

Edward L. Baker, M.D., M.P.H.
Research Professor
Health Policy and Management
UNC Gillings School of Global Public Health
University of North Carolina at Chapel Hill
Chapel Hill, NC
ed_baker@unc.edu

J. Alan Baker, M.A.
Former Chief of Staff
American Public Health Association
alanbaker09@verizon.net

Ron Bialek, M.P.P.
President and Chief Executive Officer
Public Health Foundation
Washington, DC
RBialek@phf.org

Diana M. Bontá, Dr.P.H., R.N.
Vice President, Public Affairs
Southern California Region
Kaiser Permanente
Pasadena, CA
Diana.M.Bonta@kp.org

Tim Brookes, M.A., P.C.G.E.
Director
Professional Writing Program
Champlain College
Burlington, VT
brookes@champlain.edu

E. Richard Brown, Ph.D.
Professor, UCLA School of
    Public Health
Director, UCLA Center for Health
    Policy Research
Principal Investigator, California
    Health Interview Survey
UCLA Center for Health
    Policy Research
Los Angeles, CA
erbrown@ucla.edu

**Frankie Byrum, R.N.C., B.S.N.,
    LMBT, CNMT**
Retired Public Health Nurse
    Manager
Denver, NC
byrumjr@aol.com

Virginia A. Caine, M.D.
Director
Marion County Public Health Department
Associate Professor of Medicine
Division of Infectious Diseases
Indiana University School of Medicine
Indianapolis, IN
vcaine@hhcorp.org

**Esther D. Chernak, M.D., M.P.H.,
     FACP**
Director
Center for Public Health
     Readiness & Communication
Drexel University School of
     Public Health
Medical Specialist in Infectious Diseases
Division of Ambulatory Health Services
Philadelphia Department of Public Health
Philadelphia, PA
echernak@verizon.net

Martin D. Cohen, M.S.W.
President and Chief Executive Officer
MetroWest Community Health
     Care Foundation
Framingham, MA
mcohen@mchcf.org

Donna R. Dinkin, Dr. P.H., M.P.H.
Global Health Leadership Consultant and
     Action Learning Coach
Past Director, National Public Health
     Leadership Institute
Faculty Advisor, Southeast Public Health
     Leadership Institute
Greensboro, NC
drdinkin@hotmail.com

Cheryl E. Easley, Ph.D., R.N.
Dean and Professor
College of Health and Social Welfare
University of Alaska Anchorage
Anchorage, AK
ceasley@uaa.alaska.edu

Jonathan E. Fielding, M.D., M.P.H.
Director and Health Officer
Los Angeles County Department
     of Public Health
Los Angeles, CA
jfielding@ph.lacounty.gov

Robert García, J.D.
Executive Director and Counsel
The City Project
Los Angeles, CA
rgarcia@cityprojectca.org

Joyce R. Gaufin, B.S., CPM
Executive Director
Great Basin Public Health
     Leadership Institute
Salt Lake City, UT
gaufin646@yahoo.com

Kristine M. Gebbie, Dr.P.H., R.N.
Adjunct Professor
Flinders University School of
     Nursing & Midwifery
Adelaide, South Australia
kristine.gebbie@flinders.edu.au

**Audrey Gotsch, Dr.P.H., M.P.H.,
     MCHES**
Professor, Health Education and
     Behavioral Science
Past Founding Dean
UMDNJ-School of Public Health
Piscataway, NJ
gotschar@umdnj.edu

Robert M. Gould, M.D.
President
San Francisco Bay Area Chapter
Physicians for Social Responsibility
San Francisco, CA
rmgould1@yahoo.com

Michael R. Greenberg, Ph.D.
Professor and Associate Dean of the
    Faculty
Edward J. Bloustein School of
    Planning and Public Policy
Rutgers University
Director
National Center for Neighborhood
    and Brownfields Redevelopment
Director
Center for Transportation Safety,
    Security and Risk
New Brunswick, NJ
mrg@rci.rutgers.edu

Diana Halper, B.A.
Managing Director, Communications
    and Media Services
Southern California Region Public Affairs
Kaiser Permanente
Pasadena, CA
Diana.Halper@kp.org

Paul Halverson, Dr.P.H., M.H.S.A.,
    FACHE
Director of Health and State Health Officer
Arkansas Department of Health
Professor of Public Health and Medicine
University of Arkansas for Medical
    Sciences
Little Rock, AR
Paul.Halverson@arkansas.gov

Norman S. Hartman, B.A.
TMT Worldwide, Inc.
Gold River, CA
normh@tmtww.com

Lyndon Haviland, Dr.P.H., M.P.H.
Lyndon Haviland & Company
Lyme, CT
lyndon@haviland.net

Ida Hellander, M.D.
Executive Director
Physicians for a National Health Program
Chicago, IL
ida@pnhp.org

Vonna J. Henry, R.N., B.S.N.,
    M.P.H.
Assistant Professor
State Cloud State University
St. Cloud, MN
rvhenry@aol.com

Darrin K. Hicks, Ph.D.
Associate Professor
Department of Communication Studies
University of Denver
Denver, CO
dhicks@du.edu

Omar A. Khan, M.D., M.H.S.,
    FAAFP
Clinical Assistant Professor
Department of Family Medicine
University of Vermont
Omar.Khan@vtmednet.org

Kenneth W. Kizer, M.D., M.P.H.
Distinguished Professor
University of California Davis
    School of Medicine and
    Betty Irene Moore School of Nursing
Director
Institute for Population Health
    Improvement
UC Davis Health System
Sacramento, CA
Kenneth.Kizer@ucdmc.ucdavis.edu

Linda Landesman, Dr.P.H., M.S.W.
Assistant Vice President
New York City Health and Hospitals
    Corporation
New York, NY
LindaLandesman@aol.com

Carl E. Larson, Ph.D.
Professor Emeritus
Department of Communication Studies
University of Denver
Denver, CO
clarson@du.edu

Robert S. Lawrence, M.D.
Center for a Livable Future
    Professor in Environmental
    Health Sciences
Johns Hopkins Bloomberg
    School of Public Health
Baltimore, MD
rlawrenc@jhsph.edu

Barry S. Levy, M.D., M.P.H.
Adjunct Professor
Department of Public Health and
    Community Medicine
Tufts University School of
    Medicine
Sherborn, MA
blevy@igc.org

John Loretz, M.A.
Program Director
International Physicians for the
    Prevention of Nuclear War
Somerville, MA
jloretz@ippnw.org

John W. Moran, M.B.A., Ph.D.
Senior Quality Advisor
Public Health Foundation
Washington, DC
Senior Fellow
School of Public Health
University of Minnesota
jmoran@phf.org

**Carmen Rita Nevarez, M.D.,
    M.P.H.**
Vice President for External Relations
and Preventive Medicine Advisor
Public Health Institute
Oakland, CA
CRNevarez@phi.org

Patricia A. Nolan, M.D., M.P.H.
Adjunct Associate Professor
Department of Health Services,
    Policy and Practice
Public Health Program
Alpert Medical School
Brown University
Providence, RI
Patricia_Nolan@brown.edu

Mary E. Northridge, Ph.D., M.P.H.
Assistant Professor
College of Dentistry
New York University
Professor of Clinical Sociomedical Sciences
Mailman School of Public Health
Columbia University
Editor-in-Chief
American Journal of Public Health
New York, NY
men6@nyu.edu

Magda G. Peck, Sc.D.
Professor and Associate Dean for
        Community Engagement and
        Public Health Practice
Director
Great Plains Public Health
    Leadership Institute
College of Public Health
University of Nebraska Medical Center
Omaha, NE
mpeck@unmc.edu

Fern Percheski, M.B.A., CPHQ
Development Director
HealthInsight
Las Vegas, NV
fpercheski@healthinsight.org

Giorgio A. Piccagli, Ph.D., M.P.H.
Better Multi-Party Decisions
San Francisco, CA
gapiccagli@gmail.com

Robyn Powers, B.A.
Director of Development and
    Alumni Relations
College of Liberal Arts
University of Nevada, Reno
Reno, NV
rpowers@unr.edu

Shailendra Prasad, M.D., M.P.H.
Assistant Professor
Department of Family Medicine and
        Community Health
Investigator, Rural Health Research Center
University of Minnesota
Minneapolis, MN
shailey@umn.edu

Charlotte Roberts, Ph.D.
Executive Consultant
Blue Fire Partners, Inc.
Sherrills Ford, NC
charlotter@mindspring.com

Margie Schaps, M.P.H.
Executive Director
Health & Medicine Policy Research Group
Chicago, IL
mschaps@hmprg.org

David J. Sencer, M.D., M.P.H.
Deceased
Former Director
Centers for Disease Control

Melvin D. Shipp, O.D., M.P.H., Dr.P.H.
Dean and Professor
The Ohio State University
    College of Optometry
Columbus, OH
mshipp@optometry.osu.edu

Victor W. Sidel, M.D.
Distinguished University Professor of
    Social Medicine
Montefiore Medical Center
Albert Einstein College of Medicine
Bronx, NY
Adjunct Professor of Public Health
Weill Cornell Medical College
New York, NY
vsidel@igc.org

Sylvester Taylor, M.S.
Director
Assessment, Tools, and Publications
Center for Creative Leadership
Greensboro, NC
taylorsy@ccl.org

Tricia Todd, M.P.H.
Assistant Director
Health Careers Center
Instructor
School of Public Health
University of Minnesota
Minneapolis, MN
todd0002@umn.edu

Walter Tsou, M.D., M.P.H.
Adjunct Professor
Center for Public Health Initiatives
University of Pennsylvania
Philadelphia, PA
Walter.Tsou@verizon.net

Quentin D. Young, M.D.
Chairman
Health & Medicine Policy
    Research Group
Chicago, IL
info@hmprg.org

Part One

COMMUNICATION

1

Communicating with the Public

Diana M. Bontá and Diana Halper

As a public health worker, you often need to communicate with the public for many reasons—to convey knowledge to people about threats to their health and well-being, to inform them about measures that they can take to prevent illness and injury, to warn them about hazardous exposures or unsafe products, or to motivate them.

To communicate effectively, you need to:

- Know your organization, its brand (Box 1-1), and how it is perceived
- Know the purpose of your communication
- Develop clear messages that engage and resonate with your intended audience
- Understand your audience as completely as possible
- Decide which communication strategies and tools will most likely be successful
- Use evaluation tools to measure the success of your communication, and then adjust as needed

Getting Started: Developing a Communications Plan

A communications plan helps you to define your purpose, focus and prioritize your work, meet timelines, stay within your budget, and ensure overall success. When you develop a communications plan, you need to ask the following questions:

What am I communicating?
Why am I communicating?
To whom am I communicating?
What do I want to accomplish through communication?
How will I know that I have successfully communicated?

Box 1-1: **What Is Your Brand?**

Whether you know it or not, your organization already has a brand identity. It's what the world sees and hears about your organization. Kaiser Permanente, for example, has a brand that has resonated with people for many years. One of the strengths of its brand is its belief in preventive health. This is how Kaiser Permanente health-care providers approach health—to keep people healthy, and, when they are sick, help them back to health and a quality life. Kaiser Permanente, through research among its audiences (members, patients, employees, physicians, and employers), realized that this commitment to health was how its audiences perceived it and how it perceived itself. It embraced this aspect of its brand, which remains the foundation of its brand strategy and all of its communications.

Your communications plan should contain the following:

- Situation analysis/overview/purpose
- Research
- Goals
- Audience
- Messages
- Strategies
- Tactics
- Budget
- Implementation plan
- Measurements and evaluation

You will not always need to develop a comprehensive communications plan; sometimes an outline of a plan will suffice (Box 1-2). However, whether you develop a complete plan or an outline, include all of the above elements because they will ensure that your communication remains focused, on target, and achievable. Let's explore each of these elements.

Elements of a Communications Plan

SITUATION ANALYSIS/OVERVIEW/PURPOSE

Explain the current situation, the purpose of the communication, and results to be achieved. Demonstrate how the communications plan is tied to your organization's mission, goals, strategies, and brand.

Box 1-2: **Sample Communications Plan Outline for Launch of a Web Site on Healthy Eating**

Situation Analysis/Overview/Purpose:
There is a high incidence of both diabetes and obesity in the Latino population of the local community, which includes many working parents and young children. Many people eat at easily accessible fast-food restaurants, even though the community has small grocery stores that sell fresh produce. The local health department aims to change food and nutrition behaviors of the population. It will soon launch a "Healthy Eating" Web site in both Spanish and English, with food facts, enjoyable and simple recipes, a blog by a local bilingual Latino chef, and breakfast, lunch, and dinner menus. The blog also features guest bloggers, including a nutritionist, a diabetes specialist, and the mayor. The Web site is designed to encourage daily visits, educate visitors, answer questions, and solicit feedback about families' successes in, and obstacles to, healthy eating.

Research:
This includes: (a) working with a local school to conduct a phone survey of Latino families to determine baseline community use of fast-food restaurants and perceptions about healthy eating, and (b) conducting follow-up surveys every 6 months via the Web site.

Goal:
To motivate Latino families to use healthy recipes and to reduce consumption of fast food through information presented on the Web site about affordable food options and the adverse effects of fast food on their health.

Audience:
Local Latino families

Messages:
1. Healthy families eat a nutritious and balanced diet.
2. Healthy eating can be both more affordable and better tasting than fast food.
3. Involving the whole family in good cooking has lifelong health benefits.

Strategies:
1. Use local chef with media relations to promote Web site to target population.
2. Implement "teaser" campaign via social media that highlights latest recipes, affordable food options, and the blog.

3. Promote interactive component of Web site and food events that provide answers to residents' questions.
4. Use community groups, such as churches and schools, to distribute information about new Web site and food events.
5. Use social media tools to expand usage of Web site and attract attendees to food events and the Web site.

Tactics:
Develop timeline with specific tactics tied to each strategy.

Budget:
Recipe cards, chef appearance fees, and chef blogging fee. (Note: May be able to negotiate chef's fee as "win–win" with chef receiving free publicity.)

Implementation Plan: (Consider using an Excel spreadsheet or other type of grid format to prepare your plan.)

Phase I: (a) Design and build Web site and develop content. (b) Develop survey. (c) Arrange for staff members at school to conduct survey. (d) Engage in the project the mayor and owners of local grocery stores.

Phase II: (a) Pilot-test the Web site and adjust accordingly. (b) Pilot-test the survey and make any necessary adjustments. (c) Conduct the survey to establish baseline measurements on community use of fast-food restaurants and perceptions about healthy eating. (d) Engage local Latino chef and other spokespersons. (e) Develop talking points and train spokespersons. (f) Link social media sites to Web site. (g) Launch social media "teaser" campaign.

Phase III: (a) Plan event to launch Web site. (b) Invite media representatives to event at a local grocery store. (c) Hold the event with the mayor, the local chef, and others.

Phase IV: (a) Develop a flyer with the URL of the Web site and a recipe. (b) Distribute flyers via local grocery stores, schools, and churches. (c) Update Web site daily.

Phase V: (a) Conduct follow-up survey to evaluate the impact of the project. (b) Analyze results of survey. (c) Plan next steps.

Measurements and Evaluation:
Conduct follow-up surveys and modify strategies, as needed. Track data on Web site use, including number and length of visits, specific pages visited, and number of recipes downloaded. Review comments in response to blog.

RESEARCH

Research provides critical information that establishes the roadmap for your strategies and tactics. It will help you to avoid communication pitfalls, such as making false assumptions that can derail you and creating materials that are culturally insensitive. Research also helps you establish a baseline for measuring the success of your communications.

In primary research, you gather—or a contractor gathers—information, such as by performing phone or mail surveys or through interacting with focus groups. Secondary research uses existing information, such as census reports or national polls. While this information is easily accessible and often free, it may not answer key questions and you may still need to perform primary research to fill in the gaps (Box 1-3).

Primary research can be quantitative or qualitative. Quantitative research, generally used for larger groups, often includes interviews with uniform questions and multiple-choice responses to enable you to easily obtain and tabulate data. This format excludes asking open-ended questions. Quantitative research is performed, via the Internet, by telephone, or in person, with surveys that can, for example, measure perceptions of your organization, gauge the effectiveness of your communications program, and gather specific information about important issues. The usefulness of a survey depends largely on the quality of the questionnaire. You should pilot-test it on a sample of the target population to find any problems with it and fix them.

Qualitative research allows people to share emotions, explain their thoughts and opinions, confirm areas of concern, and uncover issues you may not have previously recognized. It includes live and online focus groups, face-to-face meetings, and phone calls. While this research is time-intensive and does not typically provide quantitative data, it nevertheless yields much valuable information.

Box 1-3: **Guide to Performing Research on a Limited Budget**

- Use your Web site. Create a chat room.
- Conduct an online survey. For a small fee, services such as Survey Monkey provide an easy-to-develop and easy-to-administer survey that you can e-mail to your audience. Develop a phone survey that you or your co-workers can administer.
- Include your survey in regular mailings, such as newsletters.
- Create an informal focus group by inviting small groups from your target audience to a meal—a great way to test a new logo or slogan.
- Because social media tools can easily provide feedback that will be publicly accessible, this method won't always be appropriate.

Focus groups are effective tools for testing new publications, marketing programs, and advocacy campaigns. However, you need to be sure that members of the focus groups represent the audiences you will be targeting with your communications.

GOALS

Be specific. Avoid generic goals such as "raise awareness" or "increase media coverage." You can avoid overly general goals by adding a measurement or specific outcome. For example, if your goal is to improve the public perception of your organization by increasing media coverage, then specify which media and how much more coverage, such as "increase coverage in local newspapers by 10% compared to the previous year." If your program's purpose is to increase immunization rates in a specific population within the community by educating parents about the importance of vaccines, then your goal should reflect this: "Increase immunization rates in immigrant children under 5 years of age by 15% compared to baseline."

AUDIENCE

Any group of individuals affected by your organization is an audience—the people whom you serve, donors, government officials, community leaders, employees, and others. Audiences may include communities, customers, stakeholders, and constituents. Your audiences comprise the individuals and groups that you want to reach. If you are communicating on behalf of a public health department, your audience may be as large as the population of your city or county—or it may be a segment of the population, such as teens of new immigrant parents. If you want to change public policy, your audience may be a combination of residents of your community, local business and community leaders, and government officials.

Know each of your audiences well—their cultures, their languages, where they live, what they read and watch, how they learn and gather information, and who they look to as leaders and authority figures. By deeply understanding what motivates people in each of your audience segments, what influences them, how they get information, and whom they trust (and don't trust), you will be able to segment and develop strategies and targeted, motivating messages to reach each group. You'll also be armed with information that will help you strategically select the channels or media outlets most likely to disseminate your message to your selected audiences. With social media tools, you can develop channels to receive feedback and more deeply engage your audience. If there is more than one audience, segmenting the audiences will help you develop strategies to reach and engage each group.

Each audience has specific needs. For example, the California Department of Public Health has held forums with representatives of ethnic-specific media to discuss that, due to an increase in pertussis cases, it was expanding communication with communities of color to increase their immunization rates. The representatives from the ethnic-specific media said that they would need to feature expert spokespeople from these communities to improve their stories.

MESSAGES

To develop strong messages, think of the most important points that you want your audience to remember. Relate these core messages to your organization's mission and purpose. To help your audiences remember your core messages, make the messages simple, catchy, and memorable. And use these key messages consistently in all of your written, verbal, and visual communications.

Once you have developed your core messages, you may want to reframe them slightly so that they resonate with each of your targeted audiences. For example, for health plan members, it may be "Preventive care keeps you healthy and active," while for employers, it may be "Preventive care keeps your employees healthy and at work." Any artwork or photos should reflect the audience and its community.

STRATEGIES

Storytelling is a superb way to convey your message (see Chapter 3). Messages stick when they are communicated through compelling stories. Storytelling can help teach, entertain, and reinforce memories of historical events. If you can explain how people are positively affected by a situation that you are addressing, you can personalize your mission and goals and make them memorable. People remember a message to which they can personally relate or with which they have an emotional connection. Uncover personal stories to support your communication message. Sometimes your story may not be positive and you may need to make difficult choices, such as whether to use in a media communication the story of a parent whose child died of a vaccine-preventable disease.

Your messages should not use jargon. Testing your message for clarity with your intended audience can help you avoid the use of words and acronyms that are unique to your discipline and not widely recognized. For example, instead of saying "Establishing a medical home for transient individuals is a high priority for the safety net clinics," say "Free clinics in the area provide homeless people with ongoing health care."

Translating your message into another language may present a challenge. For example, Spanish may be the language of choice for your target population, but subsets of your audience may have different Spanish accents and slang terminology. Literal translations can also cause disconnects with an audience. Have your materials reviewed by members of the target audience for accuracy and intent. You may need to change your communications approach to meet the needs of geographically diverse audiences (Box 1-4).

Box 1-4: **Adjusting Communications to Meet Realities**

The National Farm to School Network (NFSN) conducted extensive research into marketing and communications needs with input from key local, regional, and national stakeholders to determine how best to address its burgeoning constituency and diverse target audiences. It found that to meet the needs of the communities served, it needed to simplify its messages and tactics, inform its audiences, and connect its audiences with each other.

NFSN simplified all communication, using "how-to" statements and shorter, targeted information. It established a tagline: "Nourishing kids and communities." It developed topical fact sheets and an overview brochure on "Farm to School" that was disseminated to all of its regions. It also made all of its materials available by free download from its Web site.

NFSN has become a nationally recognized source of information and education. Its Web site (www.farmtoschool.org) is a one-stop portal for farm-to-school resources and information with daily updates to program profiles, policies, events, funding opportunities, and news. It distributes a monthly e-newsletter, posts regularly on several blogs, places thousands of farm-to-school articles, and develops template presentations. NFSN created an introductory video on "Farm to School," hosted a video contest for students from kindergarten to college, co-developed the videos "Lunch Encounters of the Third Kind" and "Priceless" to initiate its One Tray campaign, and co-hosted a national "Cooking Up Change" contest to get high-school students involved in improving food served in their schools.

TACTICS

Tactics are specific methods or tools you will use to communicate your message. Typical communication tactics include use of online tools, such as Web sites; hard-copy and online newsletters; hard-copy and online annual reports; and videos. Depending on your audience and message, other tactics to consider include developing a program that incorporates events, collaborating with like-minded organizations, developing a media-relations strategy, and establishing a speakers' bureau that places expert speakers in the community (Box 1-5).

An example of collaboration is when Kaiser Permanente in Southern California partnered with the American Lung Association (ALA) during the devastating wildfires that caused poor air quality in large parts of the area. Kaiser Permanente provided funding as well as design and production for the ALA messages about poor air quality and how residents could prevent exposure by limiting outdoor activities. Public service announcements (PSAs) in newspapers and on radio directed people with further questions to the ALA hotline for more information in multiple languages.

Box 1-5: **Orange County Health Care Agency Tweets Save Beach Days**

The communications team of the Orange County Health Care Agency in California wanted to make it easier for beachgoers to find out which beaches were closed due to public health problems. It was already posting information about the closed beaches, but that wasn't helpful as it required the public to come to its Web site or beach. Most people on the way to the beach don't think about first checking with the local health department for any advisory warnings. If the beach is closed when they arrive, then they are disappointed.

Orange County established a "tweeter handle" posted on its Web site. By following this handle, one can receive the latest updates on beach closings on one's laptop and cell phone.

Sample tweets have included: (a) "OC Health removes warning signs @ North Beach in Doheny State Beach—bacteria levels meet health standards. Visit: http://ocbeachinfo.com *about 21 hours ago* via web"; and (b) "Ocean Water Warning—bacteria levels exceed health standards @ Three Arch Bay in Laguna Beach. Details: http://www.ocbeachinfo.com *2:49 PM Jul 16th* via web."

BUDGET

Your communication plan should match its budget (see Chapter 7). Be realistic about how much you can achieve with the resources you have—something that is especially difficult during challenging economic times, when there are budget cuts. Be creative in seeking ways to keep your budget lean. Use social media to expand your reach and avoid expensive printing and mailing costs. An annual report doesn't have to be glossy, slick, and expensive. You can disseminate it in a condensed format on recycled paper or post it online. Create a unique holiday message online and e-mail it to your constituents. Use viral communications, enhanced with Twitter, to promote your messages and events.

IMPLEMENTATION PLAN

Be prepared for success. Have a distribution plan for each of your communications. Be prepared for increased feedback from communication by phone, mail, and social media. Think through all the steps from developing your concept, to planning to reach your intended audiences, to handling their subsequent responses or actions. Include timelines. Prioritize your tactics.

MEASUREMENTS AND EVALUATION

Before you launch communications, choose how you will evaluate the success of your plan. Embed this evaluation in your communication plan. Measurement tools to consider include pre- and post-communications perception surveys, media tracking, and online traffic and activity. If the purpose of your communications is to support an advocacy or education program, choose how you plan to evaluate whether your message has changed behavior and in what ways. Have internal processes to review your plans and your communications before they are released to the public.

Media Relations: The Fundamental Strategy of Communication

One of the most important strategies your organization can use to reach its audience is media relations—working with various media to inform your audiences about your organization. Positive coverage in the media—through a trusted news source, such as the nightly news, the morning newspaper, an online magazine, or a popular radio station—is more credible than paid advertising (and less expensive). While you may not personally implement media relations if you work in a large organization, you may be called upon to address the media if you work in a small one. And, if you work in a large organization, you will need to interact with your media-relations department or an external media-relations agency.

Media relations refers only to work with print, broadcast, and electronic media. Public relations (or public affairs) includes not only media relations but also corporate communications, community relations, and government relations.

You cannot control representatives of the media. They will decide if your communication or story reaches a wider audience—and also how it will be told.

A reporter's job is to get the facts and tell the story in a compelling manner. Traditionally, journalists have been neutral and have not informed their audiences of their opinions—letting the facts tell the story. However, today journalists often allow their opinions to inform their stories. News organizations often lean to the left or the right politically.

Understand each media outlet. Learn when reporters are available, what their deadlines are, how they prefer to receive information, and what their areas of responsibility and interest are.

As you form long-term relationships with reporters and facilitate their coverage of your stories, you are more likely to receive coverage. When a reporter relocates to a new media outlet, continue the relationship.

Media events are important. Box 1-6 describes a successful media event.

Today, media relations have expanded to include nontraditional media outlets, such as blog sites. Know the online sites that host content related to your organization's work, including relevant blog sites and bloggers and those that your stakeholders/customers/constituents may be following. If you work for a public health agency, you need to be familiar with (a) government online sites, (b) bloggers who write about public health issues, (c) political sites that comment

---

Box 1-6: **Ingredients for a Successful Media Event**

Summer pool programs in Los Angeles were suffering from budget cuts. So were city youth, many of whom were "latchkey" kids susceptible to the influence of gangs and at risk for other inner-city threats to their health and safety. Many were facing the prospect of a long, boring, hot summer. Kaiser Permanente gave grants to the city's parks and recreation department to provide for pool chlorine, swimming lessons, and lifeguards so more pools could serve youngsters.

The city government and Kaiser Permanente wanted to let the public know about the summer pool programs—timing of communication and the right elements were critical. The program was announced at a well-organized media event on the last day of school that included the mayor, children in swimsuits, hot weather, a synchronized swim team, and messages about obesity prevention and sun safety—a perfect media event. Called "Operation Splash," it made a big splash with all the major media outlets in the city. And the media event continues to be successfully repeated every year.

---

on and follow public health issues, (d) health and medical sites aimed at the public, and (e) sites directed to health professionals.

Once you have determined your message and the best media outlets to reach your audience, you need to choose what tools to use. Traditionally, these tools include news releases, "pitch letters," media alerts, video news releases, and phone calls. Today, almost all public health communications to reporters are delivered online, either from public health workers or through wire services, such as Business Wire.

Media Tools

NEWS RELEASE

A news release (or press release) follows an "inverted pyramid" structure, with the most important information first. It answers in its first paragraph the key questions of who, what, when, where, and why—the "5 Ws."

When you write a news release, include all of these crucial 5 Ws. Have multiple people review it before you disseminate it. Most reporters will scan your news release headline and lead paragraph, and, if the release doesn't engage them, they will discard it. Some media outlets, especially those online, may use your news release intact; others may shorten it, so be sure that all of your important information is in the first paragraph (Box 1-7).

Box 1-7: **A Sample News Release**

2007/10/15
CONTACT:
Name
E-mail address
Phone number
FARM-TO-SCHOOL PORTAL ON THE MENU FOR NATIONAL SCHOOL LUNCH WEEK:

New tool provides innovative approaches to tackle childhood obesity and loss of family farms
October 15, 2007
LOS ANGELES: As a means to support community-based food systems, strengthen family farms, and improve student health by reducing childhood obesity, the National Farm to School Network launched its new and improved Web site, www.farmtoschool.org. This timely release coincides with National School Lunch Week from October 15 through 19.

Farmtoschool.org is a portal for farm-to-school information in the U.S. and includes extensive content with easy access for submitting information about programs, upcoming events, funding opportunities, and online discussion forums to dialog on issues facing farm-to-school programs.

The portal showcases the great work of innovative farmers, teachers, food service directors, parents, and others involved in farm-to-school programs. "It's the first stop for anyone looking to promote future events, discuss timely topics on the forum pages, and share lessons learned across the nation," said Debra Eschmeyer, National Farm to School Network Marketing Manager.

An exciting new feature includes a state profile for each of the 34 states with active farm-to-school programs. For example, click on California on the map, and you can search for policies, farmers, media coverage, funding opportunities, and involved groups specific to the state.

Highlighting key news and events across the nation and also specific to each region, the new Web site vastly improves the ability to stay up to date and involved in grassroots efforts. "Various tools and resources are available for free download to assist in starting a farm-to-school program," said Anupama Joshi, Farm to School Program Director.

The National Farm to School Network is supported in part by a $2.4 million grant from the W. K. Kellogg Foundation. The Kellogg Foundation grant enables the Network to establish a viable and sustainable mechanism to coordinate, promote, and expand the farm-to-school movement at the state, regional, and national levels. The Network is coordinated by the Center for Food & Justice at the Urban & Environmental Policy Institute at Occidental College (www.uepi.oxy.edu) and the Community Food Security Coalition (www.foodsecurity.org).

A media alert (or media advisory) calls attention to upcoming events, news conferences, or briefings. It describes the event with limited detail, providing information in a bulleted or outline form. It gives the reason for the event; provides information on date, time, and location; and lists spokespeople and their contact information.

Pitch letters or e-mails—short and focused—suggest ideas for feature stories. Explain why these are of interest to the media—and their readers or viewers. Follow up pitch letters with phone calls.

Video news releases or videos can accompany pitch letters or news releases. Using "flip-type," inexpensive, handheld video cameras, you can easily provide reporters with compelling videos, such as short interviews of your spokespeople, that tell your story. Your news release should contain a link to the video, which can be posted either on your Web site or a video hosting site, such as YouTube.

Your press kit should include your news release, a fact sheet about your organization or program, and short biographies of spokespeople. You can place hard-copy format materials in a folder and distribute it to reporters who attend press events. In soft copy, you can make materials available as PDFs and distribute or post them electronically.

SOCIAL MEDIA TOOLS

Use all appropriate social media tools to promote your organization, event, or news story. These tools include the following.

Twitter

Follow and develop a following of the Twitter handles for local reporters and news outlets. If you are providing important tweets that will help them in their jobs, they will begin to follow you. Have a network of people in your organization who tweet to help communicate about important news or upcoming events. Tweet cleverly and judiciously. Keep followers interested, but don't burn them out with irrelevant or excessive information.

Photo Sharing

Make it easy for reporters to obtain photos that help tell your news story by posting related photos on photo-sharing sites such as Flickr. Include links to the site in your news release.

YouTube

Establish a YouTube channel for your organization where videos of your events or other news can be posted. Flip-type video cameras enable you to shoot, edit, and post videos easily and quickly. Include links to videos in your e-mailed news releases.

Facebook

Via Facebook pages, provide more information, post photos, and links to other sites that support your story. As you develop relationships with reporters, they will follow your Facebook sites if they contain information that they can use to help them in their work.

Web Site

You can use your Web site to help reporters learn more about your organization. Include a link to your Web site in all your communication materials.

Getting Ready for a Media Interview

If you are launching a new program, expanding awareness about your organization, or raising funds, you may need a spokesperson for your organization—ideally a leader of your organization or an expert in the subject. Train the spokesperson to be ready for any type of media interview (Boxes 1-8 and 1-9; see Commentary 1-2).

Box 1-8: **Media Tips**

- Establish media policies and procedures for managing media inquiries.
- Make sure your story/message is newsworthy and tailor your story to the specific reporter or media outlet.
- Make it easy for media representatives to reach you.
- Rehearse anticipated media interactions—ideally in situations similar to the "real" scenario.
- Be clear and concise when speaking to the media. Avoid slang, cuteness, and over-explaining.
- Do your homework. Prepare your messages in advance and study them until they become second nature to you.
- Develop a list of "tough questions" and their answers.
- Think before you speak. If you're caught off guard, pause and take a moment to collect your thoughts. Then reply.

- Don't say anything is "Off the record"—presume everything you say is on the record.
- Don't say, "No comment." The public or the reporter may perceive this as dodging the question—or worse, as secrecy.
- Say, "I don't know" if you don't know. And if you don't know, promise to get back to the reporter with an answer. And then do so.
- Never mislead or lie to a reporter.
- Don't ignore a media inquiry—even if you must delay or decline, you must at least reply.
- Don't contact more than one reporter at the same organization about the same story without letting them know.
- Use press conferences sparingly. They are only for groundbreaking news.

Box 1-9: **Tips for Media Spokespeople**

- If you are your organization's media spokesperson, make sure you are appropriately trained. Hire a professional media trainer to provide both general training and training for crisis situations. And, if necessary, do short training sessions before media interviews and take refresher courses.
- Know your message and practice staying on message—no matter what the interviewer asks.
- Make your key points first.
- Know your interviewers. Watch or read other interviews they have done to familiarize yourself with their styles and methods.
- Speak to your audience, not the reporter. The reporter is your conduit to your audience.
- Don't hesitate to correct misstatements by the interviewer—diplomatically, but firmly.
- Never argue with the reporter. Don't be combative. Keep a positive attitude and posture.

Additional Tips for a Radio, Television, or Online Video Interview
- Speak in "sound bites"—short, concise sentences. Make your points succinctly, preferably in 15 to 20 seconds.
- Don't read your messages.
- Stand up when you talk, if possible. Your voice is heartier and you tend to be more alert and focused when standing.
- Speak in a normal, conversational tone—as though you are talking to a friend.

- Talk *to* your interviewers. Focus on them and speak to them as if you're having a private conversation. If you're not in the same room as the reporter, but rather on a live remote facing the camera, view the lens as the eyes of the interviewer. Don't let your eyes dart around the room or stray away from the camera.
- Be aware of your posture, sit slightly forward, and let your body language help communicate your message.
- Dress naturally, preferably in solid colors. Avoid white, busy patterns, and bulky or sparkly jewelry.

Crisis Communications

Crises are inevitable in public health. Whether or not a certain type of crisis can be anticipated, you should be prepared. Planning for potential crises can prevent you from being caught off guard. If your organization already has plans for communicating with the public in a crisis, understand the plans and your role in them. You may find that your organization has communication plans for externally generated crises, but none for those that are internally generated (Box 1-10).

Box 1-10: **The Benefits of Being Accountable to the Media**

Diana Bontá

I had just begun my work as Director of the California Department of Health Services when I was called by the Governor's Office to do an interview for *60 Minutes* on Medicaid fraud with Mike Wallace. I had less than a day to prepare.

Some staff members suggested that my message should blame the previous governor's administration. I weighed this option but chose instead to look forward. I stuck to simple and clear sound bites that conveyed my background as a nurse, the importance of serving persons in need of Medicaid, and eliminating fraud.

I told Mr. Wallace that he could come back in a year to see the administration's progress. As a result, my department received support from the governor and legislature to make necessary changes in computer programming and hire investigative staff members to turn the situation around.

Mr. Wallace returned a year later for a second interview. And he commended our department for the progress that we had made on reducing Medicaid fraud.

Your crisis communications plan should include these eight steps:

1. SELECT THE TEAM

Select and train members of a crisis management team. During a crisis, you may need to add others to this team. Members should be quickly available if a crisis occurs. Have members meet to brainstorm about potential crises and how your organization will address them.

2. DESIGNATE SPOKESPEOPLE

Designate spokespeople for various potential crises, including leaders from your organization and external experts on specific subjects.

3. PLAN A PROMPT RESPONSE

Prepare to respond as quickly as possible to address a crisis, since it can be reported in the media within minutes. Establishing a plan beforehand may enable you to quickly inform your organization's stakeholders—such as employees, donors, volunteers, and board members—before media outlets begin to report. Develop sample communications so you can disseminate initial messages quickly to reduce the likelihood of misinformation or rumor.

4. PREPARE ALTERNATIVE APPROACHES

Prepare for alternative means of communicating should normal channels become inaccessible, such as due to loss of electricity after a storm or earthquake.

5. DEVELOP PARTNERSHIPS

Establish partnerships with institutions in other regions that can assist your organization in an emergency.

6. TEST PLANS

Test your plans and ensure that each staff member and volunteer knows what to do during a crisis.

7. UPDATE

Continuously update your plan. Update contact information for staff members and stakeholders.

8. BE DIRECT

Be accountable and straightforward about crises caused, even in part, by your organization.

Five Key Principles in Responding to a Crisis

1. RAPID RESPONSE

Make yourself accessible to key stakeholders and the media as quickly and as openly as possible. After determining that a crisis exists, assemble your crisis response team quickly—ideally in less than 2 hours. Issue an initial statement to the media and key stakeholders with the information as it is then known and an indication of when additional information will be made available.

2. FULL DISCLOSURE

Provide clear and complete information quickly and forthrightly.

3. SPEAK WITH ONE VOICE

Select and train a spokesperson to represent your organization for any crisis that may develop—someone who communicates with honesty, integrity, and authority in both content and delivery.

4. PLAN ONGOING COMMUNICATIONS TO ALL YOUR AUDIENCES AND STAKEHOLDERS

Identify your organization's key stakeholders and audiences beforehand. Plan for crisis communication that will reach each of them, including identifying communicators, selecting modes of communication, and developing a timeline, until the crisis is resolved.

5. DEVELOP RELATIONSHIPS WITH THE MEDIA BEFOREHAND

Establish sound relationships with the media before a crisis occurs to help prevent or minimize friction if things go wrong (Box 1-11).

Social Media

Social media are activities, practices, and behaviors among communities of people who gather online to share information, knowledge, and opinions through

---

Box 1-11: **The Media as an Ally During a Crisis**

The Orange County Health Care Agency knew that there was a high potential for public confusion and panic as the 2009 flu season approached and the number of novel H1N1 influenza virus infections increased. To help to manage the potential for misinformation, the Agency's communications team asked the major newspaper in the area to work with its health reporter to provide up-to-date, accurate information to the public on influenza and flu vaccine.

The newspaper agreed, as long as the Agency would provide information quickly, make an expert spokesperson available, and respond promptly to meet the newspaper's deadlines. The partnership benefited local residents, who increasingly relied on the newspaper for their information on influenza.

Web-based applications that enable you to easily create, transmit, and share content in the form of words, pictures, videos, and audio recordings—all of which are known as conversational media.

Social media tools can be used in all aspects of your communications with the public. These tools can expand and enhance all aspects of your communications plan, including research, media relations, and community relations. Social media enable you and your organization to reach wider audiences more quickly than before—and often more effectively. But missteps can have consequences for your organization that may be much more significant. You need to understand these benefits, as well as the potentially adverse consequences of social media.

Make sure your organization has a social media policy. Because social media tools can be used by everyone, all employees, volunteers, and board members should understand this policy and how it applies to them. The policy should clearly delineate who manages social media in your organization, who can and cannot post content, what content can be posted, and who must review and approve it. Your organization should develop and disseminate rules on privacy and confidentiality, and how they apply to employees' personal use of social media.

Communicating with the public through social media is not separate from doing so with traditional media. You should incorporate social media strategies and tools into your communication plan.

A classification system categorizes tools and applications of social media by their 15 primary functions:[1]

- *Social Network:* This tool allows you to share information about yourself with your friends, professional colleagues, and others. For example, Facebook is often used by organizations as an adjunct to their Web sites, providing opportunities to post timely information easily and encouraging people to comment online. But monitoring these comments can be labor-intensive. Other examples are LinkedIn, Plaxo, and MySpace.

- *Publish*: This broad category includes tools that facilitate e-mail campaigns, blogging, and wikis. Tools include Blogger.com, Constant Contact, Wikia, Wikipedia, and Joomla.
- *Photo Sharing*: These tools enable you to organize, edit, archive, and share photographs.
- *Audio*: iPod and/or MP3 players enable people to download music as well as podcasts and other programs. You can use this tool to reach people at times that are convenient for them.
- *Video*: You have many choices in distributing videos, including posting them on your organization's Internet and intranet sites and on YouTube.
- *Microblogging*: Twitter, the fastest-growing tool in this category, can enable you and your organization to obtain or disseminate news in small increments, but with great immediacy.
- *Livecasting*: This category encompasses Internet radio and other tools that allow you to stream a live broadcast to an audience or social network. Livecasting offers a flexible means of engaging your audience with education or entertainment.
- *Virtual Worlds*: For education or marketing, some organizations are creating custom virtual worlds or are establishing partnerships with virtual-world programs (Box 1-12).
- *Gaming*: Used primarily by for-profit companies, these entertainment tools offer product placement and advertising opportunities. These tools may also be used as hooks to drive traffic to an online site.
- *Productivity Applications*: These are tools that enhance business productivity. Examples include methods for receiving news on specific topics, such as Google Alerts; conducting surveys, such as Survey Monkey; or sending and obtaining e-mail, such as Gmail.
- *Aggregators*: Tools in this category, such as Digg and iGoogle, help you gather, update, and store information for easy access. Some aggregators, such as Yelp, tell you what other people are saying about a product, service, or brand. These tools can help capture "marketing intelligence."
- *Really Simple Syndication (RSS)*: These tools automatically feed to you current content from those Web sites that are most important to your needs, such as information on an industry blog, data posted on a competitor's site, or information from a government agency's Web site.
- *Search*: Many people start online searches on Google. Other search tools include Technorati, which searches blogs; niche search engines such as IMDB, which searches films; and Pricegrabber, which searches online shopping sites. If you or your organization depend on being found by Web searches, you must learn how search tools can work to meet your organization's needs.

Box 1-12: **The Centers for Disease Control and Prevention (CDC) Uses Virtual Worlds**

CDC's National Center for Health Marketing uses an innovative electronic means of health communication known as eHealth and other electronic media to improve and protect the public's health. eHealth is an information exchange that uses Web-based communication and mobile applications to increase the accessibility of health data and to integrate health messaging into daily activities.

CDC has a presence in virtual worlds, which are Internet sites through which users can interact with one another. In these interactive, three-dimensional environments, each user can create a virtual self—in the form of a computer-generated character called an avatar—to become graphically visible to others.

Whyville is a popular virtual world for children age 8 to 11, who can log on to learn and create together (www.whyville.net). Whyville has places to go, things to do, and people to see. Whyville residents have their own newspaper, senators, beach, museum, city hall, town square, and suburbia. They even have their own economy, in which residents earn "clams" by playing educational games. Whyville's residents represent a hard-to-reach age group of children, who are often the "information conduit" into the household.

CDC has conducted campaigns to raise awareness among Whyville residents about seasonal influenza and to promote the seasonal flu vaccine. CDC has worked with Whyville to promote virtual vaccinations for seasonal influenza. Educating Whyville visitors empowers them to pass along information on the flu vaccine to others in their households. Whyville residents can be virtually vaccinated against "Why-Flu," a virtual illness characterized by sneezing and a facial rash. During a 6-week period, thousands of Whyville residents were vaccinated (see www.cdc.gov/healthmarketing).

For organizations focused on educational outreach, virtual worlds are exciting and unique opportunities to connect with their audiences. In contrast to traditional outreach tools, such as brochures and posters, educational outreach uses virtual worlds to enable customized development of places, games, and activities that engage audience members to actively experience an organization's message.

- *Mobile*: Mobile phones, especially smart phones, enable you and others to access social media. Mobile applications are integral tools in reaching many audiences.
- *Interpersonal*: These tools facilitate person-to-person communications. Webex, for example, has become an integral tool to facilitate meetings and training sessions. Skype is economical and convenient for media interviews.

Since social media are constantly evolving, develop resources that continuously provide you with updates about new tools and how to use them.

Conclusion

Almost everything you do as a public health worker involves communication. Understanding and mastering the basics of good communication will help you immensely in your public health work. By continuing to learn and use the essential skills described in this chapter, you will communicate more effectively with the public and be more successful in improving the public's health.

Reference

1. Safko L, Brake D. *The Social Media Bible*. Hoboken, NJ: John Wiley & Sons, Inc., 2009.

RESOURCES

Books

Caywood CL, ed. *The Handbook of Public Relations and Strategic Communications*. New York: McGraw Hill, 1997.
> *This book is a guide for communication professionals combining the art and science of marketing, public relations, and communications.*

Covello VT, McCallum DB, Pavlova MT. *Effective Risk Communication: The Role and Responsibility of Government and Nongovernment Organizations*. New York: Springer Publishing, 2004.
> *This book is a leading publication on risk communication.*

Parker JC, Thorson E. *Health Communication in the New Media Landscape*. New York: Springer Publishing, 2008.
> *This useful, well-organized book provides a good discussion of new information, technologies, and media for communicating various types of health information to various types of audiences.*

Parvanta C, Nelson DE, Parvanta SA, Harner RN. *Essentials of Public Health Communication*. Sudbury, MA: Jones & Bartlett Learning, 2010.
> *This book focuses on the competencies in health communication and informatics recommended by the Association of Schools of Public Health.*

Safko L, Brake D. *The Social Media Bible*. Hoboken, NJ: John Wiley & Sons, 2009.
> *A good resource on planning and implementing opportunities to communicate through social media.*

Schiavo R. *Health Communication: From Theory to Practice*. San Francisco: Jossey-Bass, 2007.
> *This book includes an introduction to current issues, theories, and special topics in health communication as well as a hands-on guide to program development and implementation.*

Solis B, Breakenridge D. *Putting the Public Back in Public Relations: How Social Media is Reinventing the Aging Business of PR*. Upper Saddle River, NJ: FT Press, 2009.
> *This book provides guidance on how to reinvent public relations around two-way conversations. It enables readers to transform the way they think, plan, prioritize, and deliver public relations services.*

Witte K, Meyer G, Martell DP. *Effective Health Risk Messages: A Step-by-Step Guide*. Thousand Oaks, CA: Sage Publications, 2001.
> *This book provides step-by-step instructions for developing effective communication campaigns.*

Wright K, Sparks L, O'Hair D. *Health Communication in the 21st Century*. Hoboken, NJ: Wiley-Blackwell, 2008.
> *This publication is an introductory book on health communication. It provides vivid examples and real-life cases to illustrate theories and concepts.*

Grammar and Style Guides

AP Styleguide. New York: Associated Press, 2010.
Strunk W Jr. *Elements of Style*. Minneapolis: Filiquarian Publishing, 2007.

Tool Kit

Cause Communications. *Communications Toolkit*. Available at: http:www.causecommunications.org

Associations

Public Relations Society of America (PRSA)
> www.prsa.org

Healthcare Communication and Marketing Association (HCMA)
> www. thehcma.org

Ragan Communications
> www.ragan.com

International Association of Business Communicators (IABC)
> www.iabc.com

Public Affairs Council
> www.pac.org

Blogs

bjFogg.com
> *B. J. Fogg, Ph.D., is an innovator and social scientist whose expertise is in creating systems to change human behavior.*

BrianSolis.com
> *Brian Solis is a digital analyst, marketing executive, futurist, and a thought leader in new media.*

Commentary 1-1: Lessons Learned from Communicating with the Public

Jonathan E. Fielding

As a public health leader, you have a core responsibility to communicate with the public. But there is no one "public." There are multiple groups with whom you need to have effective two-way communication for their health—and our collective health. You need to tailor your messages to their beliefs, their culture, their mode of acquiring information, their level of health literacy, and their prior experiences. A few examples from my experience underscore important lessons.

Developing Specific, Clear, and Tailored Messages

Your communications aimed at changing people's behavior must be specific and straightforward. To increase knowledge or change attitudes or behavior, your messages need to be clear, concise, and actionable.

Emergency preparedness illustrates some challenges and opportunities. Los Angeles is at great risk from earthquakes, fires, mud slides, and heat waves. And it faces threats of multiple forms of terrorism. Since comprehensive local emergency plans include individual preparedness, we wanted residents to have emergency supplies and family communication plans for emergency situations.

We developed messaging that was short, clear, and actionable: "Just Be Ready: Prepare Together!" We designed a multicultural, multilingual education and outreach campaign to increase public awareness of the need for emergency communication plans and to assist residents in preparing for emergencies. Targeting 12 languages and 13 cultural groups, our multifaceted campaign included public service announcements (PSAs) on TV, messages on radio and in print media, placement of messages at the community level, provision of various educational materials, and development of a Web site with tailored messages for diverse audiences.

We made available online simple and ready-to-use educational materials and tools for creating family emergency plans and assembling supplies. We enabled residents to download information about emergency planning for people with disabilities or special needs, to view PSAs in the language of their choice, and to call a multilingual hotline for more information on public health emergency preparedness. We tailored the approach and packaging of information to address the huge cultural and language diversity in Los Angeles. And the public responded. Surveys demonstrated that the proportion of families with an emergency communications plan went from 17% to 46% within 3 years.

Making Messaging Relevant to the Recipient

You need to humanize public health messages. Here's a situation for which I found this to be especially important. Many parents are reluctant to immunize their children, largely due to a study, which is now entirely debunked, that reported an association between children's immunizations and autism. An increasing percentage of parents in Los Angeles County have been signing "personal belief exemptions" that allow un-immunized or partially immunized children to enter kindergarten. To counter parents' concerns, we have used in our health messages photos of parents bringing their children to immunization clinics. In addition, whenever a serious case of a vaccine-preventable disease occurs in an under-immunized child, we have issued a press release highlighting the problem and reminding parents that timely, complete immunizations represent the best way that they can protect their children.

Working with Community Leaders

The epidemic of severe acute respiratory syndrome (SARS), which began in China in 2003, evoked much fear in many countries. Chinese communities in Los Angeles County were especially concerned when they received information from Chinese-language TV broadcasts originating from Taiwan and China. Many who watched as the number of deaths increased feared that the same scenario might occur in Southern California.

In Los Angeles, rumors started to circulate in the Chinese-American community that SARS was acquired in Chinese restaurants and that the chefs in those restaurants were the source of the disease. As a result, local Chinese people stopped eating in Chinese restaurants. Although we in the Los Angeles County Department of Public Health, in consultation with community leaders, issued a press release to dispel these inaccurate rumors, Chinese restaurants remained almost empty.

Several respected and trusted Chinese elders, understanding the potential impact and symbolism for the community, invited me to have lunch with them in a Chinese restaurant. This lunch visually demonstrated that public health officials and Chinese leaders had no concern about SARS being transmitted by food or restaurant workers. The event was widely televised and reported in the local Chinese and mainstream media. The image of me—the county health officer—enjoying a meal with community leaders restored faith in the safety of restaurant food and led people to return to the restaurants. (By the way, no case of SARS was ever confirmed in the United States.)

Using Images to Amplify Messages

Another experience reinforces the importance of finding the right image to amplify your voice and magnify impact in communicating a message. Often your displaying the right graphic or prop enhances communication by assisting viewers in processing the message cognitively and feeling it viscerally.

After an 8-year period in which the average adult in our county gained 6 pounds, we held a press conference to inform the public about the seriousness of the overweight epidemic and related increases in diabetes, hypertension, and heart disease—and the need for urgent action. To many people, 6 more pounds doesn't seem like a serious health problems. And 6 more pounds doesn't draw media attention. So we took a different approach. We estimated the total increase in weight over the 8-year period among adults collectively in the county: They had become 44 million pounds heavier. We also used a prop—a 6-pound blob of yellow gelatinous material that looked and felt like fat tissue. We attracted significant media attention from print and electronic media, which led to many secondary articles and a notable increase in public concern and support for policies to improve nutrition and increase physical activity.

Performing Evaluation

Communication in public health is infrequently evaluated. The amount of money spent and the number of people reached with messages are poor indicators of impact. Given competing priorities and limited resources, your evaluation of changes in knowledge, attitudes, and behaviors can help improve the effectiveness of future communication.

We designed and implemented the "I Know" campaign to motivate African-American and Latina women, age 15 through 25, to be tested for chlamydia infection and gonorrhea every 12 months (or sooner if symptomatic) and to increase their knowledge and awareness of these sexually transmitted infections (STIs). I Know included outdoor advertising, messages in guerilla media and print publications, online advertising, targeted cable TV ads, text messages, movie theater advertisements, and outreach activities. All elements of the campaign were produced in English and Spanish.

We evaluated this campaign with about 300 interviews before it began and about 600 interviews 2 years later. We found a 63% level of awareness of the campaign in the target population. Women who were aware of the campaign were more aware of chlamydia infection and gonorrhea as important health risks and 50% more likely to have been tested for these STIs in the previous 6 months than those who were not.

Later, an added I Know initiative was begun, offering, through the campaign's Web site, testing for these STIs with a home test kit. In the first 8 months of this program, over 2,500 kits were ordered and 1,350 specimens were sent to the public health laboratory for testing, leading to detection of 108 STIs.

Building Trust and Credibility

It is difficult for any public health professional to respond to a question from the media with "I don't know"—especially if the question is reasonable and you think you should know the answer. However, more important than having all the answers is building trust by telling the truth—even if doing so is unwelcome or ego-deflating. For example, in a press inquiry about some measles cases, I was asked about the incubation period for measles, which I couldn't then recall with certainty. I responded that I did not remember exactly the number of days and would have to call back the reporter. Such honesty is essential if you want to build trust—both with reporters and the public. Avoid making an erroneous statement because you fear embarrassment. Misstatements will erode your credibility. Just say: "I don't know."

Breaking Through the Clutter

It may be difficult for you to get the attention of traditional distribution channels, especially network TV and newspapers, and new digital media—particularly to obtain positive media coverage at the population level. In my experience, media ratings have often been driven by controversy, prurient material, and tragedies. For example, a single case of HIV in a porn star merits headlines, while a press release heralding remarkable public health advances—such as a 38% fall in the cardiovascular death rate within only 10 years—gets only a brief mention on the evening TV news. We were able to get good media coverage on a public health advance when the average life expectancy for county residents reached 80 years—a milestone even the mass media thought worthy of reporting.

Media representatives assert that they must give the public what it wants and that media content accurately reflects what the public will read, listen to, or watch. You have a responsibility to inform and persuade media representatives to use the media to give people the knowledge and the tools to improve their health and health literacy. Now, more than ever before, you and other public health workers need to be innovative, strategic, clear, and credible in communicating with the public.

Commentary 1-2: How to Prepare for a Media Interview

Norman S. Hartman

The best advice about what to do in a media interview can go right out the window when you're face to face with a reporter. Stress builds because you know that the few words the reporter chooses to use can help you or hurt you in a dramatic—perhaps even a career-changing—way.

In more than 40 years as a broadcast journalist, public relations executive, and media and crisis communications consultant, including 4 years heading media relations and public affairs for a major state health department, I've probably seen every mistake—and many successes.

If you are facing an interview, keep the following five guidelines in mind. They will serve you well and, perhaps more importantly, save you some embarrassment—or worse.

1. Interviews Are Not Conversations

Although we are naturally inclined to treat media interviews as conversations, they are not. The problem is context. In a conversation, context is present throughout. In a media interview, the reporter selects a few words from the conversation to quote and may take them out of context, even though you and the reporter knew the context of the quoted words during the interview.

Why? If something you said in your answer to her first question sets the tone for, or qualifies, something you said later, the reporter knows that because she's heard the entire communication. But if she uses the latter statement as a quote—without conveying your earlier tone or qualifications (context), you may feel you were misquoted. This seems to occur frequently.

A simple rule is this: When you answer a question, repeat or rephrase a portion of the question as you answer it. That may not always prevent contextual problems, but at least it serves as a reminder to the reporter.

Never answer with a simple "Yes," "No," "Maybe," "Never," or "Always." Instead of just a simple "Yes," try something like: "Yes, we do recommend that all children and seniors receive the vaccine because it will protect them in case we have a difficult flu season."

2. Reporters Don't Want an Education

I worked with a public health official who had extensive knowledge of bioterrorism and terrorist tactics and their consequences. The breadth and depth of his knowledge was remarkable and he wanted to share as much of it as he could without divulging confidential or classified information. He and I taped my questions and his answers to them. His shortest answers were 3 to 4 minutes long. When I reminded him that most quotes and sound bites in popular media are about 6 seconds or 21 words, he said, "I just can't get it down to that. No way." It took the better part of an afternoon to get just a few of his answers to an acceptable length for a media interview.

Public health officials naturally are inclined to offer detailed and sometimes complex—even confusing—information. But that's not what most reporters want. They are looking for the basics—just enough information to complete their stories. If you overload them with information, they may have no idea what is important and what is not. Inevitably, the unimportant stuff winds up in the story and the critical information is cut out and hits the "cutting room floor."

Interviews are not about demonstrating knowledge—they're about organizing it. Be brief and concise. 21 words. Say only what you want to be published.

3. Interview the Interviewer

This is perhaps the most important key to interview success. Before you agree to participate in the story, take the role of the reporter and ask her your questions: "What is the story about? What specific information do you want? Who else have you spoken to and what did they say? How much do you know about me and what I do?" Reporters are not required to answer your questions, but responsible ones usually will. If a reporter won't answer your questions, be cautious. Remember that you are not required to do the interview, and, if you sense that a reporter is being deceptive or has other motives, you may want to politely decline.

While preparing a public health client for an interview with a well-known network correspondent, I asked who else was being interviewed and was told that the information would not be offered. I held my ground, saying my client would not grant the interview unless we knew who else was involved in the story. After several days of negotiation, the producer agreed to our terms. And when we learned the names of others involved in the story, we quickly detected the hidden agenda and prepared for an entirely different interview. Our strategy worked!

Do not assume a reporter knows what you do—or what public health is about. Today, many experienced reporters are being replaced by younger, less experienced reporters. They may know little or nothing about public health. Help them understand your role and the goals of your program. Be simple and direct. Remember, you can be quoted even when you're giving "background" information.

4. Have a Message

There are few public health issues for which we don't have messages, and every interview provides an opportunity to deliver one or two of them. Naturally, the message should relate to the subject of the interview, but you ought to know that if you've interviewed the interviewer (see above) as you prepared. What information do you want people to have, or what behavior do you want them to adopt or change?

Messages should be short and direct—one or two sentences. Chances are the reporter will not ask you for your message. I never did it as a reporter, nor have I seen it happen in watching thousands of interviews. So you need to create the opportunity to deliver your message.

How do you do that? Bridge. After answering the question, move to your message with a phrase such as "It's important for your readers/viewers to know that..." or "The key point here is..." Don't be bashful or timid. Remember, you are the public health expert and that's the reason the reporter is interviewing you.

There is no law requiring you to answer a reporter's question. If you can't—or don't want to—answer, don't say, "No comment." Explain why you can't answer. Legal matters, proprietary or other confidential information, and HIPAA-related or personnel questions may not be answered within the bounds of your media policies. If a reporter persists—repeated questions may be a clue that you are not providing the answer the reporter wants—don't give in. Never concede a point to get rid of it.

Some years ago, I prepared a public health client for an interview on a major television news program. After the interview, we reviewed our recording of it and found that the interviewer asked the same question 15 times. He repeated the question because my client was (deliberately) not answering the question the way he wanted it answered. Despite the interviewer's persistence, my client did not surrender the point the reporter wanted him to make.

5. Practice, Practice, Practice

One of my clients, a leader in a large state health department, told me that, as she prepares for each media interview, she spends at least 20 minutes with her office door closed and her phones turned off. She said, "I review and rehearse my message. And I think about the questions the reporter might ask and how I would answer them." As a result, she has excelled in her media interviews.

I urge you, as a public health leader, to spend adequate time preparing for each media interview. You should never be too busy to do this. You will be more successful in communicating your message and less likely to be misquoted or misrepresented.

You are the person the reporter is planning to interview. Be positive. Be confident. Be brief. And be yourself. For many reporters, your personal insights—and your feelings and your state of mind—are as important as the facts you offer. Portray yourself as being sensitive, caring, and compassionate.

RESOURCES

Hartman NS. *The Media & You—Survival Guide for Public Health Professionals*. Marietta, GA: National Public Health Information Coalition, 2009. Published and distributed by the CDC and the National Public Health Information Coalition (NPHIC). Available at: http://www.nphic.org.

> *This book provides key tips for a media interview, including appropriate messages, appropriate language, building relationships with the media, and 10 mistakes to avoid.*

The National Public Health Information Coalition (NPHIC)

www.nphic.org

> *A leading network of public health communicators committed to making public health public by sharing knowledge, expertise, and resources to effectively communicate about important health issues.*

2

Persuading Others: How to Advocate

Patricia A. Nolan

Advocacy means "the act of pleading or arguing in favor of something, such as a cause, idea, or policy."[1] It usually aims "to influence public policy and resource allocation decisions within political, economic, and social systems and institutions."[2] Advocacy in public health encompasses a broad spectrum of activities to assure conditions in which people can be healthy.

Working in a public health organization—in government or the private sector—you are often asked to advocate for a specific cause: a policy change, budget, program, service, or interest. Not all of these causes are monumental: You may advocate on behalf of people to get their gas or electric service restored, or for tenants whose landlord has defaulted on utility bills. You may advocate for people in low-income neighborhoods to have pharmacists there stock necessary pain medications, or for students to improve their school cafeteria's menu.

In advocacy opportunities, even in these limited ones, you will be most successful if you (a) gather or join a coalition, (b) relate data and policy analyses to the issue, and (c) define the cause in a manner that facilitates action towards achieving your advocacy goal.

A core function of public health is developing public health policy based on both scientific evidence and democratic decision-making. *Policy advocacy*—for improving public health policy—is a critical activity. Your roles as policy advocate may include the following, among others:

- Developing and explaining the evidence base for public health policy
- Informing community members of policies that adversely affect their health
- Formulating evidence-based policy solutions to improve conditions affecting health
- Promoting adoption of new laws or regulations to protect the health of community members

In addition to policy advocacy, *program advocacy* is an integral part of public health work. Public health agencies not only design and implement programs, but also advocate for programs, ranging from surveillance of health risks and disease occurrence in communities to provision of medical care and public health services for underserved people. Your roles as a program advocate may include the following, among others:

- Formulating evidence-based programs to address barriers to health in the community
- Promoting and linking programs of other organizations that are likely to remove barriers and assure the conditions in which people can be healthy
- Working to change—and sometimes eliminate—programs that do not promote health in the community or that have no evidence to support them

Behavioral and cultural changes to assure the conditions in which people can be healthy are achieved through direct public health advocacy and through programs and services. Programs are important for assuring the conditions in which people can be healthy, but broader policy interventions are also necessary. In promoting policies to achieve behavioral and cultural changes, your roles as an advocate may include the following, among others:

- Describing behavioral and cultural factors that increase health risks in the community
- Using educational and social marketing tools to change behaviors and remove cultural barriers
- Clarifying the links among programs, policies, and behavioral changes

Public health advocacy is a political process, changing laws and regulations and getting permission to spend the public's money. Public health agencies in the executive branch of government advocate before local, state, and federal legislative bodies for their programs and for public funds to implement them. This type of advocacy is complex, with written and unwritten rules, formal and informal relationships, and idiosyncrasies of specific local, state, and federal jurisdictions (Box 2-1).

Advocating for programs and services to achieve public health goals also involves:

- Building coalitions
- Relating data and analyses to an issue
- Defining the desired outcome in ways that encourage movement or resolution

Internal advocacy for programs or services that you wish to provide can be a delicate matter when there is intense competition for resources within an

---

Box 2-1: **Advocating with Legislators**

Early in my career as a public health official, the legislative liaison for the agency where I worked gave me a short course in advocating for our programs and budget with legislators:

- Be clear about what you are advocating.
- Answer the questions that legislators ask.
- If you do not know an answer, say so; then find the answer and re-contact the legislator.
- Respect legislators.

These are not maxims for all communications, but they are very useful for public policy advocacy before legislatures and other rule-making bodies.

We were then proposing regulations for Medicaid managed-care organizations—a new concept, with little precedent to guide us. Being clear about our goals and how we hoped to achieve them left the door open for alternatives about which we might not have thought. Answering legislators' questions, we were able to hear their concerns, while avoiding raising new ones. Being honest about what we did not know raised our credibility and avoided mistakes. Our researching and reporting on new information in which they were interested raised our credibility. The law that passed the legislature was better than the legislation we had initially proposed.

---

organization or when programs or services are controversial. As an organization sets priorities and develops budgets, there are usually opportunities for internal advocacy. But if action by a governing board, elected official, or legislative body is part of the approval process, you may come to a point when it is risky to advocate further for a program or service that has already been rejected. In these circumstances, your advocating outside your organization may be perceived as a direct challenge to your superiors or to elected officials, and you should do it only with great caution. Understanding these risks, you can still empower external advocates and those being served by your programs or services, such as by making information available to them and assisting them in gaining access to decision-makers.

You can design an advocacy process that engages and involves stakeholders or community members in changing culture or behavior. In this situation, you may have less control than usual—which can be unnerving. Emotional argument may threaten to overwhelm the scientific basis for change. However, when a community "owns" a problem and generates possible solutions, there is a high likelihood for sustained success.

Defining Issues for Persuading Others

Evidence-based policy is a cornerstone of public health. You should regularly scan evidence relevant to your work in order to understand its scientific and practical significance and to translate it into policies and programs that can improve the health of individuals and communities. Since a body of evidence is never perfect or complete, you often need to make decisions with limited evidence. To persuade others to support what appears to be the best course of action, you need to state problems in quantitative and measurable terms and provide relevant measurement data to decision-makers and to the public.

One of many examples of using measurements to improve the public's health has been the campaign to make overweight and obesity a public health issue that requires a major commitment of public and private resources. Over time, public health workers have agreed on the body mass index (BMI) as a measurable definition of overweight and obesity, collected data on the distribution of BMI levels in populations, and determined the associations between BMI and specific chronic health conditions. In the past, overweight and obesity were described in terms of sedentary lifestyles, excessive food consumption, and other personal failings. They were described in a disease model, with increasing rates of diabetes, heart disease, hypertension, osteoarthritis, and other diseases. Now, overweight and obesity can be defined by a single measure. Policies and programs can be implemented to change the distribution of BMI in a population and can be quantitatively evaluated by their impact on this distribution. We therefore have an evidence base for defining overweight and obesity, and for designing and implementing ways of addressing this problem.

Sometimes brief windows of opportunity arise for you to advocate for your position on an important issue. Be prepared for those situations by developing an *elevator speech*—a simple description of a problem and what you believe is its best solution, one that you can articulate when such an opportunity presents itself. Hone your discussion points into sound bites—perhaps three points in 15 seconds. Then be able to deliver it on short notice to persuade an influential person or decision-maker. And have a more complete presentation ready when the opportunity arises.

Many factors determine the success of advocacy. You will often need more than a measurable public health problem and an evidence-based solution. Political debate may center on negotiating a compromise among competing interests, finding the best balance between perceived costs and benefits, or developing the strongest moral argument. To persuade others that what you believe is the best course of action, you need to understand both rational and non-rational—perhaps even irrational—arguments in favor of, and against, that action. Communicating with policymakers on what is needed to address a problem requires you to be clear on the desired outcome, the evidence to support your course of action, and political and emotional aspects of the issue.

Remember that advocacy is inherently political. The formative stage of your advocacy campaign is the best time for you to determine policymakers' views on the issue and the range of solutions that may interest them. What you learn may cause you to seek new information and rethink possible solutions. New understanding may lead you to widen the circle of interested people and organizations or to identify new partners in advocacy. You should always ask policymakers, "Who else should I confer with about this issue?"

Recruiting Partners and Allies

Effective advocates for change generally do not work alone but in groups, sharing tasks, influence, ideas, and credit. This requires an information system to build and maintain personal relationships. Advocacy goals are not accomplished by one persuasive person writing blogs, e-mails, pamphlets, or letters to the editor. Achieving policy change and improving the public's health require sustained collective work.

As you define a public health problem and develop possible solutions, encourage potential partners and allies to participate in the advocacy campaign. There are two important ways to find partners: (a) call on the "usual suspects"—like-minded individuals and organizations who generally support and promote public health issues, and (b) identify new and different partners, including "unlikely bedfellows" who may be passionate about a particular issue.

Invite the usual partners to be involved from the start—to define the problem, search for and evaluate relevant evidence, and develop possible solutions. If proposed partners do not respond to your invitations, their absence may indicate to others that the problem is not important to them or that your solution does not seem appropriate. Find out more. Listen to their concerns, appeal to their expertise, and offer them opportunities to participate on related issues.

Look for new partners, even though they may be less committed to public health or to your views on a problem and its solution. Why? New partners can demonstrate to those you seek to persuade that the policy or proposal you are advocating has wider support. New partners can bring fresh ideas and are often less invested in *how* a problem gets solved. They can often speak without political or organizational constraints.

New or unusual partners are often temporary allies, interested in one of your issues but probably not all of them. Some new partners have axes to grind or knives to sharpen, and they require strategic management.

We often work in coalitions to promote public health policy. Some are formal organizations with management and decision-making structures, such as (a) an agreement among agencies to pool funds to support a lobbying effort, or (b) an appointed advisory board with stipulated membership. Some coalitions run grassroots campaigns or electronic networks that share information and notify members of pending actions. Maintaining a coalition requires energy from members who feel strongly about an issue. As advocacy efforts evolve, leaders need to heed the wishes of all group members—not just the strongest or most vocal.

Planning Strategies

As your issue becomes better defined and your partners coalesce in supporting it, consider the following questions:

- What has to change for the policy or program to succeed in ameliorating the problem? (See Chapter 13.)
- What will it take to get the policy approved or the program implemented?
- How will we know that we have succeeded?

Learn about your opponents. Understand and recognize their legitimate concerns. Knowing your opponents can be more important than knowing your supporters. Listening to opposing positions carefully allows you to pose alternatives and to reframe some arguments.

When the Health Department and its partners chose to reframe the goal of smoke-free bars as an employee health issue—instead of a non-smokers' rights issue—it altered opponents' views and brought a focus on economic issues, to which many bar and restaurant owners could relate. This reframing enabled us to discuss the positive impacts of the proposed law on increasing sales and decreasing workers' compensation premiums, which were major concerns of owners. Therefore, we could be passionate advocates while providing matter-of-fact responses on economic arguments. (Box 2-2.)

Confer with your allies and prepare to address your opponents' concerns in ways that are compatible with your goals. Find out what your allies will support and what they will not. For example, tobacco-selling merchants might complain that clerks ignore procedures to prevent sales to minors, leaving the merchants punishable for the clerks' failings. In this situation, would your coalition support both small fines for clerks and large penalties for merchants when violations repeatedly occur? Are there effective worker-training programs that could reduce violations? Would the coalition support community-sponsored periodic training for tobacco salespeople or store managers? Could you recruit to the coalition a sympathetic convenience-store operator whose loved one was a smoker who died of lung cancer?

Consider both the costs and the potential to advance your goal. A strategy everyone in your coalition agrees on may not be cost-effective. Do you want to keep pursuing it, or do you want to settle on a more cost-effective, if imperfect, strategy?

Box 2-2: **Our Advocacy Campaign for Smoke-Free Indoor Air**

The purposes of our policy initiative to extend smoking bans to bars and restaurants could have included reducing customer exposure to secondhand smoke, reducing the number of indoor places where smokers can smoke, decreasing the quantity of cigarettes smoked by smokers, and/or encouraging smokers to quit. Any or all of these steps could reduce social supports for initiating smoking and could reduce cases of lung cancer, coronary artery disease, and asthma.

As we built our coalition, we looked critically at past efforts to restrict smoking in restaurants and bars in Rhode Island. Our assessment was that a strategy based on reducing the number of smokers, decreasing the amount of cigarettes each smoker smoked, and helping smokers quit had been tried but did not reduce smoking in bars and restaurants.

Instead, our core group chose a strategy built on worker protection, rather than either customer protection or reductions in other smoking behavior. We determined that for this strategy to succeed, we needed a strong evidence base about differential rates of lung cancer among employees of bars and restaurants. We thought that bars and restaurants that had already adopted smoke-free environments had relevant experiences to share, which would support our position. We knew we needed to recruit workers as supporters.

We studied how to frame our issue as a worker-protection issue. We considered the possibility that employers would need to pay higher workers' compensation premiums if nothing were done—a substantial amount of money. We focused on two outcomes of the policy change: (a) decreasing worker exposure to secondhand smoke, and (b) not increasing employers' workers' compensation premiums for worker illness caused by exposure to secondhand smoke.

It was a great celebration when Rhode Island's restaurants and bars went smoke-free—after more than a decade of advocacy on this issue. (See Commentary 13-2 in Chapter 13.)

When advocating for legislative change, stay in contact with legislative staff members and regularly communicate with the sponsors of a proposed law (or their designees) so that you can anticipate amendments or other changes needing responses from partners. As you do this, make sure that you follow the policies and guidelines set by your organization. Your consistent effort and responsiveness to many changes are necessary as bills are introduced, passed, and signed. Keep partners informed of changes, regardless of who makes them.

Do not rely on the policymakers whom you are trying to influence to communicate amendments.

Building Support in the Community

Support for public policy change and for programs in public health comes from the general public, not just from partner organizations. Successful advocacy requires attention to building and maintaining the public support for public policy goals and public health programs. You need to advocate directly with policymakers with community support behind you. Three avenues for building support are (a) through the media, (b) by direct dissemination of information, and (c) by person-to-person communication.

THROUGH THE MEDIA

In the public arena, be prepared for the media and plan to position your issue carefully. Develop the talking points and the elevator speeches and share them with all members of the coalition. Ensure that partners agree with the public information plan. If there are differences, discuss them and decide how to manage them within the group. Revisit the communication plan and its key points frequently (see Chapter 1).

In most situations, media representatives are neither your friends nor your enemies. Reporters are likely to develop their stories around controversy, finding someone with a policy contrary to yours. But reporters are often not expert in many of the subjects on which they report. This gives you, as the advocate, the opportunity to provide data and data analyses that support the policy you are advocating—and sometimes to even prompt questions that will help you to widely disseminate your message (Box 2-3 and Commentary 1-2).

Maintaining relationships with the media should not be confined to responding to crises. Immediate response through the news is not the only format to advocate for policies and programs. The news format has a tendency to highlight controversy and seek alternative views on a problem. In contrast, telling personal interest stories evokes emotion. Public affairs programming provides opportunities, in a positive framework, to raise awareness about a public health problem and to generate support for a proposed solution through stories.

Work with partners to identify connections with the media. Recruit people affected by the problem to tell their stories. Invite community leaders and other interested people to write letters to the editor of daily and weekly newspapers. Consider talk show appearances, and determine who will be the best spokespersons. Develop media releases about newsworthy events. Better yet, ask for opportunities to meet with TV and radio assignment editors to discuss your issue and proposals. See if they are interested in it as news. Contact representatives

---

Box 2-3: **Working with the Media**

Journalists have a classic story pattern of hero, victim, and villain. Identify coalition members or partners who are adept at framing situations for the media, and follow their lead. Your challenge is to frame a situation so you are seen as the hero, with a sympathetic victim and a villain. For example, in anti-smoking campaigns, public health workers can be positioned as the heroes, protecting victims (smokers and non-smoking teenagers) and challenging villains (the tobacco companies). However, others may see the situation differently. Poor people who smoke may see themselves as victims of an inequitable tax burden. Owners of convenience stores may see themselves as heroes providing goods, services, and jobs in low-income neighborhoods. Either group may see the government as the villain, as starving poor people or hurting business owners.

When advocating for public health policies and programs, human interest stories can be potent: A story about a child with lead poisoning can bring support for better enforcement of housing codes and blood lead screening programs. But negative images can be risky. Many people are unsympathetic toward obese people, so a 400-pound spokesperson is not likely to be helpful. Look to coalition partners with the best connections to key media outlets, including those that are in languages other than English. My visit to a Spanish-language radio station to discuss health policy was often a trial because my Spanish is very limited, but, with help from the show's host, I was able to give the community an opportunity to participate directly in policymaking.

---

of foreign-language media, especially if they reach audiences concerned with your issues.

DIRECT DISSEMINATION OF INFORMATION

Direct dissemination of information is increasingly important (see Chapter 1). Some members of your partnership or coalition may be especially equipped to disseminate information through Web sites, listservs, or blogs. Find ways to use these channels and to make your information and ideas accessible to the people you want to reach. Use printed brochures, bookmarks, and other traditional formats, especially to "push" interested community people toward your organization's electronic information resources. People seem to trust the data and analysis they find on the Web on their own, so think strategically about how to help people to find you. Linking to other relevant Web sites is another method for getting your message to potential supporters. Coalition partners can use popular Web sites and blogs to help you present a unified message.

PERSON-TO-PERSON COMMUNICATION WITH POLICYMAKERS

Advocates can personally interact with policymakers to help shape policy change, especially in local public health work. Not all the policymakers are in government. Some may be among your partners. Even you may be part of the policymaking structure. Members of your partnership or coalition should consider, in advance, what their minimal expectations are for policy change. When legislative progress is being made, there is often little time to consider the pros and cons of a compromise offer, so be prepared in advance for potential offers.

Partners often have constraints, so take full advantage of each partner's connections. Government employees and others are constrained in the positions that they can publicly take or the concessions that they can make. Nonprofit organizations have lobbying restrictions under federal and state laws; they can endanger their tax-exempt status by violating these limitations. Local affiliates of national organizations or others may lobby only for certain policies. Creative partnerships can often find paths that maximize each partner's contribution, respect restrictions, and preserve each person's and each organization's ability to continue to advocate. By anticipating issues, coalition partners can avoid the appearance of dissension and can strategically distribute their work.

PERSON-TO-PERSON COMMUNICATION WITH MEMBERS OF THE COMMUNITY

Advocacy in the community may involve your soliciting participation, even when it seems that no one cares about the issue. Constituency-building in the community involves (a) dividing up advocacy work among partners, (b) taking turns speaking at meetings with community constituents, (c) holding open forums where the community members can express concerns rather than listen to yours, and (d) speaking in the community's language. Working with opinion leaders in communities and asking them to build community support will often pay dividends (Box 2-4).

Plan to develop relationships with people whose support you will need when you advocate. Accept invitations to attend community events. Meet with community opinion leaders, and keep them informed about policies and programs that will affect their communities.

Assessing Progress

Advocacy for legislation and policy change is a long process. It can span legislative sessions, executive terms, and shifting organizational missions. How do you know when to alter strategies, discard plans, adopt new tactics, or modify policy positions? You need to continuously assess situations strategically.

Box 2-4: **Building a Parent Constituency for Maternal and Child Health Practice and Policies**

As the Medicaid program became the primary source of funding for medical care for low-income children, natural alliances with parents in the community shifted away from traditional programs for well-child supervision and for children with special health-care needs. Health departments found their resources declining and directed more toward medical care instead of health promotion and policy. Innovative strategies to build parent constituencies for child health policies, especially for children with special health-care needs, were necessary.

Our natural constituency for children with special health-care needs consisted of parents and families of these children. We recruited and hired parents to advise directors of health department programs about policies and services. We placed parents in clinics and pediatricians' offices to advise on provision of services. We hired these parent-consultants on a short-term basis so that they would not become "insiders," yet they would learn how things worked and whom to talk to in order to get things changed. By hiring and training parent-consultants, the maternal and child health program built a constituency of knowledgeable parents while significantly improving practices and policies.

Key components of constituency-building include identifying those in the community who should care about the issue or program, meeting them where they are, respecting the wisdom that they bring to the issue or program, and strengthening their knowledge base and access to decision-makers. Our parent-consultant program demonstrated how constituency-building can benefit both a health organization and a community.

There are advantages in being flexible, making compromises, and taking incremental steps. In contrast, there are times when you should take a strong stand on an issue.

In your drive to persuade others to adopt an important public health policy, have a good "road map" with milestones so that you can assess progress regularly. When you encounter a road block, consider with coalition partners the strategic options—not just the operational details. If your policy objective is passage of a law, discuss options around any roadblocks with lawmakers who are sponsoring the legislation. Be both realistic and strategic.

Recognize strategic advantages and use them wisely. For example, if you are advocating for a state law that would make uninsured women with abnormal mammograms eligible for Medicaid, the discussion is likely to focus on the impact of the proposed law on the state budget, since Medicaid is such a large item in state budgets. It will take an emotional hook to reset the focus on the health-policy question of making a diagnosis and then promptly choosing a course of treatment. A woman in the community who has had to wait 6 months after an abnormal mammogram before further diagnostic tests would likely work with the coalition, telling her story to help the advocacy campaign. However, there are several things you need to do. First, verify the facts of her story. It could be a disaster to find out later that it did not happen the way she portrayed it. Second, contact the sponsors of the proposed law and other legislative leaders, even if committee hearings have already occurred. The sponsors of the bill will want to be a part of the story, and they may be able to arrange another hearing. If they cannot, arrange with sponsors for her to tell her story to key legislators. Use your media connections to have her story reach a wider audience.

Sometimes you will need to make a strategic retreat. When a legislative session ends and no action has been taken on a law that your coalition has supported, assess your strategy with your partners. What were the weak points in the strategy? How can you find resources to overcome the weaknesses? Is re-introducing the legislation and working harder on the same plan likely to result in a different outcome in the next legislative session?

If so, start immediately to strengthen the coalition's resources; work with the sponsors to consider any changes in the proposed law that may improve it or help you to recruit additional allies. If not, put new options on the table. Consult with sponsors about alternatives. Analyze the potential for advancing parts of the proposal. For example, if you are trying, but not succeeding, in getting the legislature to pass a law mandating seatbelt use with primary enforcement, should you (a) try to improve enforcement of secondary seatbelt use provisions, (b) work to fund promotion of incentives for voluntary use, (c) team up with others to relieve fears that a primary seatbelt use law exposes minorities to discrimination or deportation, or (d) explore some other option? The coalition can revise its strategies more creatively by remembering that the policy goal is not primary enforcement of seatbelt use, but proper use of seatbelts by all passengers in motor vehicles.

If you have failed to persuade others that a state law is needed to ensure proper use of seat belts, you may need to change strategies or redefine the issue. In the seatbelt example, you could back up a step in the process. Your goal may be expressed as seatbelt use, or alternatively as passenger protection or crash prevention. Each of these goals frames a different possible solution.

Others may frame the same issues as (a) personal responsibility versus government mandates, (b) optional safety features versus required design features, or (c) driver responsibility versus road design and maintenance. Some may frame them as primarily issues of economics or social justice.

The public health problem is that motor-vehicle crashes cause many premature deaths and serious injuries. If you reframe the problem as an economic issue, you would want to emphasize that the state may lose federal highway construction funds because it does not enforce seatbelt laws. If you reframe it as a social justice issue, you may want to emphasize the need to limit police searches of vehicles or immigration checks when they stop vehicles solely for seatbelt infractions. Or you can work with minority groups to nurture a more receptive environment for a seatbelt law. Or you may turn to another approach to preventing death and injury from motor-vehicle crashes, such as car safety system designs like ignition locks.

Sometimes a road block exists within the partnership or coalition—maybe someone who does not attend meetings. Building and managing coalitions is challenging. People or organizations seeking to withdraw from an advocacy campaign need to be encouraged to maintain some degree of involvement. Disgruntled partners may need to be courted.

Do not burn bridges with people or organizations; you may need them later. Respect the viewpoints of others. If coalition members have insufficient resources or time, ask them for help in recruiting reinforcements. If a group decision is going to alienate some members, work together to figure out how to characterize and manage the disagreement. Be careful not to react rashly or vindictively.

Going only a little way down the road can be nearly as hard to accept as failing. Persuading others involves many incremental steps. Reward your supporters and forgive your detractors. And savor the small successes, celebrate them, and use them as springboards for the next plans and actions for advocacy.

References

1. *The American Heritage Dictionary of the English Language*, 4th ed. Boston: Houghton Mifflin Company, Updated 2009.
2. en.wikipedia.org/wiki/Advocacy. Accessed on October 14, 2010.

RESOURCES

Books

Bornstein D. *How to Change the World: Social Entrepreneurs and the Power of New Ideas*. New York: Oxford University Press, 2007.

> *Social entrepreneurship may be thought of a business model applied to advocacy in public health and social welfare. See especially Chapter 17, "This Country Has To Change." The story of Javed Abidi's work to change policy and perceptions of disability in India is inspiring and demonstrates many aspects of policy advocacy. This story offers insights into the importance of collaboration, workable communication strategies that alter perception, and ways to influence policymakers.*

Carney JK. *Public Health in Action: Practicing in the Real World*. Boston: Jones and Bartlett, 2006.

> *Vermont's health commissioner for more than 10 years, Dr. Jan Carney emphasizes persuasion by open communication and exchange of information when working within the political structure or with communities to change policies and promote healthy behaviors. Short chapters and relevant topics make this a very readable information resource.*

Articles

Parker EA, Eng E, Laraia B, et al. Coalition building for prevention: Lessons learned from the North Carolina Community-Based Public Health Initiative. *Journal of Public Health Management Practice* 1998; 4:25–36; reprinted in Brownson RC, Baker EA, Novick LF. *Community-Based Prevention: Programs that Work.* Gaithersburg, MD: Aspen, 1999.

This article describes the coalition-building processes fostered through the Kellogg Foundation's Community-Based Public Health Initiative in North Carolina. Other chapters in the book by Ross Brownson and colleagues describe additional coalition-building projects with the same model.

Niederdeppe J, Farrelly MC, Wenter D. Media advocacy, tobacco control policy change and teen smoking in Florida. *Tobacco Control* 2007; 16:47–52.

This article provides an important reminder about the value of media advocacy and the importance of advocating for the best policies by comparing the adoption of specific youth tobacco-control policies in counties with and without a media advocacy campaign. It contains an excellent bibliography.

Dobson NG, Gilroy AR. From partnership to policy: The evolution of active living by design in Portland, Oregon. *American Journal of Preventive Medicine* 2009; 37(supp 2): S436–444.

This article describes a major advocacy project that used science, cross-sector collaboration, and media advocacy to promote major changes in urban policy for healthier environments.

County Health Rankings

http://www.countyhealthrankings.org/

This is a very useful tool to help determine public health priorities. On this Web site, you can click on a county and find its health ranking relative to other counties within its state and its state as a whole. You can also determine how the county compares to national benchmarks on morbidity and mortality measures and health behaviors, clinical care, social and economic factors, and physical environment factors.

Association

American Public Health Association. *Advocacy Tips.* Available at: http://www.apha.org/advocacy/tips/. Accessed on February 16, 2011.

This section of the APHA Web site provides resources to assist public health workers in contacting policymakers and being successful in advocacy work.

Commentary 2-1: Lessons Learned from Advocacy for Health Care Reform

Quentin D. Young, Margie Schaps, and Ida Hellander

Implementing a Multifaceted Advocacy Campaign

Advocacy for reform generally confronts challenges from vested interests representing the status quo. We encountered these challenges when we advocated for establishing freestanding birth centers in which nurse-midwives or family practice physicians deliver babies of low-risk mothers in settings other than homes or hospitals. These centers had been prohibited under the Illinois hospital licensing act. Resistance came mainly from the state medical society, whose members' income depended on delivering babies, and the state hospital association, which was concerned that hospitals would lose paying customers. Both organizations considered these freestanding birth centers to be unnecessary competition and "an inferior and potentially dangerous way of giving birth."

Our advocacy campaign was ultimately successful, with the Illinois state legislature finally passing legislation that permits up to 10 freestanding birth centers to be established on a 5-year pilot basis, with an unlimited number possible if the pilot program is determined to be successful. The following eight elements were most important to our success:

1. HAVING A LONG-TERM PERSPECTIVE

Although we sometimes got frustrated and nearly gave up several times, we had a long-term perspective and kept our "eyes on the prize." Setbacks were frequent and required our birth center task force to regroup, identify new partners, and be open to creative options.

2. FOCUSING ON IMPROVING ACCESS AND REDUCING COSTS

Birth centers could offer delivery services in the many counties in the state that did not have any obstetrician-gynecologists. And births in freestanding birth centers are 45% to 70% less expensive than those in hospitals.

3. USING OUTCOME RESEARCH

We based our advocacy on strong science, including research reported in the *New England Journal of Medicine*. For example, infants born in freestanding birth centers have a neonatal mortality rate of 1.7 per 1,000 live births, compared with 6.8 per 1,000 for the United States as a whole. And mothers have a 4.6% rate of cesarean section, compared with 22.7% nationally.

4. TURNING OPPOSITION INTO SUPPORT

We successfully lobbied the American College of Obstetricians and Gynecologists to change its opposition into a general endorsement of freestanding birth centers, as long as they operated with oversight.

5. RELYING ON POLITICAL ALLIES

Over the years, we gathered politically significant allies who supported our position in the state legislature and among nongovernmental organizations.

6. DEVELOPING A BROAD BASE OF SUPPORT

We developed an "official" taskforce, which established a statewide consortium of advocates to support our proposal. We repeatedly mobilized members of this con-sortium—which included physicians, nurse-midwives, public health advocates, researchers, and lay women interested in alternative health-care-delivery options— to talk with legislators, physicians, and other opinion leaders on this issue.

7. HOLDING CONFERENCES

We held educational conferences that engaged members of the state medical soci-ety, advocates, researchers, and birth center practitioners from other states to help identify and distinguish the political, economic, and emotional barriers to birth centers.

8. BEING FLEXIBLE AND WILLING TO COMPROMISE

Over time, we needed to be flexible in modifying our advocacy strategies and tac-tics. In the end, we were willing to compromise. The state legislature passed the bill in part because we agreed that the state would have a maximum of 10 pilot birth centers, which would be evaluated by major academic institutions.

Effectively Using Research

Research can be an effective tool for advocacy, especially if you use it as one com-ponent of an integrated campaign that also includes other advocacy tools, such as media outreach, education, lobbying, and coalition-building. Research can help you communicate your message to policymakers and others. By illustrating key parts of a problem you seek to address and the solution you advocate, research can also help create a road map for future work.

Physicians for a National Health Program (PNHP) uses health services research to advocate for single-payer national health insurance. For example, PNHP leaders performed studies on the medical causes of personal bankruptcy and published them in peer-reviewed journals. The main conclusion of the studies was that private health insurance leaves families—even apparently well-insured, middle-class families—at risk of financial ruin. PNHP publicized this research through TV, radio, and the print and electronic media and disseminated the findings to its 18,000 physician members as well as to its organizational allies in the single-payer movement.

It was important to translate the studies' conclusions into sound bites for the media. Study co-author Steffie Woolhandler, MD, for example, said that gaps in coverage, high cost-sharing, and illness leading to job loss—and with it the loss of health insurance—make private insurance like "an umbrella that melts in the rain." Co-author David Himmelstein, MD, said, "Unless you're Warren Buffett, your family is just one serious illness away from bankruptcy."

PNHP members and allies wrote op-ed pieces and letters to the editor about the studies' results that were widely published. A key finding—that medical bills contributed to most bankruptcies—was widely cited by policymakers and became part of the conversation about health-care reform. Dr. Woolhandler testified before the House Judiciary Committee that 78% of those bankrupted by illness *had health insurance* when they got sick. As a result, PNHP's credibility as a source of expertise and research on health-care reform was strengthened and its membership grew.

PNHP is continuing to use research on the medical causes of bankruptcy in its advocacy work, such as research on medical bankruptcy in countries with single-payer national health insurance. It is also disseminating research findings that show that replacing the U.S.-based private insurance with single-payer national health insurance would save over $400 billion annually—enough to cover all the 50.7 million people who are now uninsured and to upgrade coverage for everyone else.

Commentary 2-2: Lessons Learned from Advocacy for the Promotion of Peace and Public Health

Victor W. Sidel, John Loretz, and Robert M. Gould

Based on our work as leaders in the International Physicians for the Prevention of Nuclear War (IPPNW) and Physicians for Social Responsibility (PSR), we have found that successful advocacy by nongovernmental or professional organizations depends on having committed members who are aligned in their vision and mission, designing and implementing multifaceted strategies to achieve their shared goals and objectives. We suggest the following 10 tactics:

1. Develop and Use Networks of Health Professionals

IPPNW, an international federation with 63 national chapters, and PSR (the U.S. chapter of IPPNW), a membership organization with 30 state and local chapters and activist groups, use their networks to build popular and political support for peace initiatives and public health. For example, IPPNW participated in the World Court Project with international lawyers and a global network of peace activists to build a single compelling case for declaring nuclear weapons illegal under international humanitarian law. As another example, PSR members have worked within other professional organizations, including the American Public Health Association (APHA), American Medical Association (AMA), and state medical and public health associations, to leverage support of public health policies on such issues as nuclear disarmament and climate change.

2. Put a Human Face on Problems

For example, Zambian Health Workers for Social Responsibility, the Zambian affiliate of IPPNW, has produced "one-bullet stories"—presentations in photographs and words that put a human face on the tragic toll of armed violence. It also designed and implemented a media campaign using messages such as "Guns are bad for people's health" and "Landmine injuries are inhumane." Similarly, many PSR chapters have worked to address gun violence in the United States by putting a human face on the devastating impact of gun violence in poor and disadvantaged communities.

3. Use Epidemiologic Data

In El Salvador, IPPNW members gathered, analyzed, and disseminated data on deaths and injuries due to small arms and light weapons. In doing this study, they redefined small arms and light weapons as "vectors" of injury and death, transforming this issue from a political problem to a health problem. They used their study as a basis to recommend strengthening the country's gun laws. Subsequently, the government limited carrying of arms in public places and added a tax on the sale of small arms and light weapons—and used this new tax revenue to support public health budgets.

4. Develop Evidence-based Policy Proposals

IPPNW and PSR have written proposals for laws or other policies to be developed, based on research they have performed or reviewed. For example, IPPNW has based its advocacy for an international convention banning nuclear weapons on strong science, and then advocated for it by (a) organizing delegations of physicians, medical students, and others to meet regularly with policymakers in nations that have nuclear weapons, (b) briefing them on new research findings on the medical and environmental consequences of nuclear war, and (c) urging these policymakers to support the proposed convention. In addition, IPPNW and PSR have developed many policy resolutions that have been adopted by APHA, the AMA, and other national and state public health and medical associations. For example, APHA has adopted policies opposing the development of nuclear weapons and militarization of space, and supporting nuclear disarmament. APHA's adoption of these policies has catalyzed the adoption of similar policies by state medical associations, which in turn has provided legitimacy for presentation and discussion of these issues at "grand rounds" and other medical conferences.

5. Hold Conferences to Highlight Issues

Conferences can advance advocacy campaigns by highlighting issues and building grassroots support. For example, IPPNW and the Royal Society of Medicine co-sponsored a conference to present research on the medical and environmental consequences of nuclear war. Media coverage focused on research presented by climate scientists that a regional nuclear war, using relatively few nuclear weapons, would have catastrophic effects on global climate. PSR has organized many regional and national conferences to address threats posed by the proliferation of nuclear weapons and the health impacts of war.

6. Strategically Use the Media

While traditional media activities, such as press conferences, op-ed pieces, and letters to the editor, remain important tools for communicating with mainstream news outlets, most nongovernmental organizations are shifting their attention to independent Web-based media, including blogs, news aggregation sites, and social networks, such as Facebook and Twitter. Writers from several countries regularly contribute news articles and opinion pieces to the IPPNW Peace and Health blog on the prevention of armed violence and other relevant topics. Twitter feeds and Google alerts notify readers of new articles, which are then posted on other blogs. PSR members have also given radio and TV interviews with health-based messages, such as advocating for reduction of greenhouse gas emissions. PSR leaders have often joined retired military officers in speaking to the media in support of treaties to ban proliferation of nuclear weapons.

7. Plan and Stage Public Demonstrations

Planning and staging marches and other demonstrations can capture public and media attention and promote your cause. For example, when the APHA Annual Meeting was held in Las Vegas in 1986, several hundred members demonstrated at the Nevada Nuclear Test Site to protest nuclear weapons testing. Subsequent demonstrations there over several years may have influenced the United States to stop nuclear test explosions.

8. Invite Prominent People to Participate in or Endorse Your Work

Enroll leading public health professionals, well-known politicians, entertainment celebrities, famous athletes, or other leaders to participate in and publicly endorse your advocacy work.

9. Provide Expert Testimony

IPPNW and PSR have provided expert testimony at state, national, and international hearings concerning legislation, treaties, and other policies concerning nuclear weapons, military expenses, and related issues. For example, IPPNW and PSR members who are experts on the potential impact on climate of regional nuclear war have presented testimony to Congressional committees, administration officials, members of the European Parliament and the Russian Duma, NATO staff members, and others.

10. Strategically Use Unanticipated Opportunities

When IPPNW was awarded the Nobel Prize for Peace in 1986, a Soviet journalist collapsed with an acute myocardial infarction. U.S. and Soviet physicians worked together to resuscitate him. The news media reported this as an example of international medical collaboration, underscoring IPPNW's international work in bringing physicians together to help prevent nuclear war.

RESOURCES

Associations

International Physicians for the Prevention of Nuclear War (IPPNW)
   www.ippnw.org
Physicians for Social Responsibility (PSR)
   www.psr.org
American Public Health Association (APHA)
   www.apha.org

Commentary 2-3: How Public Health Workers Can Be Directly Involved in Policymaking Processes

E. Richard Brown

Based on many years of working as a policy researcher who engages policymakers and advocates, I have identified three ways in which public health workers can be directly involved in policymaking processes. In addition to their own work in governmental agencies, academic institutions, nongovernmental organizations, or elsewhere, they can directly (a) engage in policy advocacy, (b) form relationships with policymakers, and (c) develop policy proposals.

Policy Advocacy

Working in a non-advocacy organization imposes constraints on your role. If you work for a public health agency or an academic institution, you cannot officially represent your employer without permission. In most public agencies, you cannot take public positions on legislative issues. In academic institutions, you should not take any action that may taint the public perception of your objectivity.

You must respect these constraints. But you can still have relationships with policy advocates that are helpful both to them and to you. For example, advocates, such as legal services attorneys, consumer advocates, and advocates for racial and ethnic groups, can be your eyes and ears for the health needs of disadvantaged populations, whom they may represent. Your relationships with these advocates can provide information that, for example, guides your educational and research work.

As an assistant professor early in my career, I was interested in improving health care services for low-income, uninsured populations. I developed relationships with legal services attorneys who represented these populations. I focused my own research on access to care for these groups in a way that informed the work of legal services advocates, such as studying ways to improve county health services that were intended to meet the needs of low-income people. Many programs of county health services had significant flaws in the ways they were operating, such as not having mandated free services or sliding fee scales. The board of supervisors of one county, for example, had adopted a policy to provide free or low-cost care to low-income people; however, the county had signs listing fees in several of its clinics but no visible information about the county's own policy of providing free care or sliding-scale fees based on need. Even receptionists didn't know that free care was available and denied it when asked. I conducted a study of this problem with a doctoral student, and published the results in a peer-reviewed journal article that was widely covered in local newspapers. That led to a lawsuit against the county, which legal services attorneys won. The court then ordered the county to implement policies to ensure that free or low-cost care was available, as required by law and the county's own official policies.

Advocacy groups deserve your support and assistance. They usually do not have the human and financial resources that they need. As an academic, or as a public health professional working in a local health department, you benefit by understanding, identifying, and articulating issues on which you want to work.

Another experience working with legal services attorneys is instructive. Some counties, because of budget constraints, wanted to close county hospitals that serve the poor. The state provided much money to counties to operate these hospitals and other health services, but it left it to the counties to decide how to serve these low-income residents. At the behest of advocates, the state legislature mandated that anytime a county wanted to significantly reduce or eliminate its health services, it first had to give public notice and hold a public hearing. Then, it needed to make a finding, based on evidence, that closing the county hospital would not adversely affect low-income people. I did a study of the advocates' policy strategies to determine which ones were most effective, in order to help other advocates develop their own strategies. This information was also used in court by legal services attorneys to show when a county was not giving adequate notice and was therefore violating a state law. Local judges blocked closures of such services and facilities if they determined that decisions were based on hearings that did not provide adequate notice in order to ensure due process. These legal proceedings gave advocates the opportunity to mobilize opposition to service cuts, a number of which were very effective in stopping the cuts.

More recently, I have worked with advocates to provide data analysis for public policy issues related to health care coverage for the population in general and for disadvantaged groups, in order to help advocates shape their arguments and proposals. My relationships with these advocates have helped me understand issues needing research.

Relationships with Policymakers

Legislatures and heads of executive agencies of government often are eager for information and thoughtful advice on how to respond to health needs, whether it be indigent health care or combating obesity or other public health challenges. There are different avenues for public health workers in governmental agencies and academic institutions, who may be constrained by the rules of their position or agency. However, policymakers are often eager to hear from people with expertise who can provide them with information and experience.

When you take such opportunities in relationships with policymakers, you need to make clear from the start that you are speaking only for yourself. In general, if you are a federal government official, it is acceptable to respond if a member of Congress calls for information or advice, but you must clearly inform the agency where you are working.

It is useful to know the members of the legislature and their staff members who are working on issues related to your work. When I know that legislators are interested, I send them a brief report, letter, or e-mail with analysis and evidence about that issue; talk to members of their staffs; or make a presentation or offer to be an expert witness at a hearing. Relationships that I have developed often lead to legislators calling me and providing additional opportunities for me to initiate contact.

As a public health worker, you may often be contacted by policymakers because they believe that you don't have an "axe to grind," an ideological point of view or policy-related interest to advance. You are not acting as an advocate for yourself or a particular interest group, but rather offering your experience and expertise.

For example, I knew that a U.S. senator was planning to visit my city and was interested in issues related to access to health care. A health-policy staff member from his office contacted me for my views on this subject. In response to her request, I organized and moderated a roundtable of experts. I also planned for the senator to tour the county public hospital and accompanied him on this tour, during which I provided a running commentary. He knew that I would be more candid than hospital administrators would be, and he was eager for this unbiased perspective. I therefore created an open channel of ongoing communication with the senator and his staff. At the end of his visit, I said that I would be pleased to send a summary memorandum with suggestions for legislation. Ultimately, he invited me to write proposed legislation on national health insurance, and I worked with his staff to get that legislation introduced, a bill that he promoted and that contributed to advancing development of health-care reform on the policy and political agenda.

As another example, I was asked by the chairperson of the state legislature's Latino caucus to speak at a retreat on access to health care. I spoke there and subsequently developed a relationship with that state assemblyman, who liked my advice and policy recommendations concerning expansion of Medicaid in the state and development of a state children's health insurance program. I provided expert advice and, at his request, evaluated proposals that had been offered by advocacy groups—for example, whether these proposals would make health insurance affordable at various income levels, and whether they were appropriate ways to expand coverage for low-income children and their parents. In this case, I refrained from putting my name on letters and other aspects of advocacy in public. I only acted as an individual and helped the legislator to answer questions and devise policy.

Although all of this took time away from my regular academic work, for which I was held responsible, it also enabled me to provide opportunities for students to gain experience. In addition, policymakers knew they could contact me to obtain data on such things as the number of uninsured people in the state or the nation or rates of obesity—and to develop an analysis of the options for public policy to address these problems.

As another example, a colleague and I performed research on the association between sugary drinks and obesity in children and adults. My colleague and I provided the results of this research to legislators, who were eager to have this information. We identified factors in the environment associated with increasing rates of obesity, such as the availability of sodas in schools and proximity of fast-food restaurants to schools. This work directly contributed to legislation and policy efforts to ban sodas from schools. My colleague's work on the relationship of obesity to the density of fast-food restaurants in low-income areas ultimately contributed to legislative proposals aimed at reducing the number of fast-food outlets, increasing access to full-service grocery stores and reducing rates of obesity. It also contributed to the adoption of zoning changes in an especially vulnerable part of a major city to ban fast-food restaurants near schools.

Developing Policy Proposals

As a public health practitioner or academic, you can be directly involved in the policy process in ways that respect the boundaries of your role as an expert. You can do this by helping policymakers to assess and develop policy proposals and letting them know the pros and cons of various proposals.

For example, from my personal research and work with advocates concerning health insurance coverage, I was able to develop proposals that were well documented with evidence—not just opinions. In the process, I also learned how to write briefs and memos with research findings focused on policy issues that were often used by policymakers and advocates.

My development of policy proposals has been informed by my perspective on single-payer health insurance—a broad policy perspective that I based on research evidence. I have helped to develop policies that have marshaled limited fiscal resources to maximize health care coverage and health services for low-income people. I have helped to find ways to reduce some of the profits and high administrative expenses in private health insurance plans. I have also developed proposals to broaden the pooling of health insurance risk, thereby reducing the volatility of health insurance premiums. For example, instead of a program for only high-risk children, I helped to design a health-care program for all children in the state whose families had incomes that were higher than Medicaid eligibility, but still could not afford health insurance.

In these roles, my effectiveness has been enhanced not only by my expertise and experience, but also by keeping my role as an academic clear—letting my values shape my choice of policy research issues, but not letting my own personal views bias the findings of my academic policy research or my advice.

3

Making a Presentation

Joyce R. Gaufin and Barry S. Levy

This chapter reviews the basics on making a presentation: determining the framework, and then developing, practicing, making, and evaluating your presentation.

Determining the Framework

A presentation has three key aspects: (a) its focus and purpose, (b) its audience and context, and (c) its format.

FOCUS AND PURPOSE

Choose the focus and purpose of your presentation. Be clear on what you want to accomplish. Are you making the presentation to provide specific information, to inspire people, or to motivate them to change their attitudes or behavior? Develop learning objectives on what attendees will be able to do as a result of your presentation, such as:

Describe the health-care delivery system in your geographic area
Identify suspected cases of food poisoning
Advocate for a specific legislative proposal

The fewer objectives, the better. Speakers frequently err by trying to achieve too much or to cover too much in a presentation.

AUDIENCE AND CONTEXT

Know your audience and tailor your presentation accordingly. Will it include the general public or only public health workers? Will audience members have fairly similar levels of knowledge and understanding about the subject? What beliefs or attitudes will they likely have about it? What presentations have they recently heard on your subject and related issues? How many people will likely attend?

Know the context of your presentation. Is there a controversy on the subject in the community or organization in which you will be making the presentation? Have you been invited to make the presentation to shed new light on an issue or to provide support to a group of people with a particular point of view? Will your presentation be used to help catalyze the development of a new program or policy initiative?

FORMAT

There are a wide range of formats for presentations, such as formal lectures, with or without slides; storytelling; and brief presentations followed by intensive discussions or question-and-answer periods. And there is a wide range of settings for presentations, such as classrooms, boardrooms, public forums, professional meetings, and government hearings. Choose the appropriate format (or formats), given the subject matter, your goals and objectives, the focus of your presentation, the audience, the context, and the setting.

Consider active learning in your presentation (see Commentary 3-1). And plan other aspects of your presentation, ranging from how you will express your passion for the subject to your use of props (see Commentary 3-2).

Developing Your Presentation

CONTENT

Based on the goal and objectives of your presentation, make an outline of its content—and then add detail.

Remember that the impact of your presentation depends not only on what you say, but also on how you say it and how you appear to the audience. Above all, be authentic (see Commentary 3-3).

The most important parts of your presentation are its opening and its conclusion. Start with something to capture the attention of the audience, such as telling a story—ideally one based on your personal experience.

Consider including in your opening a very brief summary of your presentation, like in the following three examples:

- Today, I'm going to outline the adverse health effects of lead exposure and what you can do to protect your children from this hazard.
- I'm going to present the methods, results, and conclusions of our research on the effectiveness of the new influenza vaccine.

- My presentation today will cover what we know about the health effects of climate change so that you will be able to engage your peers in strategies to prevent or mitigate these effects in your communities.

Consider including a relevant quotation in your opening. If you include one, make sure it can be easily understood. Ideally, the quotation is from a person familiar to your audience. Don't tell a joke to open your presentation—some people may not think it appropriate or they may be offended.

After you plan the content of your presentation, consider cutting it by at least one third. You'll probably have less time than you think.

For the conclusion of your presentation, plan to maintain—or recapture—the audience's attention. Plan to summarize the highlights or main points of your presentation. And consider ending with an appropriate quotation.

Your last sentence should be your strongest—your key message. Never end a presentation with: "I guess I'm out of time, so I'll end here" or "Does anyone have any questions?"

SLIDES AND VIDEOS

Slides are very helpful in many presentations. Here are some guidelines:

- Keep slides as simple as possible.
- Use outlines or bullet points rather than complete sentences.
- Use sans serif type.
- Use a consistent style.
- Place a clear, concise title at the top of each slide.
- Acknowledge sources at the bottom of each slide.
- Clearly label the axes of graphs and units of measurements.
- In tables, round off numbers.

When making slides, avoid long sentences and small print, avoid using too many colors on one slide, and avoid italics.

Use PowerPoint or other slides only to the extent that they amplify the effectiveness of your presentation. Face the audience—not the screen—when you are showing slides. Describe what each slide demonstrates. Don't read your slides verbatim.

Graphs can be very helpful in illustrating such things as relationships among key factors, trends over time and space, and research methods and findings. If you use graphs, place a title on each and read the titles to the audience. And remember:

- Clearly label and explain to the audience the x (horizontal) and y (vertical) axes and the units of measurement.

- Explain what the graph demonstrates.
- Discuss what you can or cannot conclude from it.

Consider giving attendees handouts that contain each of your slides, with space beside each for notes. You may want to provide handouts before your presentation so that attendees can prepare ahead of time. Or, you may want to provide handouts after your presentation so that attendees are not distracted by them during your presentation.

There are many situations when slides can be a hindrance to the purposes of your presentation. If, for example, you wish to engage and inspire your audience, you may want to totally avoid slides. (See Fig. 3-1.)

Consider using photographs to illustrate important points. Photographs are even more effective if you took them and you can tell stories about them.

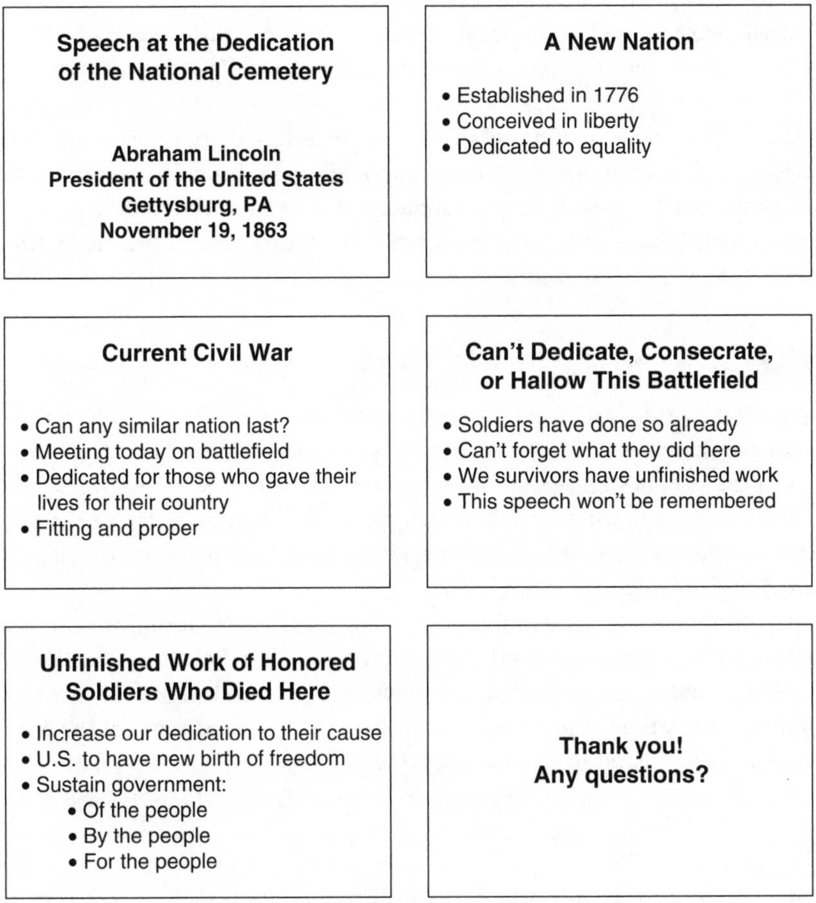

Speech at the Dedication of the National Cemetery **Abraham Lincoln** **President of the United States** **Gettysburg, PA** **November 19, 1863**	**A New Nation** • Established in 1776 • Conceived in liberty • Dedicated to equality
Current Civil War • Can any similar nation last? • Meeting today on battlefield • Dedicated for those who gave their lives for their country • Fitting and proper	**Can't Dedicate, Consecrate, or Hallow This Battlefield** • Soldiers have done so already • Can't forget what they did here • We survivors have unfinished work • This speech won't be remembered
Unfinished Work of Honored Soldiers Who Died Here • Increase our dedication to their cause • U.S. to have new birth of freedom • Sustain government: • Of the people • By the people • For the people	**Thank you!** **Any questions?**

Figure 3-1 The Gettysburg Address as a PowerPoint Presentation. (This parody was inspired by Peter Norvig. See http://www. norvig.com/Gettysburg/.)

Consider using not only slides that demonstrate ideal situations, but also those that give the audience an opportunity to answer the question "What's wrong with this picture?" Don't use artwork or photographs that do not directly pertain to your presentation; they will only distract your audience.

Videos are even better—especially if you can walk the audience through what is happening. And the presence of audio with a video can add a valuable dimension to your presentation—unless the audio drowns out your voice.

STORYTELLING

One or two relevant stories can improve your presentation. You may remember stories you heard years ago—the people or characters, the challenge or problems they faced, the villains or the heroes, any battles—and how everything turned out in the end. Similarly, members of your audience may remember your stories in great detail for years to come (Box 3-1).

Ideally, stories should be accounts of events as they actually occurred. You lose credibility if you embellish details or sensationalize events. However, you may choose to use different styles in relating stories to public health workers and to others.

Unless you are presenting to a scientific or technical audience familiar with statistical terms, limit use of statistics and clearly describe and explain the statistical terms and tests. Remind your audience that tests of statistical significance address probabilities and that the presence or absence of statistical significance does not prove or disprove an association.

INTERACTING WITH YOUR AUDIENCE

The most important and most interesting part of a presentation is often discussion with the audience. There are many ways to elicit discussion from attendees. Even at the start of your presentation, you can ask them where they live, work, or attend school, or in what area they work or study. If you ask them to raise their hands in response, ask each of those who never raise their hands to describe their area of work or study.

If you want some "give-and-take" during your presentation, prepare some questions beforehand to ask attendees, to engage them in discussion throughout—rather than only at the end. If you do so, tell attendees at the start to ask questions at any time. And let them know if you have set aside time at the end for a question-and-answer or discussion period.

HUMOR

Including humor may not only make your presentation more interesting, but it may also increase audience members' retention of information. Generally, self-effacing humor is effective. Perhaps you can relate a humorous story about

Box 3-1: **Telling a Story**

Imagine a scientist making a presentation:

> My presentation today describes a case of acute sleeping sickness in an adolescent female who lived in an isolated community with high socioeconomic status and a homogenous population. The victim apparently was infected by contact with an alternative faith practitioner of low socioeconomic status, who targeted the victim because of her physical characteristics and status. The only known cure of this disease at the time was application of direct lip-to-lip interaction from a physically fit, young adult male of similar socioeconomic status who lived in an adjacent country. Successful application of the lip-to-lip interaction resulted in immediate and full recovery. Subsequently, they established a long-lasting relationship, which was sustainable over an indeterminate period.

Now imagine a storyteller who is not a scientist recounting that same story:

> Once upon a time, a beautiful princess lived in a castle in a forest. An evil witch cast a spell upon her, causing her to fall into a deep sleep. The only cure to awaken her from this deep sleep was a kiss from a very handsome prince. The prince faced many challenges in finding the sleeping beauty. When he found her in the castle, he kissed her. And they lived happily ever after.

Which story would a lay audience rather hear?

What are the common elements in almost every great story? Characters, setting, and either a challenge that must be addressed or a problem that must be solved. Sometimes background information is also essential.

Several years ago, the U.S. Surgeon General declared that there was an epidemic of childhood obesity in the United States.[1] He noted that obese children have increased risks for heart disease, diabetes, and other serious diseases. He stated that, for the first time, children may not be as healthy or live as long as their parents. He asked parents, schools, and communities to work together to reverse this pattern. He implored health professionals and the general public to help obese children and to create an environment that will eliminate childhood obesity. He stated that everyone can help by ensuring that children have non-sedentary lifestyles, safe and accessible places to exercise, nutritious low-fat meals, and parents and physicians who track their health and their weight.

How could you make this subject more personal and more relevant to an audience? If you are presenting to staff members of a health department, you could use local data to describe the problem—possibly data on the impact of obesity on students at a specific school. You might tell the story of a child who became obese and developed diabetes and hypertension, how he becomes short of breath when playing with other children, how he dislikes sports in which he formerly participated, how he now prefers to play video games while snacking—and how he is stigmatized by other children.

How do his parents feel about his obesity? Do they know what to do to improve the situation? Are they able to change his diet and exercise pattern? What are their fears? These details will draw an audience into his story and engage them in the issue. The epidemic of obesity will become real to them.

Another approach is to think like a news reporter. Develop a story by recounting who, what, where, when, how, and why things happen, and give it "personality" by interviewing someone who is directly affected.

Reference

1. Office of the Surgeon General. *The Surgeon General's Call to Action to Prevent and Decrease Overweight and Obesity*. Rockville, MD: U.S. Public Health Service, 2001.

the circumstances in which you were invited to speak. Or maybe something humorous happened on your way to the presentation. But do not be too self-effacing—for you need to retain your credibility.

INTRODUCTION OF YOU AS THE SPEAKER

For the person introducing you, write a short paragraph that summarizes your background and experience and how it relates to the topic of your presentation. Let that person know how to pronounce your name.

Practicing Your Presentation

LEARN YOUR PRESENTATION THOROUGHLY

Practice enables you to make an effective presentation. Know the presentation so well that you can give it with few notes—or, better yet, none at all. Retain the full text or complete outline as a backup. In case you need to refer to it on paper or a computer screen as you speak, make sure the print is large enough and there will be adequate lighting. Use "bullets" or "trigger points" to help you find your place if you get lost. If you use glasses, don't repeatedly put them on and take them off during your presentation.

Gesture appropriately, but remember that your gestures, especially if you will be on a stage or at a podium, will be greatly enhanced. And if you are nervous when you speak, you may exhibit some gestures of which you are not aware. Have someone video you during a rehearsal or a presentation so you can notice your gestures; you can then learn to control them with practice and coaching. Frequent gestures include inappropriate hand and arm movements, shuffling of feet, moving from one side to the other, or hitting a pen or a pointer against a podium.

Rehearse your presentation in exactly the same way you plan to give it. If possible, practice your presentation at the venue, using the microphone, amplification system, lighting, and slides just as you plan to during your actual presentation. Get familiar with controls, such as for advancing slides, using a laser pointer, or dimming the lights. Check that your slides are in the right order. Make sure there is adequate lighting for your notes. If there are speakers before you in the program, listen to one of their presentations from the back of the room to get a better sense of how audience members can see and hear presentations. Make sure that audience members have enough light to take notes or read any handout materials.

A FINAL CHECK

Ask yourself the following questions and make any necessary changes:

- Is this the right material for this audience?
- Do I understand the context of the presentation?
- Am I clearly articulating its purpose?
- Am I pronouncing all the words—including names—correctly?
- Are all my slides correct?
- Can I define all the words and concepts?
- Will the format enable the audience to understand my key points?
- Is my presentation aligned with achieving the intended impact?
- Am I ready for any eventuality—if my slides don't work, if I have less time to present than planned, or if only a few people attend?

OVERCOMING ANXIETY OR "STAGE FRIGHT"

For many people, speaking in public is their greatest fear. If you are one of them, you can use visualization to reduce your anxiety before or during your presentation. For example, before your presentation, find a place where you can relax and sit quietly without distractions. Close your eyes. Take several deep breaths—inhaling and exhaling until you feel calm and relaxed. Imagine yourself ready to make your presentation. Think of how friendly and attentive the people in the audience appear to be. They are eager to hear what you have to say. They admire your courage and ability to speak to such a large and distinguished group of people. They give you a warm welcome as you confidently walk to the podium. You take a deep breath. You make an excellent presentation, feeling more confident as you proceed. As you do, you recognize several friendly faces in the audience. You invite the audience to ask questions. You restate each question to make sure that you have heard it clearly. Your responses are calm, deliberate, and appropriate. You notice how good you feel. As you complete the visualization, you feel calm and satisfied. Take a few more breaths and then open your eyes.

ATTIRE FOR YOUR PRESENTATION

Feel confident and comfortable. Dress as audience members will be dressing—or a bit more formal. Wear well-fitting clothing of a dark, warm, or neutral color. Consider accenting your appearance with more color—but too much may distract the audience from your message. Avoid jewelry or other accessories that may create noise or other distractions.

Making Your Presentation

When you make your presentation, speak loudly and clearly. Speak to each part of your audience. Stay within your timeframe—even if you have to omit less important parts of your presentation.

Adopt a comfortable stance with your feet—one foot slightly in front of the other—to help you be balanced and relaxed. Focus on specific members of your audience—not only on those you know. Establish eye contact with individual members of your audience; it will enable you to talk naturally and to appear sincere. And look at people all around the room.

Avoid reading your presentation. It is often best to speak from bullet points or short phrases that you have written to guide your presentation. There are four exceptions to this general rule, where you may want to read your presentation verbatim: (a) the very start of your presentation, (b) the end of your presentation, (c) direct quotations, and (d) highly technical information. If you use slides, explain or describe them completely, especially tables or graphs.

Notice if you are nervous—your voice may crack or may move to a higher pitch, or you may end sentences with upward inflections, as though they were questions. It's fine to be nervous. But if it adversely affects your presentation, find ways to control it.

Control your tempo. Speak more slowly than you normally do—but not too slowly, or the audience may become distracted. By practicing and rehearsing and getting coaching, you can improve your speaking style.

If you take questions from the audience, repeat each question so that everyone can understand it. Pause to gather your thoughts before answering a challenging or complex question. Answer questions directly and simply. Speak to the entire audience in answering—not just the person who asked the question. Often you will need to admit you don't know the answer, or that the area of the question is beyond your expertise. If questions require very detailed answers, consider asking the questioners to meet with you afterward or providing them with your e-mail address or phone number. Always thank attendees for their questions or discussion points. And end your presentation on time.

Evaluating Your Presentation

VIDEO AND REVIEW PRESENTATIONS

The most effective way to assess the totality of your presentation style is to have someone video your performance—ideally in a rehearsal or practice session, where you can control timing, lighting, and other factors. Then you can view your performance, make changes, and practice again. You can also have someone make a video of your presentation before a live audience—so you can see how you manage the stress, how the audience reacts, and how you respond to questions.

As you review a video, focus on the critical points that you want to evaluate. Limit yourself to only a few specific criticisms, since you will be your harshest critic. Acknowledge specific areas of the presentation where you excelled. Balance self-criticism and positive reflection.

Review and feedback lead to continuous improvement. Work on only a few elements at a time. Eventually, you will become a great speaker.

FEEDBACK FROM LIVE PRESENTATIONS

Capture your thoughts as soon as possible. Write yourself brief notes; you can elaborate later. In addition to your observations about how the audience reacted to your presentation, you may receive scores or comments from an evaluation form completed by attendees. If you can see this form beforehand, you may be able to plan your presentation better and suggest additional items that are important to you.

No audience will give you excellent scores on all aspects of your presentation. Look for trends or patterns that will be helpful to you for future presentations.

Ask a supervisor or colleague to attend your presentation to provide you with oral or written feedback. This can give you additional insight and suggestions for improvement. Listen to and accept feedback. Ask questions to clarify feedback. And thank those who assist you.

Conclusion

If you follow the guidelines in this chapter, you will make effective presentations—and have fun in the process.

RESOURCES

Books

Berkun S. *Confessions of a Public Speaker.* Cambridge, MA: O'Reilly Media, 2010.
   A book that presents a holistic approach to the art and science of public speaking.
Esposito JE. *In the Spotlight: Overcome Your Fear of Public Speaking and Performing.* Bridgewater, CT: In the SpotLight, LLC, 2005.
   A practical and helpful guide on this topic.
Goodman A. *Storytelling as Best Practice: How Stories Strengthen Your Organization, Engage Your Audience, and Advance Your Mission (4th ed.).* Los Angeles: Andrew Goodman, 2008.
Goodman A. *Why Bad Presentations Happen to Good Causes.* Los Angeles: Andrew Goodman, 2006. Available at: http://www.agoodmanonline.com/publications/how_bad_presentations_happen/. Accessed on July 15, 2011.
   Two valuable guides.
Koegel TJ. *The Exceptional Presenter: A Proven Formula to Open Up and Own the Room.* Austin, TX: Greenleaf Book Group Press, 2007.
   Aimed mainly at people who do not routinely speak in front of audiences, this book contains many helpful tips for beginning speakers and emphasizes the need for practice in speaking.
Monarth H, Kase L. *The Confident Speaker: Beat Your Nerves and Communicate at Your Best in Any Situation.* New York: McGraw-Hill, 2007.
   This book provides good advice for a wide variety of speaking situations and social interactions.
Olson R. *Don't Be Such a Scientist: Talking Substance in An Age of Style.* Washington, DC: Island Press, 2009.
   This is a valuable and entertaining book that calls for a focus not only on maintaining scientific accuracy, but also on the important need to hold the interest of the public.
Princeton Language Institute, Laskowski L. *10 Days to More Confident Public Speaking.* New York: Warner Books, 2001.
   This book presents a clear, concise, step-by-step approach with many useful tips.
Steele WR. *Presentation Skills 201: How to Take It to the Next Level as a Confident, Engaging Presenter.* Parker, CO: Outskirts Press, 2009.
   This book, which emphasizes the importance of planning, includes many helpful tips on how to use props, gestures, and humor properly; how to respect the timeframe of your presentations; and how to discover and eliminate unnecessarily repetitive words and phrases.

Journal

Free-Range Thinking
   This is a monthly journal of best practices, resources, and generally useful material for public-interest communicators who want to reach more people with more impact. To read back issues, to download free publications, and to learn about this work, visit www.agoodmanonline.com and www.the-goodmancenter.com.

Association

Toastmasters International
www.toastmasters.org
   This organization offers tips and techniques for learning public-speaking skills. It has local clubs in most cities throughout the United States and many other countries.

Commentary 3-1: Using Active Learning to Make Presentations Memorable

Vonna J. Henry

"What I hear, I forget;
What I see, I remember;
What I do, I understand."
—Old Chinese proverb

Many presentations involve sitting in a room and listening to a speaker lecture. It is important to recognize that we retain only 10% to 20% of what we hear after 3 days, but we remember 90% of what we do after 3 days.[1] So why don't more of us, as presenters, involve the audience? Maybe we are afraid that the audience won't participate. Maybe we fear that we may lose control or that it will take us longer to prepare. But if you want your audience to remember your main points, you need to include active learning—which involves audience members by engaging them in activities other than just listening.[2]

There are many ways to include active learning in your presentations, such as having audience members think about how they would apply the main points of your presentation to their current work situations, or encouraging each of them to repeat your message to another audience member.[3,4]

Before a session on independent contracting at a recent public health conference, there was silence as the speakers were waiting and audience members were entering the room. One of the speakers engaged audience members in active learning by asking them to introduce themselves to other people they didn't know. The room erupted into a cacophony of noise. Then, she went to the door and greeted each new audience member, introduced herself, and asked them to introduce themselves to other people. When the session began, she stated that independent contractors need to network to be effective and that her request to audience members to introduce themselves to others was practice for networking. Afterward, many audience members didn't remember what was said at the session—but they did remember introducing themselves to others.

Another example of active learning is what I call stand up/sit down, which I use in teaching about surveillance and vital statistics. I ask students a series of questions and have them stand if they fit the statement or agree with it, and remain sitting if they don't. The questions help students to learn (a) the type of information that is necessary to obtain, and (b) how to recognize patterns. My students help tally the number standing after each question and, at the end of the session, help create a profile of the class. Active learning enables the student to learn about—and even enjoy—what could be a boring subject.

Use active learning in your presentations. Your audience will be more engaged. Your presentations will be memorable—and audience members will likely remember the essence of your presentation.

References

1. Dale E. *Dale's Cone of Learning*. Available at: http://www.cals.ncsu.edu/agexed/sae/ppt1/sld012. htm. Accessed on February 11, 2011.
2. Bonwell CC, Eison JA. Active learning: Creating excitement in the classroom. *ERIC Digest*, September 1991.
3. Kinney K. *Active learning*. Available at: http://www.cat.ilstu.edu/resources/teachTopics/tips/ newActive.php. Accessed on February 11, 2011.
4. Lorenzen M. *Active learning and library instruction*. Available at: http://www.libraryinstruction. com/active.html. Accessed on February 11, 2011.

Commentary 3-2: Making Presentations with Passion and Props

Virginia A. Caine

Passion

You can move, touch, and inspire members of your audience. You can motivate them to take action—and make a difference in their lives. To do so, you need to be knowledgeable about your subject matter, be authentic, and speak with passion and sincerity—from your heart and soul.

Some of the most passionate speakers are everyday people from all walks of life and areas of interest: the pregnant woman living in an urban development community, the community grassroots worker providing outreach services, the grief-stricken mother giving testimony about the death of her son.

How you communicate is as important as what you communicate. You may need to demonstrate to your audience your knowledge and insights. You may want to show your enthusiasm for your subject. And you may wish to connect with members of your audience and engage them emotionally. The most important factor in improving your communication skills may be sharing from your personal experience and demonstrating your passion. To be a great speaker, you need to inspire your audience (see also Chapter 11).

To convey passion, vary the tone of your voice. If you speak in a monotone—literally, monotonously—your audience is likely to lose interest in your presentation. Focus on pitch and inflection of your voice. Use pauses for effect. Use gestures. All of these techniques can help you to convey your message.

Use personal experiences to which audience members can relate. Sharing your personal experience can help demonstrate the intimate knowledge you have about the subject of your presentation. For example, when I gave a speech on "Women and Heart Disease," I shared how heart-wrenching it was for me to see my mother, immediately after she had a heart attack, in an intensive care unit attached to monitors. I feared that she would never leave the hospital. As I talked about my mother, audience members saw how teary-eyed I was. As I lowered my voice, they could feel the respect, love, and reverence I had for my mother. By experiencing my emotions, audience members understood how important the subject was for me and why I am so motivated to educate women about heart disease and how they can prevent it.

Gestures can help demonstrate your passion and enhance your presentation. When I gave the opening remarks at an Annual Walk of the American Heart Association, I raised my voice to get the attention of the hundreds of participants in order to emphasize how exuberant I felt about preventing heart disease and participating in the walk. I pumped my fists in the air several times to urge participants to become physically fit and take other measures to prevent heart disease.

Props

Props can help illustrate or reinforce your points or can help listeners remember your message. Props should always relate to the content of your presentation and connect listeners to your message. Handouts can be effective props to provide additional information to your audience. You can use them to highlight important points and to provide a road map to your presentation.

I often tell public health audiences the following story that elicits their laughs—and gasps. It demonstrates how you can use a prop—together with a relevant story—to get the attention of your audience to make a point and leave a lasting impression:

> I was sitting on a plane next to a well-dressed, middle-aged woman. Thirty minutes into the flight, she began to cough and sneeze, without covering her mouth. As an infectious disease physician, I was concerned about her health—and mine! I asked if she had any allergies. She said "No."
>
> Then she sneezed onto my hand, and I became more concerned. I immediately wiped her nasal mucus off my hand with sanitizing solution. Then I got up to wash my hands. When I returned, I asked her if she would like some water for her cough. Again, she said, "No."
>
> I politely requested, "I would appreciate it if you cover your mouth, if you sneeze again." No response. Just a stare.
>
> A few minutes later, she started coughing again—still not covering her mouth. Fortunately, as a former Girl Scout, I am always prepared.

At this point in the story, I take a surgical mask out of my pocket and start to put it on while I continue telling the story:

> I pulled the N95 particulate respirator that I always carry with me out of my coat and put it over my face, covering my nose and mouth.

Then I present more specifics about what each of us can do to minimize the spread of airborne bacteria and viruses. But now I have the full attention of every member of the audience.

I have given many speeches on the importance of covering one's mouth when sneezing or coughing to prevent the spread of influenza virus and other respiratory pathogens. My using the mask to tell my story evokes a powerful image that reinforces my message. My story also illustrates the benefits of safe sanitary practice. But the mask—the prop—is what grabs people's attention and what they remember.

So, use props. But know that it takes practice to integrate props into your presentations.

RESOURCE

Public Speaking Tips: Props for Your Next Presentation. Available at: http://www.speaking-tips.com/Articles/Props-for-Your-Next-Presentation.aspx. Accessed on May 31, 2011.

Commentary 3-3: An Example of How to Accept an Award with Humility, Authenticity, and Grace

Robert García

(Adapted from remarks on receiving the American Public Health Association President's Citation, November 9, 2010, Denver).

I would like to thank Dr. Carmen Nevarez and the American Public Health Association for the President's Citation. This is the greatest recognition we have ever received for our work.

I direct The City Project, a non-profit policy and legal advocacy organization, based in Los Angeles. Our mission is equal justice, democracy, and livability for all. I am not a health professional. I am a civil rights attorney. We are making public health a civil rights issue, just like education, housing, voting, jobs, and transportation. The City Project works on public health, the built environment, and equal justice. We spend much of our time explaining how parks, schools, and obesity are civil rights issues. This is how.

Children of color and low-income children lack equal access to quality education, including physical education. They lack safe places to play in school fields. Children of color and low-income children lack safe places to play in parks in the inner city and rural communities where they live. These children disproportionately lack healthy places to eat.

All of this has profound public health consequences, including obesity and diabetes. But there is more to human health than freedom from obesity and diabetes. Public health includes the full development of the child. Physically fit students do better academically. Students who take part in after-school activities, including team sports, tend to stay in school longer. Physical activity programs provide positive alternatives to gangs, crime, drugs, and violence.

But physical education laws are not enforced, school fields are locked after school and on weekends, and there are not enough parks where at-risk children live. Their families disproportionately lack jobs to provide the children equal access to public health resources.

The lack of parks and school fields in communities of color and low-income communities is not an accident of unplanned growth. It is not the result of an efficient market allocating housing based on supply and demand. The lack of parks and school fields is the result of a continuing legacy and pattern of discriminatory land use, housing, and economic policies dating back through the 20th century.

This is why public health and the built environment is a civil rights issue—and fundamentally a human rights issue. But we are told, in the worst economic crisis since the Depression—with unemployment levels at 10% generally and much, much higher for people of color—that this society does not have the money for physical activity and healthy eating in schools and for parks and communities. That is simply wrong. That is what economic stimulus is for.

If you want justice, work for jobs. The Civil Conservation Corps (CCC) was the most successful New Deal program. It created 8,000 new parks. It created 3 million jobs—mostly for white men. It planted 2 billion trees and slowed erosion on 40 million acres of land. It was popular across the political spectrum because it created jobs and economic vitality. Other New Deal programs built 40,000 new schools. CCC is a best-practice example for economic stimulus today.[1]

At The City Project, we do not complain about a problem unless we have a solution. We are enforcing physical education law in public schools. We are creating great urban parks in underserved communities. We engage, educate, and empower communities to make concrete improvements in people's lives, give people a sense of their own power, and alter the relations of power.

Over half the school districts in California do not enforce physical education laws that daily require at least 20 minutes of physical education in elementary school and 40 minutes in middle school and high school. We persuaded the Los Angeles Unified School District to enforce education and civil rights laws by providing physical education. We are taking this best practice to other districts throughout the state.[2]

Twelve years ago, Raul Macias, a successful businessman, retired to start Anahuak, a youth sports association with 15 children in a soccer club. Today, he has 3,000 children—and their families and friends. The goal of Anahuak is not creating good soccer players; the goal is building good citizens. New Latino immigrants do not first organize politically; they first organize soccer leagues. Using the same human organizing skills they use to organize weekly games and monthly coaches meetings and sports leagues, they go on to organize politically. Today when elected officials in Los Angeles want to meet their constituents, they go to Anahuak youth tournaments and coaches' meetings.

Working to create safe places to play in parks and schools is the hardest work we have ever done. I am a former federal prosecutor. I have represented people on "death row" in Georgia, Florida, and Mississippi. I helped spring a former Black Panther leader from prison after he served 27 years for a crime he did not commit. But it has been harder to fix the built environment to serve our children.

Today we are engaged in litigation to protect human health and the environment in the heart of African-American Los Angeles. This will be the largest urban park designed in the United States in over a century. With citizens' groups, we are working against the County of Los Angeles and an oil company to protect a community and a park.[3]

At The City Project, we do not measure success by articles published or by empirical studies proving what we all know is true—although we do that work, too.

We measure success by the smiles on children's faces from playing in a park or a school field that did not exist before.

That is why I am a civil rights attorney. I was inspired to go to Stanford Law School by Thurgood Marshall, the first black Supreme Court Justice. The simple words that appear on his gravestone are "Civil Rights Advocate." I did not aspire to become a Supreme Court Justice. I aspired to be what I have become: a civil rights advocate.

It is a profoundly humbling experience to receive an award that was previously presented to Nelson Mandela and Rosa Parks. How can we possibly live up to what they have done? But Nelson Mandela brought South Africa together through sports, the World Cups in soccer and rugby. We too use soccer as an organizing tool to bring people together. Rosa Parks refused to sit at the back of the bus. We won a civil rights lawsuit in Los Angeles in which the Metropolitan Transportation Authority agreed to invest over $2 billion to keep bus fares low and improve the bus system—a victory described as "a profound moment in American urban history."[4] The simple act of providing bus service has become a profound civil rights act.

The American Public Health Association has declared that "Social justice is a public health imperative." We agree. We look forward to working with you for equal justice, democracy, and livability for all.

Thank you for this award from the bottom of my heart.

References

1. The City Project. *Economic Stimulus, Green Space and Equal Justice*. Available at: http://www. cityprojectca.org/blog/archives/1450. Accessed on December 9, 2010.
2. The City Project. *Physical Education, Student Health and Civil Rights: LA Schools Adopt Implementation Plan*. Available at: http://www.cityprojectca.org/blog/archives/3341. Accessed on December 9, 2010.
3. The City Project. *Baldwin Hills*. Available at: http://www.greaterbaldwinhillsalliance.org. Accessed on December 9, 2010.
4. The City Project. *Transportation Justice*. Available at: http://www.cityprojectca.org/ourwork/ transportation.html. Accessed on December 9, 2010.

4

Writing for Publication

Omar A. Khan and Tim Brookes

Public health does not operate in a political, social, or economic vacuum. Publication of new findings for people who are not public health workers is critical. Indeed, publication means "making public." As a public health worker, you have a variety of needs and opportunities for writing for publication—print, audio, video, and Web-based communication, including social networking.

The two main types of public health writing—that targeted to technical specialists and that targeted to the general public—are informed by the same body of research or practice, but they are expressed in different ways.

Academic writing can be extremely useful in many ways, such as a basis for advocacy or conveying technical information. However, to the general public, academic writing may not mean as much as succinct, crisp, conversational prose delivered in an accessible manner.

Audiences

The traditional audience for scientific articles in journals consists of professionals in closely related fields. This discerning and demanding audience expects new information based on sound research. Members of this audience generally speak the same professional language as the writer, so they share terminology and a base of common knowledge, allowing for a type of professional shorthand.

Professionals who share the same broad area of interest represent another audience. Widening the focus and giving up some technical specifics in order to gain a larger audience can widen readership. This audience, which may also be discerning and demanding, may be more interested in the implications of the research than in the raw data. To ensure readers' understanding, some terms may need to be explained and some background information may need to be provided. Therefore, you need to know and understand the audience for which you are writing and be adept at communicating necessary information.

Often, you can greatly affect policy through articles targeted at the educated lay public. If you are writing this type of article, you need to develop explanatory skills to present a technical subject—perhaps on specific research—in everyday language for general readers.

You can reach decision-makers, policy-makers, and many others through op-ed (opinion-editorial) pieces or letters to the editor in newspapers and magazines, or with a well-established and credible blog. Using these means of communication, you must cut to the heart of the matter, expose the central issues, and raise the crucial questions—in clear, conversational prose. You need to make issues urgent and clear without "dumbing them down" or adding extraneous detail that only an expert would appreciate.

"Telling the story" is an important form of communication. The most effective stories combine portraits of individuals and communities, clear explanations of theory and method, vivid descriptions, and quotations.

Writing for the General Public

Among the media you can use are the following:

- Newspaper and magazine articles—in print and online
- Op-ed pieces for newspapers and magazines
- Newsletters, booklets, and pamphlets
- Radio programs and other audio
- Television programs and other video
- Twitter tweets
- Blog postings
- Fliers and posters

You need to find the best medium to achieve your purpose. For example, if you want to reach a broad audience in Latin America with a message about smoking or nutrition, you might consider getting your message included in a telenovela.

The most important considerations in writing are tone and language. The ideal tone is one of respectful concern. Language should be clear, sympathetic, sincere, and not condescending. And it should not include scientific jargon.

Use the following skills and tactics of a good journalist:

1. CATCH THE READER'S ATTENTION

Use the opening paragraph—the lead—to catch the reader's attention, such as with a story that illustrates your major point.

Consider the following story from Pakistan by Dr. Romania Iqbal about rickets in children and a call for reviewing building construction policies:

> "The doctor sahib said that Ahmed has rickets," said Nafeesa, a young mother in her early 20s, glancing lovingly at her 9-month-old son Ahmed.

"He said that is why he has not been able to sit up properly as most kids do by this age."

The electric light is on in the room, even in the morning, because the high-rise apartment building across the street blocks the sun's rays from entering.

Deficiency of vitamin D ("the sunshine vitamin") can cause rickets in children. A child with rickets is restless and sleepless, skull bones are soft, and sitting, crawling, and walking are delayed. Often the legs and arms are bowed because the soft bones bend under the weight of the child's body. This condition is reversible if it is identified at an early stage and treated adequately. Typically, rickets develops in children when there isn't sufficient exposure to sunlight and/or in breastfed infants of mothers who do not have adequate vitamin D levels.

For many years, rickets was considered only an "Englishman's disease." South Asia, historically, was considered to be immune to the development of vitamin D deficiency because of plentiful sunshine. But there have been several reports of vitamin D deficiency in children in South Asia, in places such as Calcutta and Kashmir, despite ample sunshine. Crowded cities have a higher prevalence of rickets.

Dr. Iqbal has caught our attention by giving us a brief, but vivid, picture of a specific situation, one that you can see in your mind's eye—and hear in your mind's ear. Quoting conversation is a wonderful way to gain impact and immediacy. Next, the writer makes a swift transition to exposition, giving the reader information and an explanation.

In giving us this introduction to rickets, the writer is obeying another rule of journalism: Be clear and direct. When writing for a general audience with widely varying attention spans and pre-existing knowledge of your subject, avoid confusing the reader.

2. BE SUCCINCT

If possible, write short paragraphs. Avoid what's unnecessary. Lead the reader through a series of clear, logical steps, or paint a picture. Dr. Hossain Mohammad Sazzad wrote about a firsthand experience that he had while performing surveillance for diarrheal diseases in Bangladesh—an experience he turned into a very effective op-ed piece, which began as follows:

Sabina and her husband Solaiman lived in a single-room dwelling. Sabina had been living there for the last 6 months. When she came here, she was 5 months pregnant. Her husband, Solaiman, was a rickshaw puller. They came to Dhaka from Rangpur, in the northwest of Bangladesh, for work.

The floor was of polished cement. The partitions were made of bamboo mat with old newspapers pasted over it. A dirty red piece of cloth lined the ceiling. A broken mirror hung near the door. The only furniture of the room was a big wooden couch. Solaiman was sleeping on the couch, covering his head with a torn *katha*.

These visual details, usually not included in scientific writing, provide the reader with a sense of the connection between socioeconomic background and medical and social issues.

This research, put to multiple uses, was presented both as a scientific publication for a professional audience and an op-ed piece for a general audience.

3. USE JOURNALISM STYLE FOR REFERENCES AND QUOTATION

Readers of an op-ed piece in a newspaper or magazine do not want footnotes, references, or a bibliography. But they do want to know the sources of key facts and quotations.

4. USE PHOTOS, IF POSSIBLE

A picture provides one perspective, is more subjective than it seems, and is potentially sensational. But it may also be worth a thousand words.

5. BE CURRENT

When writing for the general public, you usually need to be timely, so your information must be current. Use appropriate and reliable resources to find out what is most current.

6. TELL A STORY

This may be our most valuable piece of advice.

Storytelling comes naturally in conversation—everyone tells stories. A story happens in time and space. It's a single, coherent, sequential set of events involving people. Avoid using generalities and abstractions. Recreate your experience in detail. Use real names for people and places, if possible. But if the people in the story deserve privacy or may be in jeopardy because of what you write, give them false names and let the reader know you're doing so. Describe settings. Quote dialogue. Nothing adds immediacy to a scene as readily and vividly as what people actually said. Quote only the most important parts of what people say. Write about yourself if you are the subject. Act as a video camera to move the reader through an unfamiliar setting or an event. However, it is not always appropriate for you, as storyteller, to be the focus of the story. If your thoughts, reactions, and dilemmas are the main point of what you're writing, include them. But if your focus is what is happening to someone else, tell their story, not yours. (See also Chapters 1 and 3.)

Two Examples of Writing for the General Public

Here are two examples that vividly illustrate the way in which writing for a general reader demands some significant rethinking in someone accustomed to writing for a scientific audience. For the pilot phase of our Web-based clearinghouse, The World's Children Online (www.worldschildrenonline.org), we requested stories about children's health care from Haiti and Bangladesh. We received two pieces of writing from students at the University of Vermont College of Medicine, both of whom had recently returned from Bangladesh.

EXAMPLE #1

The first, from Audrey Merriam, a fourth-year medical student, began like this:

> I spent the month of February in Dhaka, Bangladesh, doing research on "first-hour" and exclusive breastfeeding. The women we were hoping to survey [were] those who were employed, predominantly in the garments industry, which surrounded the hospital. The surveys were conducted at [the] Center for Women's and Children's Health (CWCH) with the assistance of Independent University, Bangladesh.
>
> In general, women in Bangladesh tend to breastfeed their children up to 2.5 years. However, recently trends in "first-hour" and exclusive breastfeeding have been decreasing, which is why we were interested in exploring this area. The survey consisted of questions on the economic background of the families, the women's work environment and potential for maternity leave and child care at work, their obstetrical history, their knowledge of breastfeeding, and their experience with breastfeeding. Women were asked about "first-hour" and exclusive breastfeeding in relation to their youngest and second youngest children to see if their practices changed or were consistent between children. During talks with one of the pediatricians at the clinic, he expressed to me that a large reason he hears from mothers that they stop breastfeeding is because they feel they are not producing enough milk to satisfy their children. It was due to this that questions were added to the survey about why mothers feel they have insufficient breast milk.
>
> Over nine visits to the clinic I was able to collect 114 surveys with the help of three different translators. . . .

This was a perfectly respectable—even admirable—piece of professional exposition. Audrey had identified quickly and clearly the location and subject of her research, its goals, and its methodology, and presented a paragraph of background explaining the purpose of the research. By the end of the above excerpt, she had quickly moved past the narrative of her experience and was about to discuss the data she gathered in detail, with a goal of drawing conclusions.

For general readers, this piece is fairly dry. It needs more vividness, passion, and drama—a sense that something vital may be at stake. It is, in fact, what a professional report is supposed to be: a verbal vehicle for presenting data. The principles of scientific writing have unfortunately led her to exclude almost everything that she brings to her subject. In focusing on data, she has discarded much of what might make her report more relevant and memorable for general readers, who are less interested in survey data and more interested in the broader picture of health care in Bangladesh. Consider a few phrases in her report.

"Dhaka, Bangladesh"

In her text, these are simply the names of a city and a country. Among people who haven't visited Dhaka, few know about this city, its living and working conditions, and its health care. She is observant and intelligent enough to give us a brief description of Dhaka, which is vital to the purpose and methodology of her research.

"those who were employed, predominantly in the garments industry, which surrounded the hospital"

"Garments industry" and "hospital" have different meanings in Bangladesh and in the United States. To a scientific writer of survey results, the living and working conditions of garment-makers and hospital employees are peripheral issues; for general readers, they are central. We suggested that Audrey give her readers a strong visual sense of this location and these people before describing her survey.

"nine visits to the clinic"

General readers would appreciate descriptions of these visits and this clinic. There's a risk that, in adding these descriptions, the piece would lose focus. But a good editor can help sort that out. Better to have too much life than too little.

EXAMPLE #2

Soon afterwards, we received another account of health care in Bangladesh, from Tara Song:

It is 4:00 p.m. as I enter the Special Care Unit (SCU) for afternoon rounds. It's my first day in the SCU, and I am trying to learn the ins and outs.

While each unit has its own schedule, a uniting factor is that punctuality does not hold true. The morning had been relatively uneventful, and rounds had revealed about 10 infant patients with sepsis, pneumonia, and other co-morbidities commonly associated with diarrhea, dehydration, and severe malnourishment.

I was told to return at 4:00 p.m., but when I arrive I find the room quiet, except for an occasional burst of crying from one of the tiny patients. The nurses are standing around the front desk, and I ask whether afternoon rounds are being held today. "Maybe" is the answer I get. I decide to wait around to see if a doctor appears, which usually pays off. I sit in an orange chair by the door, trying to look busy writing in my small ringed notebook that I use to record interesting facts and findings.

After a few minutes, I rise to my feet, and walk slowly from bed to bed, looking at the tiny, fragile patients and the women, some young and some old, [who] accompany them. The "beds" are not the beds we know in the United States. Rather, they are simple cots with vinyl coverings, each with a hole in the center for [stool and urine]. I scan the pieces of paper taped to the bed, reading the lists of medications and nutrition for each patient.

I stop at Bed 3, a bed I had taken note of earlier because the girl sitting on the cot with the baby looked no older than 15. This afternoon, the girl is holding a plastic ventilator mask over her patient's tiny face, and gauze is taped over his eyes to protect his corneas. The infant is suffering from sepsis, and his vacant stare is one of the presenting signs. Since he is not blinking, any pathogens or particles that get into [his] eyes can cause irreversible damage, and this is avoided by shielding [his] eyes with gauze. I can't help but notice how the gauze covers most of his tiny face, seeming to steal his identity. . . .

For general readers, Tara's piece may be more compelling than Audrey's. From its first sentence, we hear someone tell a story that matters to her—and she believes will matter to us. Her prose is conversational without being sloppy or uninformed. She tells us what she sees and hears. She explains what needs to be explained, especially to readers who have not been in a hospital in Bangladesh. She's clearly interested in specific clinical issues, but she's also interested in—and affected by—broader issues of life, death, and human nature. Yes, many sentences begin with "I," and there's a danger that she will upstage the subject. And she keeps switching present and past tenses. But a good editor can help her address these issues.

Next, Tara describes a turn in events:

As the team moved to the next bed, my gaze fell back on the patient in Bed 3. The young girl sitting on the cot with him, I had learned, was his sister, and his mother was hospitalized in Dhaka for postpartum hemorrhage. I watched one of the doctors move back to the bed to auscult the heart with the tiny bell of her pediatric stethoscope. While no one appeared concerned and rounds continued, I felt myself drifting back toward Bed 3. I could sense that something was not right. The doctor looked frustrated when she placed the stethoscope over the infant's chest, straining to hear a heartbeat. I watched as she shook her head, and beckoned to one of the medical officers. The doctor used her index and middle finger to pump the child's chest, compressing the thoracic cavity in an effort to stimulate his heart. The medical officer began [pumps of oxygen through a mask]. I suddenly realized that they were beginning CPR. I had never before seen it performed on a live infant.

The baby was handled much like the dolls I had seen in my Red Cross CPR class. There was nothing delicate about this process. This was a last attempt at saving a life. The chest compressions were violent, and the doctor flopped the infant as she repositioned herself. In the chaos, the infant's sister was standing at the bedside. No one had said a word to her. She began to cry. The incredible composure she'd maintained melted away as she watched her baby brother fade.

I realized that there was nothing for me to do but beckon the girl toward me and hug her. The intensity of the situation overwhelmed me. I tried not to manifest my own shock and sadness. I needed to keep my composure for this girl. As I squeezed her and rubbed her back, I could feel her rub my back in response. In my experience, this hospital was not a place where the staff provided physical comfort. But instinctively I knew this to be one of the most healing forms of attention. Even if the girl was not consciously aware of it, I hope she felt my support.

Once again, we can question whether the writer needs to be focusing quite as much on herself and her opinions. This story would be as strong without some of her passing comments. But this is powerful material—so vivid that at times it's almost poetic. By being powerful and memorable, it is more likely to be widely read, remembered, and discussed. And it may lead to some improvements.

Tara's account is far riskier than Audrey's. It's risky for the writer, who is prepared to show her own confusion, vulnerability, and uncertainty—qualities that are not usually encouraged in the health professions. It's also risky because the hospital and its personnel are presented with their limited resources and how they cope within these limitations. Health-care institutions generally avoid any hint that they are less than perfect. Yet these risks are worth taking.

As these accounts were revised and edited, they became more similar. Audrey became more forthcoming about her experiences, and Tara stepped out of the spotlight and let it illuminate her subject more clearly.

You need to develop different voices for different occasions and different audiences. When an oncologist and a radiologist talk about a series of x-rays, the way they talk is necessarily very different from the way the oncologist then talks to the patient and family members. Similarly, when you write, be clear about not only what you say, but also who will be reading it and in what context.

How to Write a Scientific Paper

Since much research is eventually published, you should design the research you perform, in part, with future publications in mind. This may improve both the research and the papers.

Types of publications in academic journals include:

- Original research papers
- Short reports
- Case reports
- Review articles
- Conference reports
- Editorials and commentaries
- Letters to the editor and replies from authors of articles

Each journal provides guidelines on the scope, style, and recommended length of articles. Generally, original research and letters to the editor are unsolicited, but editorials and commentaries are solicited by journal editors. (See Commentary 4-1.)

When writing for a scientific journal, be clear, precise, and concise. State the limitations of your results and conclusions. Use statistical tools correctly; consult a statistician if you are unsure. Rewrite—after putting your paper aside for a while, improve its organization and wording. Review and proofread your paper— and have a colleague do so as well. And do not delay publishing material that is current—even if it means writing just a short report.

An outline for a typical report of original research is as follows:

TITLE

Choose an appropriate title, since it is usually the first encounter a reader has with your report. Without a suitably informative and interesting title, the best research and writing may go unread. Use the fewest words that accurately describe the content of the paper. Omit phrases like "A study of . . . ," "Investigations into . . . ," or "Observations on . . ."

ABSTRACT

Concisely state the objectives and scope of your research and briefly summarize its methods, results, and conclusions. List several keywords below the abstract.

INTRODUCTION

Place your study in the context of what is already known and establish its significance, and cite key previous studies appropriately.

MATERIALS AND METHODS

Provide sufficient detail of your materials and methods, including your statistical methods, so that a competent researcher could repeat your study or perform a similar study on a different population. Use flow charts, such as for describing how subjects were chosen and how many were in each group studied.

RESULTS

Objectively present your findings. Use tables and figures, where appropriate.

DISCUSSION

Express your opinions on what your results mean in a wider context. Answer the question: "So what?" Address limitations of your study, including possible biases. Be conservative in stating the importance of your results and your conclusions.

REFERENCES

Follow the journal's guidelines for authors. Read completely the publications that you are citing—not just their abstracts. Some peer-reviewed journals have restrictions on citing Internet-based references, such as Wikipedia, or unpublished work, such as graduate theses.

ACKNOWLEDGMENTS

Recognize those who reviewed drafts and provided other assistance. Be inclusive and generous.

DISCLOSURES

Disclose any funding sources and conflicts of interest, actual or perceived. When in doubt, consult with the journal's editor.

PUBLICATION ETHICS

Appropriately cite and reference the work of others and the sources of information. Place direct quotes within quotation marks.

Clarify the order of authors and designate the corresponding author, who takes responsibility for communicating with the journal and responding to inquiries. The International Committee of Medical Journal Editors (ICMJE, the Vancouver group) has developed uniform guidelines for determining authorship. Authorship credit should be based on three criteria: (a) substantial contributions to conception and design, acquisition of data, or analysis and interpretation of data; (b) drafting the article or revising it critically for important intellectual content; and (c) final approval of the version to be published. All three criteria must be met. Acquisition of funding, collection of data, or general supervision of the research group alone does not justify authorship.

Newer Mechanisms of Publication

Open Access offers a new model of publication. Almost entirely online, Open Access is operated mainly by consortia/publishing houses, such as BioMedCentral (www.biomedcentral.com) and the Public Library of Science (PLoS). The best Open Access journals can provide quick, effective dissemination of high-quality work.

Open Access channels its funding through institutional memberships and/or direct costs to the authors—transforming the traditional model in which authors publish for free and readers pay to access. With Open Access, the reader accesses for free. The challenge for Open Access is opposite that for print journals: While many readers may not be able to afford the subscriptions to print journals, many authors may not be able to afford the publication costs of Open Access—unless their institutions are members.

Web 2.0 media, which include social networking and other Web-based communications, offer many—though often complex—opportunities. The Web changes the notion of "publication" from a uni-directional form of dissemination to a multidimensional, more-democratic form of communication. Skillful users of Web media see themselves less as writers, in the traditional sense, and more as managers of conversations. They do not ask, "What do I want to say?" Instead, they may ask: "What conversation do I want to start? On what subject? Whom do I want to involve in this conversation?" To be successful, Web postings are less likely to end with statements and more likely to end with questions. And tone becomes less authoritative and lofty, and more collegial and inviting.

The 2010 earthquake in Haiti led to many new uses of digital writing and publication, including blogs, Facebook, and Twitter. The urgency of the situation and the need to inform people throughout the world about the many dimensions of the catastrophe—including some not adequately covered by the conventional media—produced some new forms of publishing. In many instances, these reports were cited by the conventional media, including the New York Times online edition. Public health workers set up blogs, some of which were automatically forwarded to colleagues. Nongovernmental organizations created on-the-scene blogs, often with photos, to help elicit contributions.

In this situation, scientific writing blended with storytelling, case histories, conventional reporting, and memoirs. Health workers who had previously avoided using the word "I" found themselves writing "I saw," "I heard," and "I felt." The needs of time and place meshed with the opportunities of the medium.

Conclusion

You may write for publication in both media for the general public and academic publications. Your writing style, for a given publication, will be determined by the content and context of your communication and whom you have chosen as your audience. As a public health worker, your most important and valued skill may be writing effectively.

RESOURCES

Books

Strunk WJ Jr. *Elements of Style*. Minneapolis: Filiquarian Publishing, 2007.
> *The classic in its field, it covers the basics of writing.*

Cutts M. *Oxford Guide to Plain English (3rd ed.)*. Oxford: Oxford University Press, 2009.
> *This book focuses on the essential features of good writing. (See also* http://www.askoxford.com/betterwriting/plainenglish/?view=uk.*)*

Article

Sand-Jensen K. How to write consistently boring scientific literature. *Oikos*. 2007; 116: 723–727.
> *A humorous look at what features not to include in your next paper, assuming you want it to be interesting.*

Web Site

http://www.plainlanguage.gov/resources/journals/index.cfm
> *A good source of information, advice, and other resources for writing simply and well.*

Good Examples of Public Health Writing for the Lay Public

Farmer P. *Infections and Inequalities: The Modern Plagues*. Berkeley, CA: University of California Press, 2001.
> *One of Paul Farmer's first books, and perhaps his best. In it, he discusses with candor his work in Haiti and elsewhere.*

Garrett L. *The Coming Plague: Newly Emerging Diseases in a World Out of Balance*. New York: Penguin, 1995.
> *As a science writer, Laurie Garrett skillfully tackles complex medical and public health topics and makes them understandable.*

Brookes T, Khan O. *Behind the Mask: How the World Survived SARS*. Washington, DC: APHA Press, 2004.

Brookes T, Khan O. *The End of Polio?* Washington, DC: APHA Press, 2006.

Both of these books were born from the idea that a physician with an interest in writing and a science writer with an interest in medicine could collaborate to write engaging and accurate material. The first book traces the story of severe acute respiratory syndrome (SARS) from the index case in Hotel M to WHO's quarantine of Toronto. In the second, the authors write about their travels to Pakistan, Afghanistan, Bangladesh, and elsewhere to determine where polio is still present and why it is so difficult to eradicate.

Commentary 4-1: Honing Your Writing Skills for Peer-Reviewed Publication

Mary E. Northridge

While all of us who work in public health share the common goal of preventing disease and promoting health, not all of us can claim the mantle of "public health practitioner." According to Gabriel Stover and Mary Bassett, the public health practitioner is the person who conducts the daily work of public health on the front lines of federal, state, and local health departments.[1]

It is too easy to disparage peer-reviewed journals as being out of touch with the values and concerns of public health practice, and much harder to ensure that the peer-reviewed record documents the practical experience of program-building. In many cases, even when the evidence from public health research is sufficient to warrant action, not enough is known about how to translate the research findings into effective public health practice. Thus, your contributions as a public health practitioner to the evidence base of public health are vital to the field as well as to the larger global community.

Why Should Public Health Practitioners Write for Peer-Reviewed Publication?

I have previously argued that publishing in peer-reviewed journals is more than a requirement of funding agencies, organizations, and institutions: It is our ethical responsibility to the communities we serve.[2] Best practices, wisdom gained through reflection on experience (what worked, what didn't, and why), and pointers on how to sustain interventions delivered in real time—all of these are essential to changing the current patterns of disease and disability and to eliminating social disparities in health.

Gabriel Stover and Mary Bassett further believe that information conceived only as numbers denies the rightful place of field-based knowledge and hard-won experience in the published record.[1] The knowledge base of public health needs to include shared experiences and cogent observations about making programs work. In addition, such relevant information and practical knowledge needs to be grounded in theoretical concepts and real-life models, and written so that other practitioners and community partners will be able to understand and use it without advanced training. Thus, your voice from the field is essential to record in the scientific and scholarly record. The rigors of peer review will better ensure that your contributions will be as valid and accessible as possible in the service of advancing public health.

What Are the Keys to Positive Writing Experiences?

Wendy Laura Belcher has gathered lessons from the students she mentors in writing and has found that successful writers share similar attitudes and work habits.[3] Her four keys to positive writing experiences, which are adapted for practitioners, are the following:[3(pp. 5–10)]

1. SUCCESSFUL WRITERS WRITE

No matter how busy your life is, make a plan for writing. Don't wait for inspiration. Don't wait until the last minute. Don't wait for big blocks of time. Make a plan for writing and stick to it.

2. SUCCESSFUL WRITERS MAKE WRITING SOCIAL

Work to make your writing more public and less private, more social and less solitary. Start a writing group. Take a writing class. Convince a colleague to co-write an article with you. Meet a fellow practitioner at a library or café and write for an hour. Attend conferences, participate in electronic discussion boards, join journal clubs, and introduce yourself to other practitioners whose work you admire.

3. SUCCESSFUL WRITERS PERSIST DESPITE REJECTION

If you write for peer-reviewed publication, your work will be rejected. This is unavoidable. You are in august company. The important point is not to let rejection stop you. Constructive criticism is not the measure of your writing or your own worth to the field. Be persistent and revise and resubmit your work elsewhere.

4. SUCCESSFUL WRITERS PURSUE THEIR PASSIONS

Focus on the questions that fascinate you. The world is changing rapidly. You are more likely to have positive writing experiences if you follow your deepest instincts rather than passing fads. Obsess about things that interest you. Pursue your passions. Don't be bullied into writing about topics that are not core to your values and interests.

Why Is Critical Thinking Important in Peer-Reviewed Publication?

All public health practitioners are writers, but not all of the writing of public health practitioners is suitable for peer-reviewed publication. For example, reports on program activities intended for public health leaders need to demonstrate accountability, and updates intended for funding agencies tend to emphasize progress over setbacks. On the other hand, the link between critical thinking and writing for peer-reviewed publication involves identifying and challenging assumptions and exploring alternative ways of believing and acting.

According to John Bean, writing is a way of discovering, making, and communicating meanings that are significant, interesting, and challenging.[4] He asserts that if writing is merely a communication skill, then we primarily ask of it, "Is the writing clear?" But if writing is critical thinking, we ask, "Is the writing interesting? Does it show a mind actively engaged with a problem? Does it bring something new to readers? Does it make an argument?"[4 (pp. 3–4)]

Peer-reviewed publication begins with the posing of a problem. Your thesis statement is a tentative response to that problem, a "solution" that must be supported with the kinds of reasons and evidence that are valued in public health practice. You will no doubt produce multiple drafts because the act of writing is itself an act of discovery.[4]

Why Do So Few Public Health Practitioners Write for Peer-Reviewed Publication?

As with all writers, there are certain internal reasons that may hinder the process of writing and desired outcome of peer-reviewed publication for public health practitioners. The internal reasons are those that you can overcome, given sufficient guidance and commitment. Robert Boice has gained familiarity with writing problems through accounts of other people's blocking experiences.[5] These problems generally fall into the following seven categories, moving from common to fairly uncommon types, encapsulated by a representative quote from a writer who encountered each problem:[5 (pp. 22–28)]

1. *Distaste for writing*: "You probably won't like this. I hate to write. At least I do now. I'd rather clean the house. [laughs]"
2. *Lack of time for writing*: "I actually spent more time worrying about not having enough time to write and about how I'll never get caught up on my writing than I did writing. Does that make sense?"
3. *Lack of confidence*: "I just thought about writing and I realized that I have yet to build a body of knowledge, a major contribution. I'm not ready."
4. *Writing anxiety*: "I get nervous. I even started to shake a bit, kind of like stage fright, you know."
5. *Inability to start writing*: "So I knew what I wanted to do, but I wasn't sure how I would say it. I mostly sat and stared at a few sentences I didn't like."

6. *Inability to finish writing*: "Each time I think I'm finished, I see that there's a lot more to do. I always see ways to improve the writing. I worry about its going off for review with some terrible flaw in it."
7. *Other psychological disruptors (such as depression, phobias, or writing cramps)*: "What happened? I just sat there. [pause] I looked out the window, mostly. I couldn't bring myself to write."

Perhaps one or more of these accounts rings familiar to you. If so, there are practical resources at the end of this section that you may find to be useful. So, too, you may find that working with a mentor, advisor, or fellow writer is valuable. And once you have struggled over your own hurdles in writing for publication, teaching and coaching others in their writing goals is not only rewarding in and of itself, but also will help you nourish your enthusiasm for writing.

IS THERE ANY CONCRETE GUIDANCE ON EFFECTIVE WRITING FOR PEER-REVIEWED PUBLICATION TARGETED TO PUBLIC HEALTH PRACTITIONERS?

There are no shortcuts to the writing process. As with most public health endeavors, behavior change is difficult to initiate and harder to sustain. Nonetheless, there are structural interventions that may prove advantageous, including the active solicitation of practice-based work in public health journals. In addition, the following 12 strategies—born of experience—have been helpful to me. I hope they will both inspire and comfort you.[2 (p. 179)]

1. Decide on authorship up front. Choose a lead author who will be accountable for ensuring that the paper is written and published.
2. Respect the rules of authorship. List only authors who fulfill the three criteria of conceptualization, writing, and approval of the final draft, as per the International Committee of Medical Journal Editors (see http://www.icmje.org).
3. Be clear in your thinking before you begin to write, but recognize when it is time to stop talking and start writing.
4. Give credit to those who informed your ideas. Cite the seminal work of others.
5. Carve out space and time for writing in practical and sustained ways to promote reflection, creativity, and honing of writing skills.
6. Hire practitioners who are skilled writers and value their contributions as essential to the success of your program.
7. Choose appropriate formats and journals to reach your intended audience, and be prepared to respond to calls for papers that actively seek practice reports.
8. Interpret data with care and sensitivity. Uphold your duty as a socially responsible practitioner to advance the cause of underserved communities.

9. Ask for constructive feedback from other practitioners, community partners, and evaluators before submitting your writing for publication.

10. Tap your inner core to infuse your writing with passion and purpose. Then direct your energies toward careful analysis and thoughtful policy recommendations.

11. Capture the richness and immediacy of your daily work in your written reports. Avoid the "drudgery" that too often is equated with public health practice.

12. Be prepared to rethink, rework, and rewrite your paper, but never relinquish ownership or responsibility for its content.

References

References #1 and 2 constitute editorial guidance from the American Journal of Public Health. References #3, 4, and 5 are workbooks that have proven to be helpful to writers in honing their skills for peer-reviewed publication.

1. Stover GN, Bassett MB. Practice is the purpose of public health. *American Journal of Public Health.* 2003; 93: 1799–1801.
2. Northridge ME. Building coalitions for tobacco control and prevention in the 21st century. *American Journal of Public Health.* 2004; 94: 178–180.
3. Belcher WL. *Writing Your Journal Article in 12 Weeks: A Guide to Academic Publishing Success.* Thousand Oaks, CA: SAGE Publications, Inc., 2009.
4. Bean JC. *Engaging Ideas: The Professor's Guide to Integrating Writing, Critical Thinking, and Active Learning in the Classroom.* San Francisco: Jossey-Bass, 2001.
5. Boice R. *Professors as Writers: A Self-Help Guide to Productive Writing.* Stillwater, OK: New Forums Press, Inc., 1990.

Commentary 4-2: 21 Tips for Clearer Writing

Barry S. Levy and Joyce R. Gaufin

General Recommendations

1. Write in the active—not passive—voice
"The health department issued guidelines."
   Not: "The guidelines were issued by the health department."

2. Use topic sentences to start paragraphs
"There were many reasons why the immunization program succeeded. First, we assessed the needs . . . "

3. Be succinct
Avoid long sentences and paragraphs.
   Use "most" instead of "a majority of."

4. Use parallel structure
"The board was composed of physicians, nurses, and representatives of nongovernmental organizations."
   Not: "The board was composed of physicians, nurses, and nongovernmental organizations."

5. Avoid multiple nouns used as adjectives before a noun
 "The recommendations for designing the framework for the system . . . "
   Not: "The system framework design recommendations . . . "

6. Cite and reference quotations and important studies and other sources of material

7. If you use automatic spell-checking, beware of correctly spelled words that may be wrong in the context in which they are being used

8. Proofread your work and have another person also proofread it

Emphasizing Important Points

9. Use tables, graphs, and photographs

10. Use headings and subheadings to clarify organizations
As demonstrated in this commentary.

11. Use lists
"Effective ways of preventing occupational disease include the following:
- Substituting safe materials for unsafe ones
- Designing and implementing engineering measures
- Establishing surveillance systems for illnesses and hazardous exposures . . ."

12. Use italics or an "em dash"—that is, a long or double hyphen to clarify a point, like this one

13. Use numbers in parentheses
"The success of the advocacy program resulted from (1) careful definition of the issues, (2) wise choice of action items, (3) establishing a wide base of support, and (4) development of relationships with policymakers."

Grammar Recommendations

14. Ensure that nouns and pronouns match
"The committee made its recommendations."
   Not: "The committee made their recommendations."

15. When using "it" and "this," ensure that the referent is clear

16. To avoid awkward "her/his" or "his/her" pronoun designations, pluralize the noun to which the pronoun is referring
"The department gave all of its health educators their own materials."
   Not: "The department gave each health educator her/his own materials."

17. Use "that" and "which" appropriately
Use "that" with restrictive clauses, those that limit or restrict the identity of the subject. For example: "They reported on the epidemiologic study that was performed on the food-borne outbreak at the college."

Use "which" with non-restrictive clauses. For example: "They reported on the challenges of epidemiologic studies, which include developing case definitions, identifying control groups, and minimizing bias."

Practices to Avoid

18. Avoid jargon and slang
"We need to train the next employee hired."
  Not: "We need to train the next hire."
Instead of using "e.g.," write "such as."
Instead of using "i.e.," write "—that is."

19. Avoid phrases that may be unnecessary
Think twice before using, at the start of a sentence, phrases that may be unnecessary, such as "It is important to know that . . . "
  Often, the phrases "thus far," and "as yet," are unnecessary.

20. Avoid nonspecific terms
Avoid "etc." or "a number of."

21. Avoid the term "respectively"
For example, write: "Group A had 9 people, Group B had 7 people, and Group C had 5 people."
  Not: "Groups A, B, and C had 9, 7, and 5 people, respectively."

Commentary 4-3: The Evolution of Writing a Book: My Experience

Linda Landesman

Getting published was just an episodic experience until I had lunch with a colleague who understood academics. We talked about using letters to the editor as a springboard to meatier publications. Our conversation led me to think about how I might translate some of my work into such a letter.

Several years before, I suggested that the Program Development Board (now the Science Board) of the American Public Health Association (APHA) expand its activities regarding emergency preparedness. As a result, the Health Administration Section of APHA began soliciting papers on disaster-related topics for presentation at the APHA Annual Meeting. Needing material for one of those papers, I reviewed course catalogues of schools of public health to determine what, if any, disaster-related courses were being offered. My survey revealed that few courses were available.

After the massive impact on public health of Hurricane Andrew in Florida in 1992, my survey was the basis for a letter to the editor for the American Journal of Public Health in which I called for formalized public health training in disaster preparedness and response. When the letter was published in 1993, a colleague encouraged me to apply for funds to organize a conference about developing a public health curriculum for emergency preparedness. I ultimately received funding for three conferences that brought together faculty from schools of public health with leaders in public health preparedness, from which came the first Curriculum on Emergency Preparedness for Schools of Public Health. With permission, I used the content of this curriculum as the foundation for writing the first edition of *Public Health Management of Disasters: The Practice Guide*.

In emergency preparedness and response, the resources needed for public health practice are diverse, technical, and widespread. My goal in developing this book was to facilitate a basic understanding of the public health role in the various components of emergency preparedness and response, and to provide one location for the many tools needed by those performing this work.

Since the publication of my letter to the editor in 1993, academic preparation for public health preparedness and response is now widespread. Before public health workers were involved in these activities, officials of emergency management—who may have lacked the necessary education and training—often addressed the health-related aspects of a disaster response. Today, public health workers are integrated members of emergency preparedness and response teams in communities and at the state and federal levels. They participate in planning for preparedness and response. And they are often in the forefront when a disaster or other emergency situation has adversely affected public health, helping to reduce morbidity and mortality.

I learned a major lesson from this experience. Use any and all opportunities to write about subjects you're passionate about. Who knows? You may end up writing a book that will transform public health.

5

Practicing Cultural Competence

Carol Easley Allen and Cheryl E. Easley

Understanding Cultural Diversity

Cultural competence is the ability to interact effectively with people of different cultures. Achieving cultural competence is important in addressing the health needs of others; working within agencies and organizations; communicating with individuals, groups, and the general public; and advocating for evidence-based policies and practices.

Cultural competence involves examining your biases and prejudices, and developing knowledge and behaviors that enable you to provide services effectively. Cultural competence means valuing diversity and respecting individual differences, regardless of race, religious beliefs, ethnocultural background, and sexual orientation. Lack of cultural competence can have serious consequences, ranging from educational misunderstandings to complications of disease—even death.

There are four cognitive components of cultural competence:

- *Awareness*: Your consciousness of your reactions to people who are different.
- *Attitude*: The difference between awareness of cultural bias and beliefs in general, and your examination of your own beliefs and values about cultural differences.
- *Knowledge*: Your comprehension of different cultural practices and worldviews.
- *Skills*: Your cross-cultural capabilities, such as verbal and nonverbal communication, that allow you to practice cultural competence.[1]

Culture can be defined as "the complex whole which includes knowledge, belief, art, morals, law, custom and any other capabilities and habits acquired by man as a member of society,"[2] or the "systems of shared ideas, systems of concepts and rules and meanings that underlie and are expressed in the ways that human beings live."[3] Culture is a set of explicit and implicit guidelines that people inherit as members of a specific society. Culture provides people with a worldview, including how to experience the world emotionally, and how to behave in relation to other people, supernatural forces or gods, and the natural environment. Culture also provides people with a mechanism to translate these guidelines to the next generation with symbols, language, art, and ritual.[4]

International human rights documents, such as the Universal Declaration of Human Rights and the International Covenant on Economic, Social and Cultural Rights, and many statements concerning specific populations address cultural rights.

Many professional associations have codes of ethics and statements of principles that address cultural competence and respect for cultures. Review the ethical statements of your profession to be sure that cultural rights are included.

Cultural Stumbling Blocks

You need to recognize *cultural stumbling blocks*—pitfalls that hinder cross-cultural communication and may lead to the perception that others are insensitive to one's needs and points of view. These lead people to view those in other groups as inferior. Several cultural stumbling blocks are described in Box 5-1.

Categories of Diversity

RELIGION

Religion influences or defines, to a large extent, the world views of many people, and affects their system of values, ideals of right and wrong,[5] and the meanings that they attach to illness, suffering, and death. *Spirituality*, a broader concept, can include adherence to a formal religious group but goes beyond it to denote various paths to an inner sense of meaning and values, as well as connection to others, to nature, or to the cosmos. Individuals vary greatly in the extent to which they adhere or practice the tenets of their faith. You should respect people and groups who choose not to believe in any deity (atheism) or to maintain a state of uncertainty with regard to religious belief (agnosticism).

Spirituality and religion can affect health in many ways since they may influence diet (including periods of fasting), use of alcohol and tobacco, sexual activity, the role of prayer, holidays and days of rest, and other aspects of lifestyle. Most of us are aware that various faiths, for example, involve dietary restrictions or rules for fasting. Less familiar are practices without analogy in Western culture, such as rules for the proper handling of the afterbirth (placenta) following delivery.

Basic to understanding and respect of the spiritual/religious beliefs and practices of others is that you as a public health professional maintain an ongoing consciousness of your own spirituality or religiosity, related values, and biases. Be sensitive to faith-related practices that may affect health or public health, and

Box 5-1: **Cultural Stumbling Blocks**

- *Prejudice*: A hostile attitude toward individuals simply because they belong to a particular group presumed to have objectionable qualities. It is an unfavorable opinion formed beforehand, based on insufficient knowledge, irrational feelings, or inaccurate stereotypes.
- *Discrimination*: The differential treatment of individuals because they belong to a minority group. Discrimination results when prejudice leads to the unfair treatment of a group based on race, ethnicity, age, religion, or gender.
- *Racism*: A mixed form of prejudice (attitude) and discrimination (behavior) that is directed at ethnic groups other than one's own. Racism includes not only animosity against people who belong to other races, but also a belief in racial superiority. Basing decisions and policies on race subordinates people in a racial group and maintains control over them.
- *Ethnocentrism*: The inability to accept the ways that other cultures organize reality, thereby considering one's way natural and best. It is the assumption that the cultural group to which one belongs is superior to other groups—the conviction of one's own cultural superiority. One's own group is believed to be centrally important and all other groups are measured or judged in relation to one's own.
- *Cultural paternalism*: An attitude that "I know what's best for you." Health workers often practice a specific type of paternalism based on disciplinary knowledge.
- *Cultural blindness*: Ignoring differences and proceeding as if they did not exist. Denial of one's essential being is not received positively, although it may have been intended as a gesture of acceptance. People do not want their cultural group membership to be denied or ignored; they want to be acknowledged and valued for who and what they are.
- *Cultural imposition*: The expectation that everyone should conform to people in the majority, whatever their personal beliefs.
- *Stereotyping*: Categorization based on an oversimplified standardized image of a person or group, without consideration of individual differences within the group. It is the most common cultural stumbling block.

work tactfully with families and communities to find acceptable and effective accommodations in areas of conflict.

If you are seeing patients in a clinical setting or serving individuals or groups in the community, you should understand their religious or spiritual commitments and how these influence their perception of physical and mental health and disease, disability and death, and various approaches to treatment and prevention.

You should be open to learning from others how their religion should be respected in the provision of public health services and how you can build on the good health practices entailed in the various faith traditions to promote health.

ABILITY

Individuals may experience a wide variety of disabilities during all or a portion of their lives, including physical, psychological, sensory, or cognitive disabilities. Disabilities result from a wide range of genetic and environmental factors. In general, education of—and social interaction with—people with disabilities should be inclusive; they should be integrated into communities. You should be aware that people with disabilities differ in (a) their identification with other people who have the same condition, and (b) their desire to interact with those who do not have disabilities.

Some deaf persons in the United States define themselves as a distinct cultural group based on their common use of American Sign Language (ASL), taking pride in the cultural products within this language tradition. The perception of deafness as a deviation from the norm (hearing) is seen as the "clinical pathological view," in contrast to the "cultural view," which sees deaf people as a community with a primarily visual way of relating to the world.[6,7]

You should learn about disabilities among the individuals or groups you serve. Recognize that people with disabilities and their families may face health risks and challenges due to these disabilities or due to barriers to accessing appropriate health services. And recognize that people with disabilities are often stigmatized and subjected to discrimination, prejudice, and denial of human rights and equity.[8]

SEXUAL ORIENTATION AND GENDER IDENTIFICATION

Sexuality has two dimensions. Gender identity refers to the gender with which a person identifies. Sexual preference, or sexual orientation, refers to the object or objects of sexual attractiveness for a person. While many people in the United States may conceive of only two genders (male and female) and perhaps three sexualities (heterosexual, homosexual, and bisexual), historically and transculturally multiple manifestations of both of these categories exist. In U.S. culture, terms such as *transgender* and *transsexual* are used to refer to statuses that go beyond traditional concepts. In other cultures and among indigenous and immigrant groups in the United States, socially integrated and accepted ways of expressing gender identity and/or sexual preference may be found. In some cases, these categories may be biologically based in addition to having social reality.[9] Some examples are the *fa'afafine* of Samoa, the *hijra* of India, the sworn virgins of the Balkans, and the two-spirit persons in some American Indian traditions.[9-11] You should be aware of these cultural patterns and sensitive to the use of descriptive terminology that is accurate and inoffensive.

Gay men, especially younger members of this group, may be prone to sex-related activities or lifestyles that put them at greater risk of HIV and other sexually transmitted infections.[12] Homosexual persons have been found to be at increased risk for a number of mental health problems, including suicide, depression, substance abuse, and eating disorders. In some cases, these risks are related to familial[13] or societal treatment of persons who differ from the majority in gender identity and sexual preference. Transgender/transsexual youth are at greater risk of harassment and/or violent attack while at school,[14] and homosexual or trans-gender persons, in general, are more prone to being victims of verbal and physical abuse and violence.

In many instances, persons who do not fit the traditional patterns of gender and sexuality are stigmatized and discriminated against in ways that can reduce their access to appropriate health services and lead to disparities in health status. These factors may, in turn, reduce the likelihood that persons from these groups will seek health care and public health services.

Barriers to care must be eliminated, and competent and respectful health services must be publicized and made available. We should develop and maintain contact with local support and action organizations for persons of various sexual orientations in order to help gauge the efficacy of efforts to provide care. We should pay special attention to the needs of young people and school-aged youth and their families. We should advocate for the delivery of unbiased health care for all, especially for those who may face discrimination based on sexual orientation.

SOCIOECONOMIC STATUS

The significant relationship between socioeconomic status and health is often mediated through culture. The proportion of families living in poverty is higher among racial and ethnic minority groups, who often have fewer opportunities for education, housing, employment, income earning, and property ownership than those in the dominant cultural group in society. We must differentiate between culture and socioeconomic status so that we do not misinterpret behavior that is related to low socioeconomic status as having a cultural origin.

People living in poverty or those who are homeless often may not receive the respect they deserve in a society where materialism is highly valued. We must ensure that all vulnerable populations are treated with respect and afforded human dignity.

Deficit explanations of poverty and approaches to its amelioration that are based on assumed characteristics of poor people tend to blame the victims of institutional oppression for their own victimization. This perspective overlooks the root causes of oppression and instead frames the problem in terms of deficits within certain individuals and communities; it absolves the larger society from responsibility for the problems of poverty and shifts the onus to poor people and poor communities.[15]

While deficit models may have some usefulness in the identification of community needs, their negative characterization of people living in poverty disregards what is positive in such communities. By contrast, asset models emphasize positive capacities and resources in communities and accentuate coping abilities, local group decision-making, and a movement away from dependency. Public health approaches that are asset-based incorporate asset-mapping strategies that support the development of an inventory of strengths and gifts in the community before intervention.

The World Health Organization uses the term *health assets* to define a broad range of individual and community resources that protect against negative outcomes and/or promote health—that is, social, financial, physical, environmental, or human resources. An inventory of such assets provides the basis for working together with vulnerable communities to (a) identify the policy measures necessary to sustain protective and health-promoting resources, (b) involve communities as co-producers of health—rather than simply as consumers, (c) strengthen individual and community capacity to contribute to the realization of optimal health potential, and (d) involve multiple sectors of society in the quest for equitable and sustainable social and economic development.[16]

SHELTER

Closely associated with poverty and its uneven distribution among cultural groups, homelessness places individuals and families at greater risk of poor health outcomes. While homelessness is not caused by cultural differences, members of minority cultural groups are disproportionately represented in the homeless population, especially African-Americans. The association between poor health and homelessness is reciprocal: poor health can contribute to being homeless, and being homeless can lead to poor health.

Common health issues among homeless people include mental health disorders, substance abuse, respiratory infections, wound and skin infections, and exposure to temperature extremes. Homeless women are at increased risk for domestic and sexual abuse, and homeless children who witness this abuse are at risk for emotional and behavioral problems. Health problems associated with homelessness may be compounded by the disadvantages often associated with low socioeconomic status and minority status.

While the greatest concentration of people experiencing homelessness is found in several states and large cities, rural homelessness is also a significant problem. The profile of rural homelessness, however, is distinctive: typically a married, white, working woman, often with a family. Rural homelessness is also high among Native Americans and farm laborers.

In the mid-1980s, most homeless people were single men. While single adults still constitute a large share of people experiencing homelessness, the face of homelessness has changed. The fastest-growing group of people experiencing homelessness is families with children. The most likely homeless person is a single woman in her late 20s with two children, one or both under 6 years of age. The primary causes of homelessness among families include low incomes, less access to housing subsidies, and weak social networks. Domestic violence increases the vulnerability to homelessness among women and children.

Children who are homeless experience a high rate of chronic and acute illnesses, emotional problems, and substance abuse disorders. They have been disproportionately exposed to violence and experience decreased academic achievement due to repeated school mobility.

Unaccompanied youth are also among people experiencing homelessness, often leaving home due to physical or sexual abuse. Studies are inconclusive as to whether such youth are more likely to be found among ethnic and racial minorities and among gay, lesbian, bisexual, and transgender youth. Poor school performance is either a contributing factor or a result of homelessness among youth. Chronic illness, mental health problems, risky behavior, and involvement with the criminal justice system characterize youth who experience homelessness. They are at increased risk of sexual abuse and HIV infection.

The Department of Veterans Affairs reports that veterans returning from Iraq and Afghanistan are likely to experience homelessness earlier than those who served in Vietnam. This finding may be attributed to repeated deployments among this group of veterans. The causes of homelessness among veterans are same as those that affect families. In addition, homeless veterans are likely to have experienced abuse prior to military service.

In addition to the increased risk of acute and chronic illnesses and mental health problems, people experiencing homelessness are subject to lack of access to the social support system because they do not have a permanent address and often lack a photo identification card. This often leads to problems with receiving social system supports that are mailed, placing them at a disadvantage in the job market.

The new federal strategic plan to prevent and end homelessness reflects the current approach to homelessness, initiated with the Housing First program, that emphasizes moving people experiencing homelessness out of emergency shelters into stable housing as quickly as possible.[17–19]

REGIONAL ORIGIN OR RESIDENCE

You need to be aware of the regional origin and residence of individuals and groups whom you serve and the associated cultural factors that influence their health. Such cultural factors may include the importance of religion, pride, privacy, and people's desire to care for their own people and avoid accepting charity. Rural residents in the United States exhibit a pattern of risky health behaviors that David Hartley[20] has characterized as a *rural culture* health determinant. This pattern suggests the possibility of cultural and environmental factors that are unique to rural towns and regions of the United States. People in rural regions rank poorly on a number of health parameters, including health behaviors, morbidity, mortality, and measures of maternal and child health. The role of place in health outcomes for rural residents appears to be associated with their isolation and lack of access to health care.[21] While we must be careful not to give reality to a fictional "rural culture," the negative health behaviors and poor health outcomes that characterize rural residents must be met with culturally competent public health approaches to care.[20]

Problems with access to health care are especially acute in rural communities. Shortages among health-care providers are exacerbated by their getting older and inadequacies in the education of their replacements. Access issues are a special concern in rural areas. Compared to the urban population, the population in rural areas is older, has lower education and income levels, is more likely to be living in medically underserved areas, is less likely to be from a minority group, and has greater health care needs—as well as higher rates of age-adjusted mortality, disability, and chronic disease. Farm workers have an especially high occupational fatality rate, and higher rates of work-related lung diseases, noise-induced hearing loss, skin diseases, and certain cancers associated with exposure to pesticides, agrochemicals, and prolonged sun exposure.[22,23] And farm children experience high fatal accident rates.

The people who live in Appalachia, the mountain counties that stretch from southern New York State to the foothills of Mississippi, experience poorer health outcomes than the rest of the nation.[24] Unlike other rural residents, who possibly may not be conceived of as a single cultural group, Appalachian people form a mountain culture shaped by their history and geographic isolation.

There is clearly a distinguishable Appalachian culture, and place is a prominent feature in it.[24] Appalachian people tend to have poor educational achievement and lower incomes than the general population. They also tend to be older. Although seven of eight Appalachians are white, minorities—such as blacks—among them experience even worse health outcomes than other Appalachians.

We are all challenged to communicate effectively to develop trust with Appalachians and other groups of people who tend to be skeptical of health-care providers and fear being taken advantage of by "the system."

In response to the lack of access to health care in several rural counties of southwest Alabama, the University of South Alabama College of Medicine established a tele-health network with a grant from the Health Resources and Services Administration.[25] The network, which includes four hospitals, many clinic sites, and a 200-member physician practice plan, provides "virtual" health-care services to four rural sites within a 50-mile radius of the medical college. A major focus is to provide access to perinatal services to a rural population that has some of the highest rates of low-birthweight infants and infant mortality in the United States. The rural residents served by real-time interactive video access to specialists are primarily low-income people living in medically underserved areas.

Alaska Natives and other Alaskans living in "the bush"—isolated, frontier areas—are vulnerable to many health risks. These people often occupy small regional centers or even smaller villages that may be accessible only by air or water and are subject to extreme weather conditions for much of the year. Access to health-care facilities and health professionals is limited, and many places lack indoor plumbing and adequate safe water supplies. Health care is provided through the creative use of community health workers (also known as lay health-care workers) through such mechanisms as the Community Health Aide Program (CHAP), itinerant public health nurses, traveling clinics, and a well-developed telemedicine system.

Health Literacy

Health literacy is the degree to which people have the capacity to obtain, process, and understand basic health information and services needed to make appropriate health decisions.[26] People with low health literacy may have difficulty in giving informed consent, following prescribed diets and medication orders, reading food labels, or understanding health education materials. An estimated 36% of adults in the United States have low health literacy.[27]

Low health literacy is more prevalent among elderly people, people in minority groups, and immigrants, but most U.S. residents with low health literacy are white and native-born. Even among well-educated people, low health literacy may be present because of limited exposure to the complex U.S. system of health-care delivery.[28]

Low health literacy is associated with an increased risk for complications of chronic disease, hospital readmissions, and other poor health outcomes—and a lower likelihood of engaging in preventive behaviors. Many people with low health literacy are adept at hiding this problem from others—even close friends and family members—because of the stigma attached to it.

Determining a person's level of health literacy requires skillful, sensitive assessment. The Newest Vital Sign (NVS), a bilingual screening tool, can help you identify people with low health literacy in 3 minutes. This is done by asking six questions about how people would interpret and act on information on a nutrition label from an ice cream container.[29]

Another approach you can use to assess health literacy consists of three questions that can be rated on a five-point scale:

• How confident are you in filling out medical forms by yourself?
• How often do you have someone help you read hospital materials?
• How often do you have problems learning about your medical condition?

You can address limited health literacy by making assessments sensitively; providing clear, appropriate, and understandable verbal and written communication of health information; and using a variety of evaluation techniques to validate people's understanding of and ability to use information provided.

Encourage patients to ask—and get answers to—these three questions during each health-care encounter:

- What is my main problem?
- What do I need to do about it?
- Why is it important for me to do this?[30]

How to Experience Your Feelings about Diversity

To develop cultural competence, you must become aware of your attitudes about cultural diversity. Almost everyone harbors some negative attitudes about various cultural groups. Only by examining and acknowledging your attitudes can you affirm your positive attitudes and modify your negative attitudes.

List the diverse cultural groups you typically encounter in your work. Ask yourself the following questions:

- How does my agency or organization respond to diversity?
- Is diversity ignored or viewed as a disadvantage?
- Is it celebrated?
- Are there specific programs available to assist "diverse" clients, students, or communities?
- What is my gut reaction to the "diverse" people I encounter?
- Do I view them positively or negatively?
- Do I do anything special to meet their needs?

Cultural Worldviews

A *worldview*, or a *vision of life*, is a coherent set of fundamental beliefs through which each of us views the world and our place in it.[31] It is a fundamental orientation of the heart that can be expressed as a story or in a set of assumptions—which may be true, partially true, or entirely false—held about the basic constitution of reality. A worldview provides the foundation on which we live.[32] It provides us with the mental blueprints that guide our actions.[33] It provides an interpretive and integrated framework that defines order and disorder, manages reality, and informs thinking and doing. All people have worldviews that enable them to think coherently about everything from casual matters to profound questions.

Worldviews function in several ways:

- They provide guidance on who we are and what our purpose in life is.
- They give us emotional stability.

- They validate cultural norms that we use to evaluate experience and determine courses of action.
- They help to integrate culture by organizing ideas, feelings, and values.
- They monitor cultural change, helping us to search a range of new ideas, behaviors, and products for those that fit our culture, and to reject or modify those that do not.
- They provide psychological reassurance that the world is truly as we see it.[34]

The worldview of members of a cultural group allows them to communicate with each other within a shared frame of reference. Because worldviews are intertwined with social systems, they can be used by powerful people within the cultural group to oppress the poor, and by the poor to justify rebellion. There are many ways you can discover the worldview themes of a cultural group, such as folklore, myths, art, music, dance, theater, descriptions of heroes and villains, poetry, proverbs, riddles, stories, and wisdom literature.

Male and White Privilege

Privilege refers to disproportionate advantage of one group (such as white men) and a concomitant disadvantage of another group (such as women of color). Those who benefit from privilege in the short run are often unaware of, or deny, its existence. Lack of awareness or denial protects privilege from being acknowledged or ended.

If you are a member of a privileged group, assess the extent to which you enjoy privilege. What things do you take for granted as a result? Try to imagine the feelings of those who are disadvantaged by your advantage. Think of ways in which the effects of this situation can be remedied in your setting and in society at large. If you are a member of a group that does not enjoy privilege, consider your personal feelings when confronting those who are privileged. Examine the ways in which these reactions might affect your interactions with co-workers, families, or communities.

Cultural Humility

The concept of *cultural humility* was developed in reaction to the idea that one could achieve a state of ongoing cultural competence based on a supposed understanding of the cultures of others. (The dangers of stereotyping and assuming that one's own culture is the norm are discussed later in this chapter.)

You may find it helpful to perform the following exercises in self-reflection:

1. Identify the beliefs and values of yourself and your family.
2. Describe your own culture and identity, including such aspects as ethnicity, experience, education, socioeconomic status, age, gender, sexual orientation, and religion.

3. Make a list of your personal biases and assumptions about people with values that are different from yours.
4. Ask yourself if your values are the norm.
5. Identify a time when you saw yourself as being different from others.[35]

Cultural humility is based on continuous self-reflection and self-critique of one's own culture and an ongoing process of exploring with those of other cultures the similarities and differences among your perspectives. It is based on an attitude of respect, openness, and flexibility.[35-37]

Cultural Self-Assessment Tools

Even if you are committed to social justice, you may have hidden or automatic stereotypes or prejudices that can adversely affect your behavior. A group of psychologists has developed a set of online tools, called Implicit Association Tests (IATs), to measure unconscious bias.[38,39] The National Center for Cultural Competence provides instruments for cultural self-assessment for organizations and individuals, including one for health workers.[39] (See the Resources section at the end of this chapter.)

How to Learn about Cultural Diversity

CULTURAL INFORMANTS

Expert informants, people who are steeped in their own culture and are sensitive to your culture and the areas in which you lack awareness, can help you learn about their culture.[40-43] They may be co-workers, patients or clients, or members of a community you serve. They should be familiar with the goals of public health and willing to share information that will facilitate your work. They are ideally good communicators who are objective and unbiased.

CULTURAL VALUES

Cultural values in a community or society are commonly held standards of what is acceptable or unacceptable, important or unimportant, right or wrong, workable or unworkable. They refer to the enduring ideas or belief systems to which an individual, group, or society is committed.[44]

You are conscious of some of your values and value systems but unconscious of others. You may feel that your values are shared by everyone else. Values clarification can enable you to recognize and understand your values and value systems.

You can delineate your cultural values in the following framework:[45,46]

1. *Universalist or particularist*: Universalism focuses on rules, particularism focuses on relationships. Which is more important to you?
2. *Individualist or collectivist*: In individualist culture, the welfare and desires of the individual take precedence over those of the group. In collectivist cultures, family or community takes precedence over the individual. Do you function as an individual or in a group?
3. *Neutral or emotional*: How intensely do you display your emotions?
4. *Specific or diffuse*: Are your interactions direct or indirect? In specific cultures, people tend to separate personal from professional life and people are more direct, purposeful, and transparent when relating to others. In diffuse cultures, personal contact pervades every human transaction and relations with others tend to be more indirect.
5. *Achievement-oriented or ascription-oriented*: Do you have to prove yourself to receive status, or is it given to you?
6. *Sequential or synchronic*: Do you do one thing at a time or several things at once?
7. *Internal or external control*: Do you control your environment or are you controlled by it?

Cultures have also been differentiated as to whether they are high or low context. In high-context cultures, people tend to be less verbally explicit and use less formal or written communications because there is more embedded shared understanding based on long-term relationships and strong group boundaries. Low-context cultures are characterized by more rule-orientation and publicly codified knowledge. Interpersonal communication is of shorter duration and more action-oriented.[47] All cultures exhibit some high-context and some low-context characteristics.

Consider how value orientations affect your beliefs, feelings, and actions. For example, what impact could a belief in external control have on the likelihood that a family or community will trust the effectiveness of immunization for their children? How might you confront this issue?

PROVERBS

A comparison of the proverbs of cultural groups reveals values and highlights cross-cultural differences and possible areas of conflict. Exploring the meaning of proverbs can be used to begin a conversation about cultural attitudes. This conversation can be extended as relationships develop to consideration of more complex genres such as group legends, myths, and founding epics.

Examples of proverbs from cultural groups include the following from a Native American tribe and three countries (with the cultural value implied in each proverb indicated after it in parentheses):

- *Hopi*: "One finger cannot lift a pebble." (Teamwork and community)
- *Ireland*: "It is easy to halve the potato where there is love." (Relationship)
- *The Philippines*: "Laziness is the sibling of starvation." (Hard work)
- *South Africa*: "Not everyone who chased the zebra caught it, but he who caught it chased it." (Initiative and perseverance)

Pay close attention to the proverbs quoted by people you encounter in your practice, noting generational and gender differences in the values and attitudes that are emphasized within and among cultural groups. Ask clients to share proverbs they learned from their parents or that are common in their cultural group. How do these proverbs inform the values and attitudes that shape the life choices and health behaviors of clients and communities in your practice?

VALIDATION

One of the best ways to avoid stereotyping is continual *validation*. Validation simply involves asking the person or group to confirm or correct one's assumptions or beliefs about a particular cultural generalization. For example, "I know that many Muslim women prefer female health care providers. Is this true for you?"

Validation may also take the form of your seeking an accurate interpretation of what you observe in a health-care encounter. For example, "I see that your grandmother plays an important role in helping you to make decisions about your baby's care. Would you like her to be present when I discuss his care with you?"

Cultural Assessment Categories

Public health workers also need to have competence and sensitivity concerning other attributes of individuals and populations that may be related to culture. These include, but are not limited to, attributes such as older age, lower mental capacity, lower educational level, and overweight and obesity.

TIME PERCEPTION

Cultural conceptions of time are related to basic lifestyles and religious foundations of Eastern and Western experience and thought. Time in some agrarian societies is perceived as spiral or circular based on crop cycles. The religions of some of these cultures include concepts of reincarnation or an endless cycle of birth, death, and rebirth. Western cultural views are generally founded on more linear concepts of time, which are compatible with industrialized societies. They are based on the worldview of time beginning with the creation of the world.

In the Western worldview, time is considered tangible, sequential, and divisible into regular segments. Time serves to regulate life. Westerners see time as a type of currency—"Time is money"—that can be saved or wasted.

A different conception more typical of Eastern cultures and some groups in the West is that of polychronic time. Here time is experienced as more circular or flowing, and capable of involving simultaneous occurrences. From this perspective time is seen as a more elastic entity during which relationships or interactions converge, with relationships being seen as more important than adhering to schedules. Events take place when the time is right, and life is experienced as much more relaxed.[48,49]

Conflicts may arise when cultural differences in time perception exist between clients and public health workers, such as when families are late for clinic appointments or when public health workers neglect to spend time developing the personal relationships that are often crucial to collaborative work with communities from differing cultures. Think creatively and in collaboration with representatives of various communities to ensure access to health services for persons whose concepts and priorities regarding time differ from those of mainstream America.

COMMUNICATION AND INTERPRETATION

Because people differ across cultures in how they send and receive messages, cultural misunderstandings are frequent. Become aware of differences in cultural communication patterns, especially with groups with whom you frequently interact. Actively listen and frequently validate, even with people from your own culture. To increase the clarity of your messages, avoid using slang expressions and idioms, jargon, and technical terms. Consider the meanings that various groups attach to words.

Using interpreters is often necessary to achieve culturally competent practice. They may need preparation in health-care terminology. Print and audiovisual materials in the language of the patient or client should also be available.

- The interpreter should know health care terms.
- Family members are usually not appropriate interpreters, especially children of a patient. Issues of confidentiality may arise. Family members may misinterpret health-care information. Patients or clients may be embarrassed or withhold information.
- The gender of the interpreter may facilitate or hinder the interaction. In some cultures, the interpreter needs to be of the same gender as the patient or client.
- Select an interpreter who is familiar with the dialect that the client speaks; this is especially important for Spanish speakers from different countries. Chinese patients who speak Mandarin cannot understand those who speak Cantonese—although they can communicate in writing.

- Ensure that the interpreter translates accurately, without changing the message. Stress the importance of word-for-word translation.
- Participate actively in the process by careful observation of the patient's body language, facial expressions, and other nonverbal behaviors.
- Contact a video or telephone translation service if competent interpreters cannot be identified. (See the Resources section at the end of this chapter.)

Ideally, you should learn the language of the cultural group of most of your clients or patients. But, at a minimum, you should learn and use at least a few phrases, such as "How are you?," "Please," and "Thank you."

MALE–FEMALE RELATIONSHIPS

The assessment of male–female relationships is important in health-related decision making for couples and families. You can determine if a relationship is the traditional patriarchal pattern of male dominance or a more egalitarian model. The traditional model is based on the male as breadwinner and authority in the home. The man is in control of the sexual relationship, and in many cases makes all decisions about sexual issues, including the women's use of contraception. If this is the case, family planning information must be shared with the man to gain his acceptance of contraceptive methods recommended by health professionals. Even if the woman indicates understanding and acceptance of health-care recommendations, she is unlikely to implement them if the man does not consent. The traditional female role is that of housewife and mother. It is associated ideally with female modesty and deference to male authority. Traditional female functions include child-bearer, domestic worker, and caregiver. Sometimes the apparent power relationship between a man and a woman masks the real situation.

Policies that reflect increased equality for women, based on a rising concern for human rights, now characterize the governments in many countries; however, lack of full female equality continues to be an international concern, particularly as it relates to female disadvantage in the areas of health, education, economics, legal rights, and political participation. Concerning male–female interactions, you should avoid positive or negative stereotyping of families you encounter.

FAMILY STRUCTURE AND INTERACTION

Family variation across cultures has long been recognized. Previous descriptions of family structure usually distinguished between *nuclear families* (characteristic of urban, industrialized societies) and *extended families* (more common in agrarian settings and some, especially non-Western, cultures). More recently, other variations in family composition have been recognized, leading to a more nuanced view of the nuclear family. Previously, the nuclear family consisted of a married heterosexual pair and their children, who lived apart from other generations and lateral kin. Now, it is recognized that even if these children do not live with other family members, the intergenerational ties of affection, support, and sometimes frequent meetings are more common. Societal forces, such as ongoing modernization, globalization, demographic shifts, and educational advances (especially for women), are changing families throughout the world.

The nuclear family is becoming much more prevalent in areas where extended family patterns were once the norm. But the "nuclear family" now connotes a range of structures, including unmarried heterosexual couples or same-sex couples living together, or families where one of the two adults may live out of the home, even at a distance. Other family patterns, such as the one-parent family, are becoming more prevalent, due, in part, to more frequent divorces in many cultures. Also common are families of three or more generations, grandparents raising grandchildren, and other groupings related by kinship or affiliation. Family structure and relationships are dependent on economic and subsistence factors as well as cultural and religious characteristics. Changes in family structure and patterns of residence interact with the aging of populations throughout the world, raising questions about who will care for the growing number of older people.[50]

SKIN COLOR

Skin color is often used to identify a person's *race*. "Race is primarily a social classification that relies on physical markers."[51] There is much confusion about the concepts of race and ethnicity. Although race has no biological or genetic basis, people are classified, treated differentially, and given access to power and other resources based on how others perceive their race. In contrast, *ethnicity* indicates membership in a cultural group. It is based on people sharing similar cultural patterns—such as beliefs, values, customs, behaviors, and traditions—that establish a common history that is exceedingly resistant to change.[51]

The most potent indicator of race is skin color. People are typically labeled as "white," "black," "brown," "yellow," or "red." Variations in skin color serve to differentiate among people within many cultural groups as well. People from India, Japan, Mexico, and Central and South American countries, and African-Americans often favor lighter skin color. In India, where most people are dark-skinned, most people seen on television or in movies are light-skinned. Among African-Americans, there is a history, dating from slavery, of an association between light skin and social desirability. Light-skinned persons have been—and in some cases still are—favored in the job market, housing, and the distribution of other social opportunities.

CONCEPTS OF BODY-MIND AND HEALTH-ILLNESS

Cultural worldviews enable people to conceptualize body image, the body's structure and function, and its social and psychological significance. The following body-image categories can assist you to assess deeply held cultural concepts about the body:[52]

- Optimal shape and size, including clothing and decoration
- Boundaries
- Inner structure
- Functions

You can assess cultural beliefs and values regarding the body through observation, questioning, and validation. With a simple exercise, you can explore your and your clients' or patients' cultural concepts about health. Ask your mother, maternal aunt(s), and grandmothers a few simple questions about (a) their cultural and religious origins, and (b) what practices and home remedies they and *their* mothers used to maintain, protect, and restore health.

DEATH AND DYING

Cultures address dying, death, and bereavement within the *meaning structures* provided by their cultural worldviews. Among the many areas that are culturally defined are the meaning of death, what constitutes a "good" death, appropriate ways to die and to grieve, and the acceptability of suicide. You can assess attitudes and values on death and dying by asking the following questions:[53]

- What are your cultural rituals for coping with dying, the deceased person's body, the final arrangements for the body, and honoring the dead person?
- What are your family's beliefs about what happens after death?
- What does your family feel is a normal expression of grief and the acceptance of the loss?
- What does your family consider to be the roles of each family member in handling the death?
- Are certain types of death, such as suicide, less acceptable?
- Are certain types of death especially hard to handle for that culture?

TOUCH AND PERSONAL SPACE

Invasion of personal space by other persons usually leads to feelings of discomfort, anxiety, or even anger. People from different cultures vary in terms of their level of comfort with physical touching by others. There are also cultural variations regarding touching between people of the same or opposite gender.[49]

Be conscious of your own comfort levels with touching and personal space. Reflect with others on how you differ in your use of touch. Learn what cues you can use to determine appropriate use of touch and personal space in interacting with people and communities from other cultures.

FOOD

Do not overlook the cultural implications of food. Major cultural differences involve what is eaten, when, and with whom.

Gender, age, and status distinctions are symbolized by the quality and quantity of food consumed. For example, in some cultures, men are given more and better-quality food than women and children. People of high social status may be offered "prestige foods" that are rare, expensive, or imported.

The social significance of food affects when people eat and with whom. This determination may also be based on age, gender, and social status. In many cultures, men sit down first and are served by women, who eat later with the children. Women of high social status may eat with the men.

Here are several distinctions you can use to assess cultural values associated with food:

- *Is it food or not?* The definition of food varies greatly among cultures.
- *Is food sacred or profane?* Foods defined as sacred may be eaten only by certain people or by all on special occasions.
- *Is food hot or cold?* In some cultures, foods are designated as *hot* or *cold*. Such foods are either prescribed or prohibited in order to achieve balance in the body, treat or prevent illness, or manage pregnancy, postpartum care, and breastfeeding.
- *Is food medicine or is medicine food?* Foods considered as appropriate for medicinal use in some cultures may actually have adverse health effects.
- *Is it a social food?* Social foods are foods eaten in the presence of other people that have symbolic significance.[52]

Because many immigrants to the United States do not adopt a U.S. diet, you may need to assess dietary patterns of individuals or families you encounter and provide appropriate nutritional counsel.

How You Can Learn More about Cultural Issues in Personal and Organizational Public Health Practice

RECOGNITION OF, AND RESPONSE TO, DIVERSITY IN PATIENTS AND COMMUNITIES

You can learn about cultural groups by:

- Interacting with cultural informants
- Reading scholarly and popular books and articles, including histories, contemporary analyses, novels, accounts on folklore, children's books, and plays
- Visiting ethnic neighborhoods, shopping areas, and playgrounds

- Attending public cultural events and celebrations as well as performances of drama and music
- Attending art and crafts exhibits
- Participating with families and communities in religious services and rites to mark special occasions

There are several culturally competent practices that you can use to appropriately address diversity in individuals, families, and communities, including the following:

- *Cultural preservation:* Actions that help retain and preserve traditional values to maintain promote or restore health
- *Cultural accommodation:* Actions that enable people to adapt to or negotiate with you to achieve satisfying health care outcomes
- *Cultural repatterning:* Actions that help people to make a beneficial change or modification in a cultural practice. This requires you to respect cultural values and beliefs as you work with individuals, families, and communities toward the mutual development of new patterns.
- *Cultural brokering:* Actions that you may take to advocate for an individual in relationship to the biomedical health-care culture[51]

Natural gathering places or events among cultures can provide you with opportunities to engage communities in health-related discussions and education. These include community organizations, places of worship, barbershops, and hair salons.

CULTURAL CONSIDERATIONS IN TEACHING AND LEARNING

Your use of a variety of teaching/learning modalities helps to ensure cultural competence in health education and accounts for different learning styles among individuals. Effective teaching depends on accurate assessment of the understanding and comprehension by learners of what is being communicated. This assessment is especially important if teacher and learner are from different cultures. Restate important concepts in the learner's own words. Ask if what has been taught has been understood. However, when teaching people from cultural groups that defer respectfully to teachers, don't ask, "Do you understand?" The answer will almost always be "Yes" because saying "No" is disrespectful to the teacher—whether the learner understands the information or not.

Consider variations among cultures in terms of body language, amount of eye contact or nonverbal feedback, cultural concepts of time, and withholding information or questions. Make accommodations for learners who speak English as a second language.

CULTURAL ISSUES IN CONDUCTING COMMUNITY-BASED RESEARCH

Eliminating disparities in health status and access to health care depends, in part, on culturally sensitive and inclusive research in community settings. Unfortunately, the foundation of trust between health researchers and diverse communities has been complicated, over many years, by exploitation and harm done in the name of scientific progress.

Collaborative research models, such as community-based participatory research (CBPR), offer opportunities to rebuild trust necessary for useful research. The ultimate goal of research in diverse cultures is to involve persons from these cultures not only as participants, but also as members and leaders of research teams.

Elicit meaningful participation by community members from the start of a study, when its focus and design are determined. Work with community leaders to identify and elicit the participation of people who are qualified to serve as partners or consultants in planning or performing the study. Involve young people to spark their interest in careers in health care or research. Develop a community advisory committee to provide guidance and consultation. Employ cultural informants to help ensure that cultural values are understood and respected and that analysis is accurate.[42,43]

Learn about the formal and informal processes to gain approval and access for studies within the community. In some communities, this is done through local churches. In others, it is done through village or tribal elders. You may need to work with an intermediary who is known and trusted in the community. Ensure that all communications and research instruments are culturally appropriate and, if necessary, accurately translated.[54]

Methods of data collection should be compatible with cultural norms. Who in a family should be asked for information? Are data best obtained from interactions with individuals or groups? Protect confidentiality in interviewing and reporting of findings, especially when communities are so small that respondents may be easily indentified.[55]

Work with communities in reporting the results of your research. Provide opportunities for community representatives to co-author research reports.

Consider ways in which research can benefit the community. Avoid exploiting the community to meet the needs of the research team for publications and professional recognition, without giving back anything to those who made the study possible.

PUBLIC HEALTH ADVOCACY AND CULTURAL DIVERSITY

Advocacy is a key public health function (see Chapter 2). Concern for human rights, equity, and social justice is basic to public health. As you serve and interact with individuals or groups who differ from mainstream culture in various ways, you will find prejudice, discrimination, stigmatization, marginalization, violation of human rights, and denial of justice and equity—all of which lead to reduced access to quality health care and reduced health status. You may choose to advocate on behalf of others for positive change, taking care not to be paternalistic. As outsiders to a community or culture, you should act in supportive—or consultative—roles rather than in leadership roles. Members of the community or culture—not you—need to set the agenda and determine goals and priorities.

Meaningful advocacy can involve anything from working for the passage of needed legislation at the national, state, or local level to working to ensure that the voices of a cultural group are heard or that denial of human rights is protested.

STANDARDS FOR CULTURAL COMPETENCE

The National Standards for Culturally and Linguistically Appropriate Services in Health Care (CLAS) were developed by the Office of Minority Health (OMH) of the U.S. Department of Health and Human Services to ensure culturally and linguistically appropriate practice. The 14 CLAS standards are used by federal and state health agencies and other health-related organizations, but they are primarily recommended for use by health-care providers to make their practices more culturally and linguistically accessible.[56,57] Some of these standards are mandates (requirements for all recipients of federal funds), some are guidelines (activities recommended by OMH for adoption as mandates by federal and state government agencies and national accrediting agencies), and some are recommendations (suggested by OMH for voluntary adoption by health-care organizations). The CLAS standards should be integrated throughout health-care organizations in partnership with the communities they serve. They are organized by theme: Culturally Competent Care (Standards 1–3), Language Access Services (Standards 4–7), and Organizational Supports for Cultural Competence (Standards 8–14).[57]

References

1. Martin M, Vaughn BE. Strategic Diversity & Inclusion Management Magazine. San Francisco: DTUI Publications Division, 2007.
2. Tylor EB. *Primitive Culture*. New York: J.P. Putnam Sons, 1920 [1871].
3. Kessing R. *Cultural Anthropology: A Contemporary Perspective (2nd ed.)*. New York: CBS College Publishing, 1981.
4. Helman CG. *Culture, Health and Illness (2nd ed.)*. Boston: Butterworth Heinemann, 1990.
5. Adamczyk A, Pitt C. Shaping attitudes about homosexuality: The role of religion and cultural context. Social Science Review 2009; 38: 338–351.

6. American Deaf Culture. Perspectives on Deaf People. Available at: http://www.signmedia.com/info/adc.htm. Accessed on July 23, 2010.

7. Information and Resources related to American Sign Language (AS), Interpreting and Deaf Culture. Available at: http://www.aslinfo.com/deafculture.cfm. Accessed on July 23, 2010.

8. Human Rights Education Associates. Human Rights of Persons with Disabilities. Available at: http://www.hrea.org/index.php?vase_id=152. Accessed on May 4, 2010.

9. Vasey PL, VanderLaan DP. Birth order and male androphilia in Samoan fa'afafine. Proceedings of the Royal Society, June 7, 2007. Available at http://www.ncbi.nlm.nih.gov/pmc/articles/PMC2176197/. Accessed on July 27, 2010.

10. Weston K. Lesbian/gay studies in the house of anthropology. Annual Review 1993; 38:339–367.

11. National Geographic. Sworn Virgins. (Video) Available at: http://video.nationalgeographic.com/video/player/places/culture-places/beliefs-and-traditions/albania_swornvirgins.html. Accessed on July 27, 2010.

12. Stolberg SG. Identity crisis: Gay culture weighs sense and sensibility. New York Times, November 23, 1997. Available at: http://www.nytimes.com/1997/11/23/weekinreview/identity-crisis-gay-culture-weighs-sense-and-sexuality.html. Accessed on July 27, 2010.

13. Ryan C, Huebner D, Diaz RM, Sanchez J. Family rejection as a predictor of negative health outcomes in white, Latino lesbian, gay, and bisexual young adults. Pediatrics 2009; 123: 346–352.

14. Greytak EA, Kosciw JG, Diaz EM. Harsh Realities: The Experiences of Transgender Youth in Our Nation's Schools. A Report from the Gay, Lesbian and Straight Education Network, 2009. Available at: http://www.glsen.org/binary-data/GLSEN_ATTACHMENTS/file/000/001/1375-1.pdf. Accessed on December 29, 2010.

15. Education.com. Characteristics of the Cultural Deficit Model, 2010. Available at: http://www.education.com/reference/article/cultural-deficit-model. Accessed on November 29, 2010.

16. Morgan A, Ziglio E. Revitalising the evidence base for public health: an assets model. Promotion & Education Supplement 2007; 14:17–22.

17. Main Street, a project of Working America. The Changing Face of Homelessness. Available at: http://www.workingamerica.org/blog. Accessed on November 29, 2010.

18. National Law Center on Homelessness & Poverty. Homelessness & Poverty in America, 2010. Available at: http://www.nlchp.org/hapia.cfm. Accessed on November 29, 2010.

19. United States Interagency Council on Homelessness. Opening doors: Federal Strategic Plan to Prevent and End Homelessness 2010. Available at: http://www.ich.gov/PDF/OpeningDoors_2010_FSPPreventEndHomeless.pdf. Accessed on December 29, 2010.

20. Hartley D. Rural health disparities, population health, and rural culture. American Journal of Public Health 2004; 10:1675–1678.

21. Rural Assistance Center. Rural Health Disparities. Available at: http://www.raconline.org. Accessed on July 29, 2010.

22. Bailey JM. No. 9 Health Care Reform, What's in It? Rural Communities and Rural Medical Care. Center for Rural Affairs, July 2010 Available at: http://files.cfra.org/pdf/Rural-Communities-and-Medical-Care-brief.pdf. Accessed on November 29, 2010.

23. Jones CA, Parker TS, Ahearn M, et al. Health status and health care access of farm and rural populations. United States Department of Agriculture. Economic Research Service. Economic Information Bulletin, Number August 57, 2009.

24. Behringer B, Friedel GH. Appalachia: Where Place Matters in Health. Preventing Chronic Disease, 2006. Available at: http://www.cdc.gov/pcd/issues/2006/pct/06_0067.htm. Accessed on July 27, 2010.

25. Telehealth Rescues Isolated Patients–University of South Alabama's telehealth network provides rural areas with medical expertise. Health Management Technology, December 1999. Available at: http://findarticles.com/p/articles/mi_m0DUD/is_11_20/ai_55811692. Accessed on November 29, 2010.

26. Institute of Medicine. Health Literacy: A Prescription to End Confusion. Washington DC: Institute of Medicine, Board on Neuroscience and Behavioral Health, Committee on Health Literacy, 2004.

27. Vernon JA, Trujillo A, Rosenbaum S, DeBuono B. Low Health Literacy: Implications for National Health Policy. Available at: http://www.pfizerhealthliteracy.com/pdf/Low-Health-Literacy_Implications-for-National-Health-Policy.pdf. Accessed on August 1, 2010.

28. Sand-Jecklin K, Murray B, Summers B, Watson J. Educating nursing students about health literacy: from the classroom to the patient bedside. Online Journal of Issues in Nursing. 2010; 15;3. Available at: http://www.nursingworld.org/MainMenuCategories/ANAMarketplace/ANAPeriodicals/OJIN/TableofContents/Vol152010/No3-Sept-2010/Articles-Previously-Topic/Educating-Nursing-Students-about-Health-Literacy.aspx#IOM04b. Accessed on July 28, 2010.

29. Pfizer Clear Health Communication Initiative. Available at: http://www.pfizerhealthliteracy.com/physicians-providers/newest-vital-sign.html. Accessed on August 1, 2010.

30. Partnership for Clear Health Communication. Available at: http://www.npsf.org/askme3/. Accessed on August 1, 2010.

31. Olthuis J. On worldviews. In Marshall PA, Griffioen S, Mouw RJ (eds.). *Stained Glass: Worldviews and Social Science*. Lanham, MD: University Press of America, 1989.

32. Sire JW. *The Universe Next Door (5th ed)*. Downers Grove, IL: InterVarsity Press, 2009.

33. Geertz C. *The Interpretation of Cultures: Selected Essays by Clifford Geertz*. New York: Basic Books, 1973.

34. Hiebert PG. *Transforming Worldviews: An Anthropological Understanding of How People Change*. Grand Rapids, MI: Baker Academic, 2008.

35. California Health Advocates. Are you practicing cultural humility? The key to success in cultural competence, 2007. Available at: http://www.cahealthadvocates.org/news/disparities/2007/are-you.html. Accessed on July 29, 2010.

36. Trevalon M, Murray-Garcia J. Cultural humility versus cultural competence: A critical distinction in defining physician training outcomes in multicultural education. Journal of Health Care for the Poor and Underserved 1998; 2:117–125.

37. Hixon AL. Beyond cultural competence. Academic Medicine 2003; 6:634.

38. Implicit Association Tests. Project Implicit, 2002. Available at: http://implicit.harvard.edu. Accessed on July 29, 2010.

39. Teaching Tolerance: A project of the Southern Poverty Law Center. Test Yourself for Hidden Bias. Available at: http://www.tolerance.org/print/activity/test-yourself-hidden-bias. Accessed on November 29, 2010.

40. National Center for Cultural Competence. Available at: http://www11.georgetown.edu/research/gucchd/nccc/. Accessed on July 10, 2010.

41. Godar SH, Rimsane I. Utilizing a native informant to gain cultural competence. International Business: Research, Teaching and Practice 2009; 3:21–31.

42. Marshall MN. The key informant technique. Family Practice 1996; 13(1): 92–97.

43. Center for Substance Abuse Prevention's Northeast Center for the Application of Prevention Techniques (NECAPT). Key Informant Interviews. In the online course "Data collection methods: Getting down to basics." Education Development Center, 2004.

44. Ludwick R. Ethics: Nursing around the world: Cultural values and ethical conflicts. Online Journal of Issues in Nursing, 2000. Available at: http://www.nursingworld.org/MainMenucategories/ANAMarketplace/ANAPeriodicals/OJIN/Columbus/Ethics/CulturalValuesandEthicalConflicts.aspx. Accessed on May 6, 2010.

45. A model of culture in seven dimensions. Available at: http://egginger.nethead.at/downloads/content/25/webdoc.html. Accessed on July 29, 2010.

46. Dunn P, Marinetti A. Cultural adaptation: Necessity for global elearning. Organizational Readiness in Turbulent Times. Available at: http://www.linezine.com/7.2/articles/pdamca.htm. Accessed on May 4, 2010.

47. Domitorio I. Edmonton 2008 cultural profiles. In Mobilizing for Action: A Report to Help Create Culturally Responsive Pathways for Isolated Immigrant Seniors. Available at: http://www.seniorscouncil.net/uploads/files/Issues/Mobilizing_Action_Report/Cultural%20Orientations%20and%20putting%20the%20cultural%20profiles%20in%20in%20context.pdf. Accessed on May 4, 2010.

48. Helman CG. *Cultural aspects of time and ageing*. EMBO (European Molecular Biology Organization) Reports, Special Issue, 2005.

49. LeBaron M. Culture-based negotiation styles. In Burgess G, Burgess H, eds. *Beyond Intractability*. Boulder, CO: Conflict Research Consortium, University of Colorado. Available at: http://www.beyondintractability.org/essay/culture_negotiation/. Accessed on July 29, 2010.

50. Georgas J. Family: Variations and changes across cultures. Online Readings in Psychology and Culture. Available at: http://www.ac.ww.edu/~culture. Accessed on July 29, 2010.

51. Degazon CE. Cultural diversity in the community. In: Stanhope M, Lancaster J. *Public Health Nursing: Population-Centered Health Care in the Community (7th ed.)*. St. Louis, MO: Mosby, 2008.

52. Helman CG. *Culture, Health and Illness (5th ed.)*. Boston: Butterworth Heinemann, 2007.

53. National Cancer Institute. Cross-Cultural Responses to Grief and Mourning. Available at: www.cancer.gov. Accessed on July 29, 2010.

54. Rahman A, Iqbal Z, Waheed W, Hussain N. Translation and Cultural Adaptation of Health Questionnaires. Available at: http://www.jpma.org.pk/full_article_text.php?article_id=115. Accessed on August 4, 2010.

55. Clyne ID. Finding Common Ground: Cross-Cultural Research in the Muslim Community. Australian Association for Research in Education. Available at: http://www.aare.edu.au/01pap/don01569.htm. Accessed on May 4, 2010.

56. Spector RE. *Cultural Diversity in Health and Illness (7th ed.)*. Upper Saddle River, NJ: Pearson Prentice Hall, 2008.

57. Office of Minority Health. Assuring Cultural Competence in Health Care: Recommendations for National Standards and on Outcomes-Focused Research Agenda, 2001. Available at: http://www.omhrc.gov/CLAS/cultural1a.htm. Accessed on July 29, 2010.

RESOURCES

Books and Other Documents

Center for Health Leadership and Practice, Public Health Institute. *The Principles of the Ethical Practice of Public Health*. Available at http://www.phls.org/home/section/3-26/. Accessed on June 1, 2011.

This public health code of ethics is a useful document.

Fadiman A. The Spirit Catches You and You Fall Down: A Hmong Child, Her American Doctors, and the Collision of Two Cultures. New York: Farrar, Straus and Giroux, 1997.

A profoundly moving account of the cultural collision between a Hmong family and the U.S. health care system that teaches important lessons in cultural competence.

Health Resources and Services Administration. Indicators of Cultural Competence in Health Care Delivery Organizations: An Organizational Cultural Competence Assessment Profile, 2002. Available at: http://www.hrsa.gov/culturalcompetence/indicators/. Accessed on May 4, 2010.

This cultural assessment guide provides general knowledge about various cultural and national groups, and provides a basis for observation, questioning, and validation of assumptions with the individual, family, or community.

Warrier S. Culture Handbook. Family Violence Prevention Fund, 2005.

This handbook was developed by the Family Violence Prevention Fund for use by advocates and professionals who work with those who are victims of domestic and sexual violence.

Organizations and Web Sites

Office of Minority Health Cultural Competency
www.minorityhealth.hhs.gov/ (click on "Cultural Competency")
The National Center for Cultural Competence (NCCC)
www11.georgetown.edu/research/gucchd/nccc/

Implicit Association Tests

    www.implicit.harvard.edu

    Implicit Association Tests detect the strength of an individual's automatic association between mental representations of objects or concepts in memory

The California Endowment. Culturally Competent Health Systems.

    www.calendow.org/article.aspx?id=1378

The Center for Cross Cultural Research at Western Washington University

    www.wwu.edu/culture/

The University of Washington Medical Center.

    depts.washington.edu/pfes/CultureClues.htm

    This Web site has end-of-life care tips for various cultural groups.

Language Access Network. My Accessible Real-Time Trusted Interpreter (MARTTI) languageaccessnetwork.com/

    A system available in some hospitals in which medically trained interpreters assist health care providers and their patients (and their families) with video-assisted real-time interpretation.

AT&T. Language Line

    http://languageline.com/page/industry_healthcare/.

    A service to assist people with limited communication skills in English.

ToolKit

Elliot C, Adams RJ, Sockalingam S. Multicultural Toolkit http://www.awesomelibrary.org/multiculturaltoolkit.html.

    A toolkit for cross-cultural collaboration.

Commentary 5-1: Two Examples of the Importance of Cultural Competence

Carmen Rita Nevarez

As a physician in training years ago, I encountered a fellow intern who did not understand the situation that he faced with an agitated and weeping new mother. She was inconsolable because her husband had, in anger, just left her, soon after this intern had circumcised their newborn son. She had given her written consent, but she was not literate in English and barely literate in Spanish. Her husband, who believed that their son had been turned into a homosexual by the circumcision (a common belief in his village), walked out, leaving his wife terrified about the future of her family.

The intern might have avoided the situation if he had (a) not assumed that this circumcision was routine, (b) asked the mother's nurses about her ability to understand the choices she was being offered, and (c) asked her and her husband about their wishes. A culturally competent provider would have understood the importance of asking these kinds of questions and not making assumptions.

Often I am faced with unique assumptions that I have made as a Latina of Mexican descent, a member of a large extended family, and a product of the Catholic education system. Frequently I experience clashes of culture that catch me off guard, when I fail to understand others' attitudes or behaviors.

The tools of cultural competence enable me to understand and sometimes to speak the language of others with whom—or for whom—I serve. Some of my work has been aimed at understanding and reducing the high rate of births to teenagers in California. I learned that Latino parents, who are very concerned about their children's health, strongly wish that their teenage daughters be vaccinated against human papillomavirus (HPV). I better understand this desire when I realize that Latinos living in California are primarily from Mexico, where childhood vaccination is seen as a right—a right that is reinforced at civic events throughout that country. Vaccinations in Mexico are made available free of charge and vaccination rates are very high—even in rural areas. In fact, the government of Mexico uses these events to reinforce the culture of prevention and the belief that health is a right. I also learned that Latino parents in California, who were very uncomfortable in directly addressing sexuality with their children, nevertheless strongly promote comprehensive sexuality education in the schools.[1] This led me to think about how to approach Latino parents as partners in protecting their children's health.

I have also learned that cultural competence is important in understanding the foods people eat and how they perceive that these foods affect their health. People have deeply embedded cultural beliefs and behaviors about food and eating. In many cultures, meals nurture relationships—sometimes expressed through extended mealtime conversations that create bonds and preserve family harmony.

As Mexicans have migrated to the United States, their second- and third-generation family members have become overweight, in part due to the U.S. diet and decreased opportunities for physical exertion at work. Public health workers can trivialize the importance of mealtimes and erroneously assume that over-weight Mexican-Americans do not know how to prepare food properly. They can also fail to appreciate that lower-income people cannot easily afford lean meat, often cannot access fresh fruits and vegetables, and frequently eat "fast food." So public health workers can erroneously assume that poor people just don't know better—or simply don't care about their diets.

My co-workers and I have worked in a collaborative project to improve the qual-ity of food at an ethnic food court. Initially, our team spoke with food vendors there about why there was a need for them to offer healthier food items. Then technical assistance was provided to help them offer food items that were more nutritious—and still tasty. A bicultural nutritionist who worked with us spent time with the vendors to understand the values that had been influencing their choices of food items to offer. She saw that they regarded their work as a community service—as a responsibility—and that they were using treasured recipes passed down to them from their mothers and grandmothers. Although she found it challenging to get the vendors to modify their recipes, she ultimately succeeded in enabling them to see the benefits of offering healthier food items by reducing calorie counts and increasing the variety of vegetables. As a result, the vendors now offer more nutri-tious—and still tasty—food, and they are proud of this achievement. In addition, they see the benefits of this change on their own improved personal health.

As a part of this project, we asked patrons—most of whom have low incomes and speak mainly Spanish—about their interest in receiving information about the nutritional value of menu items. Overwhelmingly, they expressed a strong desire to know more about the nutritional value of the food items they purchase.

Cultural competence is not a static set of facts to be memorized and then recalled when seemingly appropriate. The values, beliefs, and family structures of populations are always in flux. For example, the population in a community served by a clinic where I worked for 10 years changed during that period from a fairly homogenous African-American population to a heterogeneous population of Vietnamese, Chinese, and Latinos.

We need to always be deeply aware of our own cultural footing. Unless we know our own cultural biases and remain aware of the value systems with which we ourselves have been raised, we are destined to continually fail to serve our patients, clients, and communities. To practice public health competently, we must know what the people whom we serve believe, value, and desire for themselves and their families. And to know, we must ask—with humility and sensitivity.

Reference

1. Public Health Institute. Center for Research on Adolescent Health and Development. No Time for Complacency Policy Review: California Parents Overwhelmingly Support Comprehensive Sex Education. Available at: http://teenbirths.phi.org/2007PolicyReview. pdf. Accessed on December 15, 2010.

Part Two

ADMINISTRATION AND MANAGEMENT

6

Working Within an Organization

Tricia Todd and Shailendra Prasad

Introduction

A new assistant to the director of a fairly large public health agency was asked by her boss to bring together people from various departments within the agency to begin strategic planning—something she had experience doing, but in another sector. She contacted department heads and told them that she needed them to attend a meeting that was set strategically for a Monday morning—before people would be too far into their busy week.

Much to her surprise, only one third of the expected number of people came. And of those who did, most were not invitees, but stand-ins with little authority. The assistant was upset. She told those present that the key decision-makers she needed at the meeting were not present, and therefore she was canceling the meeting because of low turnout. She suggested that the blame rested with her boss; if her boss had more authority, then the key leaders would have come.

Because she was concerned that she would be blamed for the poor turnout, she assured her boss that the blame rested with the other leaders of the agency and their lack of commitment to strategic planning.

This story reflects several mistakes made by people trying to work effectively within an organization. This chapter will highlight the challenges of working effectively in an organization, along with some strategies to help address these challenges. This chapter has been organized around the "Four Cs" of working effectively in an organization: Context, Content, Connections, and Careers.

In the above story, the assistant was new, but not entirely inexperienced. She had worked in another organization, where the norm or culture was to hold important meetings early on Monday mornings. In her new organization, Monday was considered a sacred day, preserved for getting organized for a busy week ahead. Since Tuesday was when most local board meetings were held, Monday was reserved as preparation time—except for an emergency meeting, which could be called only by the director.

Therefore, when the assistant invited people to attend a meeting on a Monday, it was not seen as an important meeting, so most division directors delegated other staff members to attend. She would have been more successful if she understood the agency's culture and protocol—and the way things had previously been done. In addition, instead of using the opportunity to build connections with other staff members who did attend the meeting, she dismissed them as powerless, rather than appreciating their informal power. She failed to recognize that content knowledge and experience from one setting does not always translate directly into new settings, because culture shapes how things get done. Finally, she made many assumptions and failed to accept responsibility for her own thoughts and behaviors, which ultimately could hurt her career and make it very difficult for her to get things done in the agency in the future.

Context: Understanding the Environment in Which You Work

Organizations develop and maintain cultures—like personalities—that create the context for your work. To work effectively in an organization, you must learn about its culture: "the way things are done here." Culture defines what is and what is not acceptable. You must understand the boundaries of acceptable behavior, and either work within these boundaries or understand how to strategically change them. How you manage the relational and power dynamics within this framework will likely determine whether or not you are successful at getting things done (Box 6-1).

The culture of an organization is created over time and influenced and maintained by the people who work in it, along with its leaders. There are various ways to learn about the culture of an organization, such as paying attention to symbols, including language. Language includes not only words, but also acronyms. If you do not take the time to learn your organization's language, including its acronyms, you might remain a cultural outsider and, therefore, possibly ineffective. Pay attention to how you and others use acronyms, especially when trying to work with people outside your organization.

When you are new to an organization, it can take a long time to truly understand its culture—and any subcultures. Key to learning about its culture is looking for patterns—how things are typically done, how decisions are made, how information flows, and how meetings are conducted. Also key are more personal cues, such as what people wear and the type or amount of food or drink that is served at organization functions. For example, public health organizations will often practice what they preach and offer healthful food options at meetings and

---

Box 6-1: **Leadership and Culture**

A new state health commissioner developed her leadership style while working in a health care setting that was a command-and-control environment. She used this approach when she began serving as commissioner. From her perspective, she was very successful; she told people what to do and they did it. What she did not realize was that most of her employees did not trust her, many avoided working with her, and some even tried to sabotage her.

At one of her first presentations to staff members, she spoke about the importance of health care and having a strong workforce that could perform the necessary acute care functions needed in the 218 hospitals in the state. Most of the staff members were dumbfounded; she seemed entirely unaware of the state and local public health agencies and their core public health functions. She did not understand the context, culture, or language of public health.

---

events. When they do not, it may be noticeable to a newcomer and appear as counter-cultural (Box 6-2).

It is possible for you to get things done working within an existing culture; however, sometimes you must challenge the existing culture—the status quo—to make things happen. Culture does not change easily because people do not change easily. Those with a stake in the status quo are often powerful in maintaining an organization's culture. But change is often necessary for organizations to grow. There are times when breaking boundaries and moving outside the existing

---

Box 6-2: **An Exercise on the Culture of Your Organization**

Make the following five requests to your colleagues:

1. Identify three to five words or phrases that describe the culture of our organization. (Pay attention to those words that show up time and again.)
2. Tell me five things I should never do if I want to be effective in this organization.
3. Identify five people who are important to have on my side when I need to get things done.
4. Identify three to five successful outcomes that this organization has achieved.
5. Explain what made each of these outcomes successful.

Their responses will provide you with a picture of the organization and how to work effectively within its culture.

---

culture is the only way to produce change and get things done in an organization. Before you decide to take on the role of a change agent, learn how to do so successfully and keep your focus on proactive change, rather than reactive change.

MISSION AND VISION OF AN ORGANIZATION

An organization's mission describes its purpose—or why it exists. Its vision describes its intended future. An organization's mission and vision shape its culture—and, in turn, are shaped by the culture. To work effectively in an organization, you need to explore, with your colleagues, their understanding of the organization's mission and vision. Pay attention to the way the mission and vision are promoted. Are they printed and posted? Do you hear co-workers talk about the mission and vision when new projects are discussed? In an organization that is driven by its mission and vision, there will be clear guidance on how your work fits within the organization. If you can describe how your work is central to the mission and vision of the organization, you will increase your effectiveness.

In an organization that is not driven by its mission or its vision, it is more challenging to get things done. What gets done in those organizations is often driven by historical cultural patterns, strong personalities, and funding streams. Recognize when you are in this type of organization, because your ability to be effective may rely even more on relationships.

UNDERSTANDING YOUR ORGANIZATION'S ROLE IN THE COMMUNITY

In addition to understanding your organization from the inside, you must understand it from the outside—its external reputation, its place in the community. External influences can shape the internal culture of an organization. This understanding is especially important if your work requires you to interact with people from other organizations or the community. While the reputation of your organization is not solely your responsibility, your ability to be effective requires that you understand its reputation. Whenever you interact with people outside of your organization you help shape its reputation for good or ill. Your ability to represent the best of the organization will benefit both you and your organization.

UNDERSTANDING AND LEVERAGING POWER

Power dynamics are part of an organization's culture. Power is the ability to make things happen—to bring people together, to promote important discussions, to make essential decisions, to shape behavior. Power can be positional or personal. Knowing your own positional and personal power—and when and how to use it—will help you to be effective in an organization. People who do not hold powerful positions can exert personal power by paying close attention to others' needs and wants and learning ways to meet them.

Understanding other people's power is also important because your power to get things done will increase when it is combined with other people's power. To work effectively in an organization, you must understand where the positional and personal power exists and how to align your programs, projects, and goals with others to increase your own power.

MANAGING AMBIGUITY BY ASKING GOOD QUESTIONS AND CLARIFYING PROBLEMS

Some cultures are highly structured with clear rules, expectations, and boundaries. Others are less structured and require you to work well with ambiguity. Problem-solving in a highly ambiguous organization requires adaptability, flexibility, and creativity as well as the ability to ask good questions.

Albert Einstein said: "If I had an hour to solve a problem and my life depended on the solution, I would spend the first 55 minutes determining the proper question to ask, for once I know the proper question, I could solve the problem in less than five minutes." Asking the right questions is an art and a skill necessary for identifying problems and creating solutions.

Asking yourself questions about your beliefs and assumptions will help you to understand your biases in any given situation, clearing the way to seeing possible solutions. A powerful question may take you past the obvious and unveil unstated assumptions that stand in the way of solving a problem. Powerful questions such as "What if?" and "Why not?" open opportunities and create discussions. Powerful questions provoke relevant curiosity. Asking powerful questions helps you work effectively in an organization and creates a culture of potential.

How often have you been given a job without a job description? How often have you been asked to respond to a problem, see what you can do, and come up with some answers? Public health challenges are often complex and without easy solutions. When you find yourself needing to solve problems in an ambiguous situation, ask good questions, such as the following:

- How do I know there is a problem?
- Who is seeing and experiencing a problem?
- What does the problem look like for them?
- Why do they believe it is a problem?
- Who is affected by the problem?
- Who needs to be part of the problem-solving?

These types of questions help you learn about the nuances or culture surrounding a problem and make it less ambiguous. Understanding who is affected is essential. (See Chapter 8.)

If the problem is actually not yours, but rather one that is perceived by the stakeholders of your organization, it will eventually become your problem. Ask people from different perspectives about their understandings of the problem. Ask open-ended questions, which do not require a "yes" or "no" answer. Be careful not to make assumptions. Before taking action, validate your and others' understanding of the problem. Understand their perceptions and their expectations about what should be done to address the problem. Without getting broad understanding and input, you run the risk of solving the wrong problem and angering or alienating others, neither of which are productive in getting things done (Box 6-3).

Content and Process: Understanding What You Need To Know and Do To Be Effective

Being able to navigate the culture of an organization is one thing, but effectively getting things done in an organization also requires content and process knowledge. Content knowledge is the information you need to perform your job. For example, an epidemiologist needs to know the science of epidemiology. Content is constantly changing; new content comes at you daily. You need to determine and obtain the content that is important or essential to do your work.

Process knowledge is what you gain when you apply content knowledge in "real-life" situations. Experience is gained as you repeat the cyclical process, in which the experience either reinforces the content knowledge and process used or requires an adjustment for the future when faced with similar situations. It takes time to acquire experience. If you have little knowledge or experience, begin by finding people in the organization who are effective and ask them for guidance. Ask them to mentor you.

Box 6-3: **An Exercise on How to Address a Problem or Situation**

When faced with a problem or situation that needs to be addressed, write down every possible question you can think of related to the situation. Do not judge or limit yourself. Do not try to answer any of the questions initially. See how many different ways you can look at the problem or situation.

When your list is finished, organize or group your questions together. Identify those that seem duplicative, and determine if they should be combined or kept separate.

Then, use these questions to address the problem or solution. Pose questions to both the powerbrokers and the stakeholders. Get as much perspective as possible on the problem or situation before you begin trying to address it.

BASIC SKILLS FOR WORKING EFFECTIVELY IN AN ORGANIZATION

There are some basic skills that you need to get things done effectively in an organization. In addition to problem-solving, these skills include communication (writing, speaking, and listening), facilitation, planning, and prioritization. Being effective and acquiring a reputation for being able to get things done is important for your future career. Spending time to build the skills that help you is time and money well spent.

Communication

Effective communication is essential in working with people. Keep in mind that clear communication follows clear thinking, and that thinking is a learned quality. Pay attention to your thinking, how and what you observe, how you intepret what you observe, your ability to question what you see and what you think, and your ability to reflect on the whole and the parts of what you think in a synchronous way. Pay attention to what you say and how you say it. Pay attention to how others may perceive your communication differently than intended.

There are many tools available to help you communicate well. Choose and use your tools appropriately and carefully. Match the communication tool with the purpose of the communication. Telephone and face-to-face conversations may be best when a longer conversation is needed. This is especially true if you are about to communicate disappointing information—a face-to-face conversation may lead to a better outcome.

When communicating using e-mail, think about the purpose. Do you want to provide information, ask a question, or request an action? Think of the information you are providing from the receiver's perspective. Compose the subject line with the recipients in mind—both to get their attention and to easily locate the filed e-mail at a later time. Be clear of your expectations, be concise, and be organized. Keep e-mails brief—often one paragraph in length. Have one subject per e-mail and put the most important information first, with supporting information later. Send only information relevant to the subject line. Also, consider if an e-mail is the best way to communicate; for example, if you change the location of a meeting on short notice, a phone call is usually preferable.

Facilitation

Arranging and running meetings effectively is an important skill. Before bringing people together face to face, make sure the meeting is actually necessary. Determine what needs to be discussed or accomplished and why you need to convene a meeting. (Sometimes a conversation with just one other person will suffice.) Know the purpose of the meeting and design it to meet this need. If the purpose of a staff meeting is to increase interdepartmental communication and the only person who talks is the director, you have not properly designed the meeting to meet your goal.

For any meeting—be it a face-to-face meeting or a conference call—a key question is, "What is the best use of everyone's time?" If, for example, you want to ensure everyone is aware of a policy change in the organization, you may not need to meet. Instead, it may suffice to send the policy change to all staff members, asking each of them to answer a series of questions about it, and confirm that they understand and will abide by it—and know the consequences if they do not.

In contrast, if you want to discuss the possibilities for a new policy and get others' thoughts and ideas, then a meeting is important. But just bringing people together and asking for their input is not sufficient. You will need a facilitated process to ensure that everyone's input is obtained and acknowledged.

As a meeting facilitator, you are like an orchestra conductor. Although you are not playing any instrument, it is your responsibility to ensure that every instrument—or voice—is heard at the appropriate loudness and in harmony with other instruments—or voices. A meeting facilitator can create effective conversation, just as an orchestra conductor creates beautiful music.

Planning

Once you decide a meeting is necessary, determine who needs to be present to accomplish your goal. Use appropriate software to establish a mutually convenient time for a meeting. Then, follow up with e-mails or phone calls to confirm with everyone when and where the meeting will take place.

Planning skills are essential, and planning a meeting is just one example of where those skills are used. In planning a meeting, determine your goals—precisely what decision or action you need to have accomplished by the end of that meeting. If you need to make a decision as a group, then you collect, assemble, and disseminate the necessary information and make sure that everyone has it before the meeting.

An agenda should identify the goals for the meeting and provide logistical information. Distribute it beforehand, and ideally obtain input from those attending—before or at the meeting. Everyone attending should understand the purpose of the meeting and what is to be accomplished before the meeting begins. Ideally, the meeting facilitator should have an annotated agenda that details the flow of the meeting, time allotted for each agenda item, strategies for dealing with unexpected developments, and other necessary information.

Prioritization

Prioritization and decision-making are often a part of meetings. Your capacity to facilitate the discussion and help the group prioritize is tied directly to a clear goal. When a group of people meet and need to make a decision, the decision-making process and timeline should be agreed upon beforehand and adhered to during the meeting.

Ground rules help keep a meeting on schedule, control the conversation, and ensure that everyone's voice is heard. Meetings involve human dynamics. In some meetings, the attendees know each other beforehand—their personalities, reputations, and behaviors. Ground rules can help orchestrate interpersonal dynamics. On the other hand, if a group of people is coming together for the first time and no one knows each other, there are entirely different dynamics. A new group may need time to build trust by having an opportunity to get to know each other, and jointly choose the ground rules and decision-making process.

Rarely do meetings go according to plan, so having a backup plan is essential. Some examples of backup plans include:

- "Parking lots": Have a location, such as a piece of paper on a wall, for issues that may be important, but not relevant. This allows you to track them, and to either return to them at the end of the meeting or contact the person who brought up the issue after the meeting to explore what, if anything, needs to be done.
- Impasse strategies: Have at least three strategies available to address a discussion during the meeting that appears to be at an impasse, such as the following:
  - Ask the meeting participants to address the impasse: "We appear to be at an impasse; how do you want to move forward?"
  - Take a break: "Let's take a 5-minute break and then come back to talk about this topic." Sometimes taking a short break is all that is needed to either refresh participants' creativity in addressing the impasse, or resolve tension among participants. If, for example, one person is causing the impasse, a break offers you an opportunity to ask that person what it would take to get him or her to help resolve the impasse.
  - Put the agenda item aside and return to it later. If the rest of the meeting agenda is not dependent on resolving the impasse, move on to another item and return to the issue of the impasse later in the meeting.

Connections: Building and Managing Relationships

Almost everything you do in a public health organization requires that you work with others. Learn whom to approach for assistance. Which people have the knowledge, skills, and talents you need to help you achieve your goal? How and when should you approach them? Can you contact them directly or do you need to work through their supervisors?

You need to consider that they are already busy with their own work. Your challenge—and opportunity—is to negotiate to get their time and attention on your work. What are you willing to provide them in exchange? What can you do to support their work since you are asking them to contribute to yours? When working with other people, you must understand their perspectives and their needs, especially if you want them to work with you.

Relationships are built on respect—the ability to recognize and honor differences without judgment. People have varying perspectives, values, beliefs, and experiences. Your ability to recognize these differences and value them enables you to be more effective in working with others.

Building relationships with others requires you to have a good relationship with yourself. You need to develop self-awareness and a balanced level of self-appreciation. Having a high level of self-awareness enables you to look objectively at yourself, and to recognize your role in an interpersonal interaction. Your ability to do this without judgment or defensiveness allows you to work more effectively with others. You need to understand your own style of interaction—and recognize when your style is a strength or a weakness in interacting with others.

Understanding your own emotional intelligence helps you to be more effective in interpersonal relationships. Emotional intelligence enables you to recognize emotions, both your own and those of others. It enables you to manage your emotions, especially in response to those of others, and to recognize and control your thoughts and behaviors as a result of your emotions.

Once you understand yourself, you can more easily build relationships with others. Professional relationships are the foundation of professional networks. To be successful, you need to build a diverse network of colleagues whom you can count on for support and assistance. At the same time, you must keep clear professional boundaries at work to protect yourself and your position. A strong network will have allies and confidants.[1] *Allies* are those people with whom you build relationships to serve a common purpose or achieve a common goal. You have allies in other parts of your organization and in other organizations. Your allies might shift over time, such as when you work with others to advocate for legislation. In these relationships, you build trust in working towards a goal—not by sharing personal information. In contrast, *confidants* are people with whom you can share personal information. Choosing the right people to be your confidants is important and challenging. Confidants should be people who are far enough removed from your professional position that they do not have conflicting relationships or objectives (Box 6-4).

Career: Mastering Your Professional Future

Learning how to build a professional reputation and to design a career path that takes you where you want to go enables you to be effective in your career. Your professional reputation is built on both what you do and how you do it. You are judged by your performance and the outcomes you help to create. When you are given responsibility for a task, large or small, people will judge you on whether you complete it and on how you performed.

Self-awareness helps you to understand your motivations. Developing a professional career requires a balance between serving yourself and serving your organization—goals that are not mutually exclusive. If your actions focus solely on feeding your ego or your résumé, you will likely not achieve your organization's

---

Box 6-4: **Confidants**

A program director and a project coordinator had worked their way up in an urban public health department. Over many years, they developed a strong working relationship. The program director considered the project coordinator to be her friend and confidant. When a high-level position in the department opened, she shared with the project coordinator her intention to apply for the position—and her strategy for getting it.

She eventually learned indirectly that the project coordinator had also applied for the position—and he ultimately got the job. She felt hurt, angry, and betrayed and left the department because she did not think she could work for him.

In retrospect, he treated her as an ally, while she was treating him as a confidant.

You always need to be clear about mutual roles and expectations in any professional relationship.

---

goals because your personal goals have become more important. When you build your career, performing well for your organization will mean you are also building your professional reputation.

It's up to you to determine the professional reputation you want to have. Following are some of the qualities necessary for developing a good professional reputation:

- Conscientiousness
- Reliability
- Respectfulness
- Responsiveness
- Trustworthiness
- Diplomacy
- Being principled
- Positivity
- Curiosity
- Intelligence
- Sensitivity
- Confidence
- Humility

Choose those qualities you want others to use in describing your professional reputation. Then determine how you will develop these qualities.

Make a list of words that describe the type of person you would like to be. Use this list to begin reflecting on which qualities you believe you already possess—and to what degree. List also evidence for the presence of these qualities—often a challenge. Find a mentor or coach who will help you explore your qualities, both those that are strong and those where you have room for improvement. A mentor or coach can also help you build your skills and your career. This person needs to be honest and direct with you, and to help you gain an understanding of what you do and why you do it. A mentor or coach does not need to be your friend—but often will become your confidant. Choose your mentor or coach wisely. And be clear on the purpose of this relationship.

Building a successful career requires building skills through experience. Jobs offer us one set of experiences. But often you need to find experiences outside of the job setting to build your skills further. You can acquire some of these skills through volunteer work for a professional association or through your community outside of work—such as for community associations, faith-based organizations, or schools. Recognize skills you want to develop and link them to your volunteer work, such as by chairing a committee to gain experience in bringing people together to achieve a goal as a team.

While skills are important, having the right attitude is equally as important. Recognize and understand your attitude. Pay attention to the way you think and talk. Observe the relationships among your feelings, thoughts, and behaviors. Develop a strong sense of self-awareness that allows you to recognize and, if necessary, change your attitude.

Having a positive "can-do" attitude is central to being effective in an organization. Begin every opportunity with a sense that improvements can be made. But recognize that change is very difficult for most people (see Chapter 13). Change generally causes fear of loss, such as the loss of the familiar way of doing things or a perceived loss of power and reputation. Recognize this fear of loss as very real. Those affected should feel as though they have been heard and dealt with respectfully. You may need to reframe your message so all affected clearly understand the benefits of the intended change. Your positive attitude can help you and others manage change more effectively.

Conclusion

Being effective in an organization means getting things done. Getting things done requires that you know how to work within and across a wide range of cultures, and that you can adapt content knowledge appropriately in varying situations. Knowing yourself, recognizing the skills and qualities you need, being adaptable, and building your capacity to work with and through others will help you to be effective. Your reputation is built and maintained upon both what you choose to do and the ways you do it. There is a synergy between building a successful career and working effectively in various organizations. Learning from the past and being flexible and adaptable to personal and organizational change will help you build your career—and will help you work effectively within an organization.

Reference

1. Heifetz R. *Leadership Without Easy Answers*. Cambridge, MA: Belknap/Harvard University Press, 1994.

RESOURCES

Books

Bradberry T, Greaves J. *The Emotional Intelligence Quickbook: Everything You Need to Know*. San Diego, CA: TalentSmart, Inc., 2003.
> To assist you in being effective in working within an organization, this book describes emotional intelligence and four unique skills that can enable you to recognize and understand emotions of yourself and others.

Brandt R, Kastl T, eds. *Business Leadership*. San Francisco: Jossey-Bass, 2003.
> This book is a compendium of articles from leading authors on leadership and organizational development on such topics as ethics, dealing with change, creating visions, and the roles of a leader.

Deal TE, Kennedy AA. *Corporate Cultures: The Rites and Rituals of Corporate Life*. Harmondsworth: Penguin Books, 1982.
> Defining organizational culture as "the way things are done here," this book reviews the common cultural practices that are established as processes within organizations.

Heifetz RA, Linsky M, Grashow A. *The Practice of Adaptive Leadership: Tools and Tactics for Changing Your Organization and the World*. Boston: Harvard Business Review, 2009.
> This book provides practical tools to use in an organization when working towards adaptive change.

Kotter JP, Garvin DA, Roberto MA, et al. *HBR's 10 Must Reads on Change*. Boston: Harvard Business Review, 2011.
> Each chapter provides great advice for adapting and managing change.

Pfeffer J. *Power: Why Some People Have It and Others Don't*. New York: HarperBusiness, 2010.
> This book describes the role of power in getting things done and building a successful career.

Schein EH. *Organizational Culture and Leadership* (4th ed.). San Francisco: Jossey-Bass, 2010.
> This book examines the relationship of leadership to the culture of an organization.

Chapter and Article

Heifetz R, Grashow A, Linsky M. *Build an Adaptive Culture: Key Tactics for Improving the Organization's Ability to Tackle Adaptive Challenges*. Harvard Business Review, May 18, 2009.
> This chapter provides concrete strategies for enabling an organization to adapt to challenges.

Hammond JS, Keeney RL, Raiffa H, Hammond JS. *Hidden Traps in Decision Making*. Boston: Harvard Business Review 2006; 84: 118-126.
> This article discusses roadblocks to quick and sound decisions.

Web Site

govleaders.org/
> This is a free online resource designed to help government managers cultivate a more effective and motivated public sector workforce.

Commentary 6-1: Lessons Learned from Working in Organizations

J. Alan Baker

In my experience, several personal skills have been essential to being able to work successfully in an organization: working well with others, being persistent, effectively communicating, using resources wisely, and developing technical abilities.

Working Well With Others

The most important interpersonal skill is the ability to work well with others—being respectful and cooperative, and knowing when and whom to ask for assistance or guidance. Your ability to call on resources and personal connections to get things done is critical to your success. Not everything can be done by e-mail. Often in-person communication is most effective.

A negative example makes the point. When I was the chief budget analyst for a state health department, one of my unofficial duties was to talk to the assistant superintendent of one of the state hospitals for chronic disease. My boss, the budget director, who had worked with him in their previous capacities as personnel officers, had lost all patience with him and assigned me to be the contact. I initially thought this was unusual, but soon I learned that everything the assistant superintendent told people had to be double-checked. He went beyond trying to put his facility in a good light to selectively choosing the facts to make a positive—but inaccurate—version of a situation. Now, his reduced access to the budget director was a disadvantage to him and to his hospital. Because people didn't trust him, even his legitimate requests were delayed.

In contrast, here is a positive example. When I was an executive assistant to the state secretary of health, I worked closely with one of the deputy secretary's special assistants. We talked every day about our assignments and jointly solved problems. Later, when her boss became the secretary, he required that all outgoing grant proposals arrive for his review at least 2 weeks before the application deadline—and that he personally sign them. Yet, we often received requests for proposals for small grants less than 2 weeks before they were due. I would always alert her as soon as we learned about these requests and promised to have them sent to his office for his review and approval as soon as possible. I also kept in close contact throughout the process. Sometimes it was not possible to get the application finished until the day it was due. However, because of my credibility and prior communication with her, she was able to get the necessary signatures—even when the secretary was not available.

Positive connections not only accomplish project goals, but they also build personal resources that can be used for other projects and your career advancement. Similarly, creating negative impressions or not being viewed as being able to work well and credibly with others can limit your success and the success of your projects.

Being Persistent

The second most important interpersonal skill is persistence. Bureaucracies have an inherent resistance to change—it is always easier to do things the way they have been done for years. Since doing things the same way and expecting a different outcome is foolish, program improvement and innovation are essential. Your priorities may not be shared by co-workers, which can present a challenge when you need assistance from Personnel, Finance, Procurement, or Legal Counsel. While having established personal relations can help immensely, you also have to be persistent—even if it means being a "nudge" or a "squeaky wheel."

Our state health department looked for the best value in buying baby formula for the Women, Infants, and Children Supplemental Nutrition Program (WIC). Baby formula companies offered huge discounts to get our state's contract, since that strongly influenced its shelf location in food stores. In some small groceries, the only formula that would be stocked was the WIC program's baby formula. When it came to the end of the initial contract period, it was always a complicated discussion to determine if we should renew the contract for the option years or have it rebid. States carefully monitored the bids received by other states in the preceding months.

When our state let its current contract expire and joined a consortium of states to benefit from a larger group discount, the baby formula company that did not get renewed complained to officials in our state, pointing out it had submitted the low bid in the previous bid cycle. This was true, but it obscured the fact that bids had been decreasing to even lower levels in recent years and the consortium that our state joined had much larger volume and lower prices.

Officials in our state, due to a reasonable-sounding complaint by a prominent local lobbyist, initially refused to allow the new contract and required our health department to meet with state officials to consider all options. It would have been easy for us to agree to a 2-year renewal with the same baby formula company, but the higher cost would have resulted in fewer families being served. So the WIC director and I attended many meetings, reviewed the entire history of the program, and looked at all bids in other states for the previous 2 years.

Finally, state officials discovered that we were right. They interceded by speaking to the state comptroller and treasurer, with whom they had good relationships, while we made sure the governor was briefed. This enabled us to reject the former company's bid and join the consortium of other states so we could serve more families at a lower cost per family.

At the national public health association where I worked for several years, there had been interest in a pilot program in which members could join both this national organization and their state affiliates at reduced combined rates. This program was not initially implemented because of competing priorities, the failure of a similar program years before, and the complexity of dues structures, membership categories, and duration of membership. When we finally embarked on this program, it was largely due to the persistence of several key volunteer members, who thought there was great potential in this program, at least for the affiliates. But even then, it took a senior project leader and many meetings with external stakeholders and internal staff members to work through all the issues and implement the program. This required us to have constant vigilance, weekly meetings with tangible outcomes, and a clear sense that this was a priority project.

Often, there are so many needs and competing projects that address these needs that your persistence is required to bring a project to completion. This requires a critical eye toward deciding which ones are important and which are simply desirable. Important projects may be organizational imperatives or simply the right things to do.

Effectively Communicating

A third personal skill needed to work successfully in an organization is effective communication. Communication about your work is critical, but that doesn't always mean that you are its key spokesperson. Appropriate spokespersons will differ, given different situations or audiences. Sometimes a technical, programmatic, or clinical person is best. At a legislative briefing, it may be best to have the highest-ranking official make the presentation. In choosing the right spokesperson, you need to think strategically.

Just as it is important to have the right spokesperson, it is essential to use the right communication vehicle. These vehicles range from an oral report from a workgroup at a staff retreat to a formal decision memo that provides the background, issues, and rationale for a recommended course of action. But you must remember your audience. I have worked for secretaries of health who loved long detailed analyses. And I also worked for a governor who never wanted more than a one-page analysis of an issue. In trying to gather material from program staff members, I learned that some people cannot condense what they know to just one page. They are too proud of their programs and think that everything is critical. Yet our sending 40 pages of material to the governor would have ensured that it would not be considered. Your ability to take much technical material and reduce it to three or four key points in a written or spoken presentation is essential for personal and organizational success.

Using Resources Wisely

A fourth critical personal skill is to know how to use resources wisely—which requires knowledge, organizational expertise, and at least some financial resources.

There are rarely enough resources to adequately fund programs or projects. Use resources wisely—use all of them, but no more. The odds of getting additional resources are greatly reduced if budgeted money was not spent or if there were cost overruns.

In the public sector, procurement rules can be both complex and contradictory— "Get the best price, but give preference to in-state companies." Knowing the rules and having a trusted guide can help you navigate to avoid delays and have your initiative succeed.

If you are successful, you may be promoted into a supervisory or managerial position. Find a mentor or develop a relationship with someone who can help train you in the skills you need.

Even with inadequate funding, you can be successful by being creative and innovative. Sometimes development of new policy, such as passing a no-smoking ordinance, may not require money, but rather scientific evidence, political will, and relationships built over time.

Here's another personal example. In the early 1990s, handgun violence was the leading cause of death for African-American males 14 to 19 years of age in our state. Yet even the health secretary did not see it as a public health problem, but rather as a law enforcement issue. We built our case by developing data on handgun deaths by jurisdiction, time trends in these deaths, and comparisons to other causes of death, such as motor vehicle crashes. We also lobbied extensively within the state health department, looking for allies for support. We persuaded the deputy secretary to have the health department testify in support of a gun control bill. The following year, legislation passed that supported progress toward gun control, funding data collection and policy development.

Developing Technical Abilities

Several technical abilities can help you succeed in an organization. You should have a working knowledge of personnel management (Chapter 10); procurement, budgeting, and expenditure management (Chapter 7); grant writing (Chapter 9); and information-technology software and systems.

The need for familiarly with information technology (IT) is highly dependent on the specific position you have. But you should be proficient with word processing, making spreadsheets, and performing basic research on the Internet. Establishing relationships with IT staff members can help you meet deadlines, when something crashes or new software is introduced in the middle of a priority project.

Conclusion

A final example illustrates most of the skills I have outlined. When I became the human resources director for the health department, I had an opportunity during budget preparation to propose new initiatives, including one for a leadership and management development institute. We succeeded as a result of our persistence, clear communication about the potential benefits of this institute (such as training existing staff members to fill challenging vacant positions), well-established working relationships, and our credibility for bringing new initiatives to fruition and for using resources well.

7

Planning and Budgeting

Walter Tsou

Planning

Planning is both a necessity and a luxury in public health. In the short term, people rightfully expect that public health agencies and organizations will be prepared to protect them in an emergency. Such preparedness does not happen without careful and thoughtful planning. In addition, for the long term, strategic planning is important for public health agencies, which try to balance competing priorities in an often-changing fiscal and political environment. However, for most public health agencies, finding the time to plan while addressing daily crises with shrinking resources is a major challenge.

State and local public health departments plan for and implement the 10 essential services of public health (Table 7-1). Whether you work in a large public health agency that is responsible for all 10 essential services, in a small agency, or in a nongovernmental organization, you can use these services as a framework for planning.

When I served as the city health commissioner in Philadelphia, I evaluated our department by how it was providing the 10 essential services in relation to expectations of city residents. When we fell short of expectations, we elicited community input into planning to improve services, within budgeting constraints.

SWOT ANALYSIS

All public health agencies and organizations make planning decisions on a regular basis, some of which can have long-term consequences. To effectively use planning time, you can use a "quick-and-easy" method of strategic planning that includes a *SWOT analysis*, named for its component parts: *S*trengths, *W*eaknesses, *O*pportunities, and *T*hreats. A facilitator can help you and others conduct a SWOT analysis by guiding discussion as well as by synthesizing and reporting major findings. The success of a SWOT analysis generally depends on the active participation

Table 7-1: **The 10 Essential Services of Public Health**

1. *Monitor* health status to identify and solve community health problems.
2. *Diagnose and investigate* health problems and health hazards in the community.
3. *Inform, educate, and empower* people about health issues.
4. *Mobilize* community partnerships and action to identify and solve health problems.
5. *Develop policies and plans* that support individual and community health efforts.
6. *Enforce* laws and regulations that protect health and ensure safety.
7. *Link* people to needed personal health services and assure the provision of health care when otherwise unavailable.
8. *Assure* competent public and personal health care workforce.
9. *Evaluate* effectiveness, accessibility, and quality of personal and population-based health services.
10. *Research* for new insights and innovative solutions to health problems.

of critical-thinking staff members with differing perspectives—since they will ultimately implement its recommendations.

Our health department's SWOT analysis identified needs for better informing, educating, and empowering people in preventing chronic diseases. It led us to getting funds to hire health educators and to reassign existing staff members to better prevent these diseases.

While valuable, SWOT analyses performed by staff members may lack engagement by or support from key external stakeholders or the public at large. Therefore, you should initiate a strategic planning process with broader input for planning that affects most of the community or has major financial implications.

PLANNING FOR AND WITH THE COMMUNITY

A community needs assessment and asset-mapping can help you identify who is providing what services in your community. You should convene major stakeholders to determine who delivers public health services and how. If you work in a small agency or organization, consider how it fits within a larger community plan for public health, and which of the essential public health services it provides.

Your development of public health plans defines a community's vision of health and can justify the necessary public support to sustain that vision. For example, if your community has strong hospitals but few public health agencies engaged in prevention, you can begin by identifying your community's strengths, overlapping services and gaps, opportunities to fill these gaps, and obstacles to overcome in doing so. Your challenge may be getting the community to recognize that essential community resources include an outreach program for prenatal care or an advocacy organization for those without health insurance.

There are many choices you have to make as a public health worker that make planning and priority-setting difficult. If you have limited funds, you may have to choose whether to invest them in immunizations, lead poisoning abatement, primary care services, or air pollution control.

In addressing such challenges, your developing a strategic plan can engage stakeholders and seek input from the community in the planning process. Inevitably, you will need to make choices together concerning difficult social, moral, or ethical issues. For example, a state health department created a strategic plan to limit Medicaid funds, basing its choices on evidence-based studies and priorities developed from input at town meetings and from focus groups. Although this strategic plan restricted access of Medicaid patients to some expensive health-care services, it provided more funds for other important services. Especially during times of fiscal austerity, difficult choices can be made easier and justified by strategic planning that has broad community input.

Community-based participatory research (CBPR) is a form of strategic planning relevant to public health that enables community organizations and residents to help plan a research project. Community residents help formulate the research questions, participate in the planning and implementation of the project, help draw its conclusions, and evaluate it. A good strategic plan—like CBPR—provides a framework for community input.

COMMUNITY-BASED STRATEGIC PLANNING

Mobilizing for Action for Planning and Partnerships (MAPP), developed by the National Association of County and City Health Officials (NACCHO), is a community-based process for public health strategic planning. It is generally performed over several months, with many community stakeholders and often a facilitator. Driven and owned by the community, it draws on the collective wisdom of community members to strengthen local public health systems. It uses quantitative and qualitative data on the essential public health services and identifies opportunities for community members and local public health officials to work together.

The Minnesota Office of Public Health Practice has developed a 5-year strategic planning process called the Community Health Assessment and Action Planning (CHAAP) process, which all local health departments in Minnesota are expected to use to comprehensively assess community health needs. Its key elements are (a) assessment and prioritization of the health needs of communities, (b) assessment and prioritization of the capacity of each local health department to meet these needs, and (c) development of an action plan. CHAAP identifies essential public health services, conducts needs assessments with community input, prioritizes local needs, and weighs addressing these needs within available resources. It supports a limited role of the local health department, based on its resources and capacity to provide services.

Another strategic planning approach is Future Search, a 3-day program that brings together key stakeholders on an issue, and then, through a series of exercises, develops a workable, realistic plan that can be implemented in both the short and

Table 7-2: **A Checklist for Developing a Strategic Plan**

1. Engage the community and key stakeholders.
2. Create a mission statement.
3. Create a needs assessment based on the 10 essential public health services.
4. Identify gaps in services.
5. Use SWOT analyses for making time-limited, important decisions.
6. Keep politicians "in the loop."

long term. It identifies local, state, federal, and international factors that influence resource allocation and priorities. Future Search is especially valuable for smaller organizations who seek to identify their roles in their communities and to develop long-range strategic plans.

Table 7–2 provides a checklist for developing a strategic plan.

MISSION STATEMENT

A strategic plan begins with a mission statement that clearly and succinctly reflects the aspirations of an organization. The culture of the organization and the political environment help shape its mission.

Once a mission is agreed upon, you can develop goals and measurable objectives. Goals reflect both the aspirations and achievable aspects of the mission. Objectives are steps that, taken together, help achieve a goal. The framework for the mission and goals comes from the strategic plan. For example, a goal for a county health department could be "To reduce smoking." Measurable objectives could be "To reduce to under 10% the percentage of merchants who sell cigarettes to minors" or "To increase by 20% the number of phone calls to the smoking cessation quit line."

Creating Innovative Programs

After establishing a mission statement, goals, and measurable objectives, you will need to plan the activities needed to achieve these objectives. This can be a very creative process—a true joy of public health. There are multiple ways to achieve any objective. Social media and the Internet often provide innovative opportunities, but there is no substitute for "hands-on" demonstrations and live education programs, such as the following:

- Promoting in supermarkets fat-free milk by offering blinded tasting events and providing recipes that use fat-free milk
- Including the smoking cessation quit line number in rap songs for young smokers
- Promoting walking by encouraging residents to adopt a dog

Each creative activity has to legitimately advance the mission and goals of a public health strategic plan.

NEEDS ASSESSMENT AND MAPPING

Your organization's strategic plan requires an understanding of the assets and essential public health services in your community. Many activities of public health departments are related to needs assessment, such as collecting vital statistics and communicable disease reports, or monitoring the quality of and access to medical care—as well as obtaining "denominator" data on the population. These data are necessary for planning.

Illustrating trends or associations on graphs and maps can facilitate interpretation of data. Geographic information systems (GIS) can be helpful in analyzing data and educating the public and policymakers on such matters as plans for distributing medications in an emergency, for matching health-care resources to areas of high disease prevalence, or for determining the health effects of environmental hazards.

Your ability to use GIS to show elected officials important public health data, analyzed by political district, can help ensure funding of public health services. The public generally finds mapped data in newspapers, on TV, or on Web sites useful in understanding public health information about their communities.

Use great care when using maps to show incidence or prevalence of disease in an area. We once presented a map showing infant mortality data in our county, which led to disagreements and accusations among hospital representatives and government officials, who questioned our data.

By using graphics, you can help enlist community residents and other stakeholders in your organization's strategic plan, raising its profile and making it politically stronger. Engaging the community in developing your strategic plan increases the likelihood of the community being engaged in its implementation. You can elicit community participation by advertising in local newspapers and on community listservs.

You can present your draft strategic plan with graphics and other visuals at meetings of community members and political leaders to gain their input and support. Press releases and information placed in newspapers and on the Internet can facilitate community input.

LONG-TERM PLANNING DURING CHALLENGING TIMES

Long-term planning during difficult times or crises is essential for the following four reasons:

1. Political leaders need to understand and appreciate public health. In challenging economic times, they may want to cut funds for surveillance, preventive

services, environmental protection, and access to medical care. You need to powerfully assert that these services are essential (see Chapter 2). If you are a government worker, you likely will not be permitted to lobby on these issues, so you must work with nongovernmental organizations who can advocate for funding of your programs or services (see Chapter 15).

2. Even if political leaders severely cut services, public announcements need to be made about what government services have been suspended and what alternatives, if any, exist.

3. You need to develop a plan on how suspended services can be restarted once funding is restored. (Unfortunately, some key staff members may never return once services are suspended.)

4. Some public services are essential, unduplicated, and expensive. For example, services for prison health, community mental health, health care for the homeless, animal control, and primary care for the uninsured cannot be suspended. Since those served by such services generally are disenfranchised, do not vote, and cannot advocate for themselves, advocacy organizations who work in public health need to represent and advocate for them (Table 7-3).

Implementation translates plans into reality. Measurable objectives require concrete activities, for which personnel, supplies, and other resources have to be budgeted and allocated. A reasonable timeframe to perform these activities needs to be estimated. Developing a budget is where "the rubber meets the road." When a budget is developed and approved, plans can be implemented to advance an organization toward its goals and objectives.

Table 7-3: **What to Do and What Not to Do When Budget Cuts Threaten Services of Your Health Department**

DO:
Work with service providers and nongovernmental organizations to advocate against cuts.
Write a press release explaining the cuts and offering alternative sources of services.
Perform SWOT analyses to prioritize services.
Plan how to restore essential services, if cuts are partially restored, such as by keeping key personnel in other roles.
DON'T:
Lobby publicly against your own administration.
Release press information without clearance from the administration.
Close essential and unduplicated public services, if possible.

Budgeting

THE BUDGET AS POLICY

The primary policy document for a government public health agency is its budget. Public health policies need to be funded—budgeted for—to be implemented.

Budgets define the sources of revenue and the broad categories for capital expenditures. Because government funds almost all public health services directly or indirectly, public health budgets are developed for geopolitical areas, such as states and cities.

A budget reflects the priority programs and services of the government agency. It also reflects policies and interests of elected officials and other opinion leaders who, in turn, are influenced by lobbyists, advocates, and the public at large. Many lobbyists and advocates have interests that may be in conflict with public health.

Even if you do not develop your organization's budget, you still need to be an effective advocate so that the budget reflects public health policies that you wish to promote (see Chapter 2).

BUDGETING AND POLITICS

For most state and federal government agencies, budgets have to be approved annually or semi-annually. They are frequently described in multi-year cycles that correspond to the terms of political leaders. Newly elected executive branch leaders, such as mayors, governors, and the President of the United States, generally have a very short period—from November (when they are usually elected) to early February (when they have to present their budgets to the city council, state legislature, or Congress)—to develop budgets that reflect their campaign promises and other priorities.

The best opportunity for executive branch leaders to advance bold changes is with their inaugural budgets, since legislators are more likely to give them a chance to advance their campaign goals. Therefore, an important time to advocate for a budget is during an election campaign.

As Election Day approaches, many incumbent elected officials and others running for office call for more austerity in budgets. Public health programs and services may be threatened by proposed spending cuts, unless there are constituencies supporting them.

Shortly after Election Day in November, our county health department used an influenza immunization campaign to convince the public that the newly elected county commissioners were committed to public health. We used goodwill from that campaign to advance other public health programs and services. We also spent money on implementing programs and services early in the political cycle to demonstrate the many things that our public health department could—and should—be doing.

BUDGET BASICS

Each government system has its own template and format for budgets. Budgets have "line items" that clearly show where revenues and expenditures are anticipated. Many agencies have computer-generated programs that can address standard increases and decreases, such as a 3% cost-of-living (COL) salary and benefit increase or a 5% across-the-board decrease.

Major revenue sources for city or county government entities are taxes, bonds, fees, grants, interest on held funds, and federal and state funds. Most public health departments contribute to this revenue stream with inspection and license fees, grant funds, and payment for direct services, such as immunization and home care.

Major expenditure categories are personnel, pensions, fringe benefits, employee taxes, contracts, materials, supplies, equipment, debt service, and capital budget. In large budgets, line items frequently represent best estimates of expenditures, based on incremental budgeting. Detailed expenditures, especially travel expenses, are frequent targets of inquiry and criticism and therefore need careful justification.

Capital budgets are separate because they cover multiple years and represent large expenditures over longer timeframes. Expenses for constructing or renovating buildings are subject to zoning laws and availability of construction workers. These expenses generally span multiple annual budgets.

Government officials appreciate budgets that are funded largely from external grants because they reduce demand on general tax revenue. In general, local health departments are highly dependent on funds from state and federal grants. Occasionally, foundations or other private funders will develop partnerships with local governments to advance a public health cause. You should develop and maintain strong relationships with potential funders to identify and coordinate opportunities for financial support of programs and services (see Chapter 9).

Each public health agency needs to have a process that allows leaders to regularly monitor the expenditure of funds. All leaders and managers should become familiar with the budget process to translate agency priorities into action. An agency leadership team should regularly review all categorical and general spending to ensure that no funds are left unexpended and that no overspending occurs. Unspent funds may provide justification for a legislative body to reduce your agency's budget for the following year, so most agencies try to spend exactly what is available in each account category.

Even with the best planning, some unforeseen situations will occur that require unanticipated expenditures—generally from the current budget. Most governments have mechanisms to transfer money from one budget category to another, but these transfers usually must be approved by legislative bodies. In smaller jurisdictions with less bureaucracy, budget transfers can be approved by the town manager or chief operating officer.

INCREMENTAL AND ZERO-BASED BUDGETING

Incremental budgeting relies heavily on the previous year's budget, with program managers and directors requesting and justifying any changes that are needed in the following year's budget in order to implement programs. Most incremental budgeting maintains the status quo, with only small incremental changes. The main advantage of incremental budgeting is that it helps maintain successful programs, for which budget justifications are usually easier to explain. However, its main disadvantage is that it tends to maintain the status quo. For example, it may maintain a budget line item that is no longer relevant, given changing priorities reflected in the strategic plan. Therefore, incremental budgeting often begins with keeping employees' jobs—rather than asking if the jobs are the appropriate ones to implement the strategic plan.

Zero-based budgeting assumes nothing about previous budgets. Instead, it builds the budget from zero and requires justification for each activity, which is linked to achieving the objectives and attaining the goals of the strategic plan. The main advantage of zero-based budgeting is that it is tied to the strategic plan, with a justification for every line item in the budget. If developed well, it ensures a better use of taxpayers' money. The main disadvantages of zero-based budgeting are the following:

- It is difficult to write justifications for all line items.
- It takes much more time than incremental budgeting.
- It requires special training for managers for implementation, especially since it depends on an up-to-date strategic plan that is meeting the needs of those served.
- It is often unrealistic to implement when there is a labor–management agreement with regulations concerning hiring and firing of employees.

CREATING A 5-YEAR PLAN

The permanency of large governmental agencies offers some stability to public health functions. A 5-year budget offers many advantages, including long-range planning. It enables government leaders to support short-term spending in order to achieve important health objectives in the longer term. In addition, a 5-year budget can transcend political terms, since 5 years goes beyond the usual 4-year election cycle.

Many achievable outcomes in public health are inherently long-term. For example, investments in prevention might reduce medical expenditures within 5 years, but more likely 10 or 20 years. Reducing the long-term impact of childhood obesity may take decades, but interim measures may demonstrate progress towards this goal.

DEVELOPING THE BUDGET

Writing a budget involves balancing priority public health needs with resources, in the face of political pressures. With a strategic plan that clearly identifies goals and objectives, it is easier to identify activities to achieve them and develop a budget to support these activities. Early in the process, program directors need to agree on which activities will be funded and what amount of money each requires.

How do you choose which activities to support? The U.S. Task Force on Community Preventive Services, composed of public health experts who review the literature to find public health programs that work, has published its recommendations in the *Guide to Community Preventive Services*.[1] This guide can help you plan activities that can be implemented locally and can help you justify budgeting expenditures for these activities.

Because the personnel line item is the largest expense for most governmental programs, it is often a target for reduction by some elected officials who may question the number of employees in a public health department. In areas where public employees are unionized, civil-service, merit-system, and union rules have a strong impact on hiring and firing decisions. For example, in some cities, government employees hired under civil service regulations are classified in a budget line item separate from contract employees. In these cities, since government employees are paid from general tax revenues, this line item is closely scrutinized because it represents the largest expenditure in city government.

An important line item in public health is anticipating unforeseen circumstances. Contingency or "rainy-day" funds should be built into budgets to allow for a quick and effective response to emergencies.

INDIRECT AND OVERHEAD EXPENSES

Government agencies have major overhead expenses for such line items as rent, utilities, administrative support, and supplies. When these overhead expenses are accounted for in grants, they can be recovered as *indirect costs* (those not identified with a specific project or activity, but used to benefit multiple projects and activities). With tight budgets, indirect costs are an important part of grant revenue. (See Chapter 9.)

The federal government negotiates with each grantee an agreed percentage of grant funds that can be allocated for indirect costs—now called *facilities and administrative (F & A) costs*. For new grantees, the calculation of F & A costs, which is a complex calculation based on audited expenses, is best performed by staff members in the finance office of your organization. This amount is then submitted, usually as a percentage of the grant award, for approval by the funder, such as the federal government. Most academic institutions have negotiated rates for indirect costs; however, government entities are increasingly developing their own rates and negotiating for better deals on indirect costs.

DEALING WITH BUDGETS IN DIFFICULT TIMES

Because of reductions in revenues, you cannot generally rely on previous budgets when developing new ones. In times of tight budgets, your organization must have a prioritized strategic plan for providing essential public health services.

Cutting services in lean times is extremely painful—for public health workers, for elected officials, and especially for people who depend on these services. Here is some advice:

1. Be clear on the core essential services that your agency uniquely provides in the community. These services should be preserved at all costs.
2. Have good lines of communication with the political leaders and advocacy groups, who should know about the consequences of major budget cuts. Advocacy groups can serve as vocal advocates for your programs and services if you are a government employee who may be restricted from advocating for programs and services.
3. Arrange for letters to the editor and op-ed pieces to be written by opinion leaders in the community to explain the importance of programs and services.
4. Invite reporters to attend budget hearings. Their reports may influence political leaders about the personal and community costs associated with cuts and help to restore funding.
5. Involve staff members in the decisions on what cuts need to be made.
6. Anticipate budget cuts, recognizing that they may lead to unfilled staff positions and difficulties in fulfilling requirements of grant-funded programs.
7. Inform community members on the reduction or elimination of programs and services so they can find ways of meeting needs.
8. Inform elected officials about the consequences of cuts in programs and services on the lives of those served through their testimony and the presentation of relevant data.

You should always be looking for new sources of funding, such as local and community-based foundations, private family foundations, state agencies, and federal grants. (A good source to find and apply for federal grants is www.grants.gov.) Many foundations do not fund government agencies but will occasionally fund programs that are designed and implemented by collaboration among non-governmental organizations and government agencies (see Chapter 9). Table 7-4 highlights some things to do and not to do in budgeting.

In conclusion, translating mission and vision into achievable goals and objectives requires effective planning and budgeting. Strong leaders articulate mission and vision, but also are skillful in addressing long-term goals and short-term objectives as well as inevitable emergencies and crises as they occur. Mastering the skills discussed in this chapter is essential for anyone leading an agency or organization or managing a program.

Table 7-4: **What to Do and What Not to Do in Budgeting**

DO:
Clarify public health priorities in a strategic plan.
Build trust with political leaders and funders.
Explain budget challenges to staff members.
Budget conservatively and anticipate cuts.
Inform political leaders about the public health consequences of cuts.
Look for new funding sources.

DON'T:
Fail to have a strategic plan.
Forget to seek input from staff members.
Make overly optimistic assumptions on future revenues.
Fail to work with nongovernmental organizations, advocacy groups, and the media.
Fail to inform residents who will be affected by budget cuts.

Reference

1. The Task Force on Community Preventive Services. *The Guide to Community Preventive Services.* Available at: http://www.thecommunityguide.org. Accessed on July 22, 2010.

RESOURCES

Planning

Bryson JM. *Strategic Planning for Public and Nonprofit Organizations: A Guide to Strengthening and Sustaining Organizational Achievement* (3rd ed.). San Francisco: Jossey-Bass, 2004.
> *This book is a valuable resource for strategic planning for policymakers and planners in public agencies and nongovernmental organizations. It presents key steps in using a strategy change cycle to think and act strategically.*

Edwards R, Brown JS, Hodgson P, et al. An action plan for tobacco control at regional level. *Public Health* 1999; 113: 165–170.
> *This article describes a regional action plan for tobacco created based on a SWOT analysis.*

El Ansari W, Russell J, Ryder E, Chambers C. New skills for a new age: leading the introduction of public health concepts in healthcare curricula. *Public Health* 2003; 117: 77–87.
> *An example of a SWOT analysis on whether and how public health principles should be integrated into the training of health professionals and specialists.*

Janssen R. Evaluation of the organization and financing of the Danish health care system. *Health Policy* 2002; 59: 145–159.
> *This article provides a SWOT analysis offers insights on improving the Danish health care system.*

Lanzotti LM. Staff participation in a SWOT analysis. *Journal of Nursing Administration* 1991; 21:67–69.
> *This article describes how a home health care agency used a SWOT analysis to create department goals and objectives and to build staff cohesiveness.*

Lyons S, Zidouh A, Ali Bejaoui M, et al. Implications of the International Health Regulations (2005) for communicable disease surveillance systems: Tunisia's experience. *Public Health* 2007; 121: 690–695.

> *This article presents a SWOT analysis of the capacity of a communicable disease surveillance program.*

Mastorovich MJ, Drenkard KN. Nursing Future Search. Building a community of nurses in an integrated healthcare system. *Journal of Nursing Administration* 2000; 30: 173–179.

Wilson LB, Carroccio J. Using the Future Search process for senior volunteer service in long term care. *Journal of Volunteer Administration* 1995; 14: 33–38.

> *These two articles provide additional examples of using the Future Search process.*

Minnesota Department of Health. *Community Health Assessment and Action Planning (CHAAP).*

> *A full discussion of the program, including a handbook on conducting this planning process, can be found at http://www.health.state.mn.us/divs/cfh/ophp/system/planning/chaap/.*

Morrisey GL. *Morrisey on Planning, A Guide to Long-Range Planning: Creating Your Strategic Journey* (Vol. 2). San Francisco: Jossey-Bass, 1995.

> *This book provides step-by-step instructions for developing one model of a strategic plan for long-range goals.*

Morrisey GL. *Morrisey on Planning, A Guide to Tactical Planning: Producing Your Short-Term Results* (Vol. 3). San Francisco: Jossey-Bass, 1995.

> *This book provides a model for developing short-term objectives, such as for an annual plan and an annual budget.*

National Association of County and City Health Officials (NACCHO). *Mobilizing for Action through Planning and Partnerships (MAPP).*

> *This program has extensive resources, including publications, manuals, and training materials. Further information is available at http://www.naccho.org/topics/infrastructure/mapp/index.cfm.*

Weisbord M, Janoff S. *Future Search.* San Francisco: Berrett-Koehler Publishers, 2000.

Weisbord M, Janoff S. *Future Search: Getting the Whole System in the Room for Vision, Commitment, and Action.* San Francisco: Berrett-Koehler Publishers, 2010.

> *These books provide guidance on and successful examples using the Future Search methodology.*

Budgeting

Novick LF, Morrow CB, Mays GP. *Public Health Administration: Principles for Population-Based Management.* Sudbury, MA: Jones and Bartlett, 2008.

> *A good general reference book on public health administration, including a civics lesson on the federal budget and on public health financing mechanisms.*

Fallon LF, Zgodzinsi EJ. *Essentials of Public Health Management.* Sudbury, MA: Jones and Bartlett, 2005.

> *A practical book on public health management, including budget preparation.*

Commentary 7-1: How to Plan and Budget in an Emergency Situation

Esther D. Chernak

Emergency Preparedness

Public health agencies have vital roles to play during emergencies that have the potential to cause widespread injury, illness, and death. Each type of emergency requires a specific set of responses that are best planned in advance. However, there are common principles and considerations that should guide planning for all public heath emergencies. The material in this commentary can be used as general advice. You should consult the guidelines of your agency or organization for more specific direction.

INCIDENT COMMAND SYSTEM AND COMPLIANCE WITH THE NATIONAL INCIDENT MANAGEMENT SYSTEM

The incident command system (ICS) has become the standard framework used by emergency responders to ensure that they have an effective management-and-command structure during an emergency. The ICS requires the designation of a single or unified command position—an incident commander—and clear assignment of responsibility for logistics, operations, financial oversight, responder safety, and public information. Important characteristics of the ICS, such as a clear chain of command, accountability, and delegation of responsibility with a manageable span of control for specific functions, should guide public health agencies as they use it in preparing for emergencies.

Government agencies at all levels coordinate their emergency response activities through the National Incident Management System (NIMS), which is based on the ICS. NIMS ensures that response agencies in all disciplines at local, state, and federal levels have a consistent, coordinated approach to emergency response. NIMS ensures that all participating agencies and organizations rely on a core set of concepts, principles, terminology, and technology (see http://training.fema.gov/EMIWeb/IS/ICSResource/assets/HSPD-5.pdf).

AN APPROACH FOR MULTIPLE PURPOSES AND ALL HAZARDS

Because public health emergencies may arise from a wide range of threats, preparedness should be directed to all possible hazards. For example, while there are specific control measures for various infectious agents, efficient use of public health resources involves developing overarching plans to deal with any type of infectious disease threat. Critical components of strategies to address these infectious diseases—such as mass immunization, isolation and quarantine, preparation for depletion of the workforce, and dissemination of information to the public—might be required during other emergencies, such as an extreme weather event or a release of radioactive material. These basic components of emergency response provide a framework for planning for all types of emergencies.

Because the best emergency response strategies are those practiced or used frequently, agencies should integrate these strategies into day-to-day public health practice. This multiple-purpose approach strengthens agency infrastructure for responding to frequent non-emergency events, and also ensures the success of emergency responses when they are needed.

Inclusion and Collaboration

The process of emergency response planning is as valuable as the emergency response plan. Key staff members and other stakeholders critical to the implementation of an emergency plan should be engaged throughout the planning process to integrate the perspectives and capabilities of all participants. Every person, unit, and department should contribute, understand, and agree to its prescribed roles and responsibilities before an emergency occurs. It is too late to do this planning during the emergency, when communication may be limited and there may be widespread fear and confusion. The time to get to know your partners is before the crisis—not during it. Response partners who know each other and who understand each other's mission and capabilities work more effectively during emergencies than those who do not.

Continuity of Operations

Planners must determine whether and how their agency or department will continue to provide services during an emergency that disrupts their operations. In some emergencies, these services may be directly relevant to response measures, such as the provision of medical care during an epidemic. In other emergencies, these services may not be related to response measures but may be necessary for sustaining the health of the population. For example, dialysis centers must function during storms that cause long-term power outages. Environmental health programs need to assess the nature and magnitude of a chemical spill or release. Agencies that provide daily services to home-bound people with visiting nurses or nurses' aides need to continue providing these services during emergencies that disrupt transportation.

When you plan for continuity of operations, you should answer the following questions:

- What services are the most important, and how will they be provided during an emergency?
- Which staff members are most important to providing services? Who needs to work? What will they do?
- How will staff members be reached during an emergency? How will they learn that the emergency plan has been activated?
- How will work be performed if the primary worksite is inaccessible? How will staff members get there?
- What supplies and equipment are necessary to provide the core services that must continue during an emergency? Are there contingency plans for working with limited resources? Do some materials need to be stockpiled?
- How will the agency communicate with external entities and the general public during an emergency?

Planning for continuity of operations may necessitate investing in supplies and communications equipment, renting facilities, and developing options for relocation. During emergencies, resources are often scarce and communication networks that rely on sophisticated technology may fail. Continuity of operations can be facilitated by establishing simple communication chains, clearly delineating core functions and services, and designating key staff members to assume leadership positions during an emergency.

Participation in a Community-wide Emergency Response

Public health emergencies may require a wide variety of responses to contain or mitigate a serious threat. The roles of an agency will likely extend beyond its primary mission and activities during non-emergency periods. Public health activities to reduce morbidity and mortality during emergencies may include the following:

- Disease surveillance or case-finding activities to identify who has been exposed and affected
- Clinical care, including an expansion of services for medical screening and evaluation and for intensive care
- Coordination among hospitals and other medical facilities and public health agencies
- Public information to guide people to appropriate medical care or public health services

- Disease control measures, including quarantine and isolation recommendations, shelter-in-place advisories, and mass prophylaxis or vaccination
- Environmental health services to ensure that affected communities have access to safe drinking water and food and clean air

PUBLIC INFORMATION AND RISK COMMUNICATION

Frequent, clear, and frank assessments of the health impact of an emergency, with guidance and instructions for individual behavior, are critical. Inaccurate rumors emerge from an uninformed public, undermining confidence in the response effort and derailing control measures. Prompt acknowledgement and correction of erroneous information is critical to the emergency response and effective implementation of control measures. (See Chapter 1.)

PLANS TO REACH VULNERABLE POPULATIONS

Some people and communities are especially vulnerable to certain threats and may therefore be at higher risk for suffering severe health consequences. Examples include persons with limited access or mobility, people who are immunosuppressed, people who do not speak English fluently, and members of racial and ethnic minorities.[1] Specific planning is needed to ensure that all people and communities will be prepared and protected. (See Chapter 5.)

Mental Health Support

Public health emergencies can overwhelm the mental health system. Planners should consider the types of psychological and emotional support that will be needed by the general public and by those responding to the emergency. In the short term, psychological first aid, designed to reduce the initial stress induced by traumatic events, should be a priority. Ultimately, long-term counseling and support may be required. Therefore, the planning process should engage mental health professionals, representatives of disaster relief organizations and faith-based organizations, primary care providers, and members of crisis and emergency-response teams.

Training and Exercises

Training and exercises help to ensure that all staff members understand the emergency response plan. Tabletop exercises can help train staff members and also obtain valuable feedback on the content of an emergency response plan.

Functional and field exercises reinforce training and allow for further evaluation and revision of a plan.

A *tabletop exercise* is a group discussion guided by a simulated disaster. A facilitator leads participants through problem-solving sessions designed to stimulate the thinking and decision-making that would occur during a real disaster.

A *functional exercise* is designed to simulate a real emergency situation, short of moving people to a real disaster scene. Its goals are to evaluate the capability of one or more functions or responses (such as communications, command-and-control, and resource management) in the context of an emergency. Functional exercise events occur in real time, and prompt real-time reactions from participants who must then deal with the consequences of those responses. They allow participants to practice and evaluate their roles and responses in a realistic context, without the costs or safety risks of a full-scale field exercise.

A *full-scale exercise* replicates a real emergency. It takes place at a location where a real response would occur, using the personnel and equipment that would be required during a real emergency. Full-scale exercises are often lengthy and involve the coordination of multiple agencies that perform many different functions or operations.

All three types of exercises represent an essential continuum for an organization that is training and preparing to respond to emergencies. These exercise concepts are expanded in training documents developed by the Federal Emergency Management Agency (FEMA) that can be found at http://www.training.fema.gov.

Budget Considerations and Public Health Emergency Planning

It is often difficult for resource-poor public health agencies to invest in supplies, equipment, and staff members whose sole purpose is to respond to emergencies that may occur only rarely. Investments that are intended to enhance the organization's ability to function in or respond to disasters should be guided by the following principles:

- Whenever possible, the investment should have multiple purposes and should expand the organization's capacity during non-emergency events.
- Agencies should participate in a hazard-vulnerability analysis to identify the hazards or disaster scenarios they are most likely to face, given the organization's location, mission, organization, and unique vulnerabilities. The disasters that an organization is most likely to address warrant the most significant investments in capacity.
- When resources are scarce, agreements with other agencies (such as through memoranda of understanding) to share resources during emergencies are critical.

Planners should work closely with partner agencies in the nonprofit and government sectors to identify common resources and ways to manage and share assets during disasters.

- Planners at the local and state level should assess the resources available for emergency response at the federal level. The federal Strategic National Stockpile contains critical pharmaceutical and medical supplies and represents a major asset to support the response to a public health emergency. Planners should understand what they can expect should they need to request critical supplies from this stockpile, and should identify resources that might be needed while waiting their arrival.

During emergencies, the finance/administration section in the ICS is responsible for (a) tracking of all costs associated with the response to the incident, and (b) reimbursement accounting. It is important to track personnel costs, including overtime costs, in addition to other expenses that are incurred during the response and recovery phases. Following federally declared disasters, agencies may be eligible for cost recovery (or a percentage of cost recovery) from federal agencies, such as FEMA.

Conclusion

To summarize, in emergency planning:

- Plan using an incident command system and ensure that your plan and your agency are compliant with the National Incident Management System.
- Plan for all hazards, and recognize that plans that serve dual or multiple purposes are more likely to be used and used effectively during emergencies.
- Provide frank, up-to-date assessments for the public and clear instructions or guidance for what people can do during the emergency.
- Plan with staff members and stakeholders, including those outside the agency, who will participate in the plan's implementation.
- To support the plan's implementation, make key staff members and stakeholders aware of their expected roles.
- Test the plan in exercises or field situations.
- Have a backup communication plan that uses multiple modalities in case an emergency disrupts power or overwhelms communication networks.

Reference

1. The National Resource Center on Advancing Emergency Preparedness for Culturally Diverse Communities. *National Consensus Statement on Emergency Preparedness and Cultural Diversity*,

June 2008. Available at: http://www.diversitypreparedness.org/NCP/92/. Accessed on July 23, 2010.

RESOURCES

Book

Landesman LY. *Public Health Management of Disasters: The Practice Guide* (Third Edition). Washington, DC: American Public Health Association, 2012.

A valuable practical guide.

Web Sites

Centers for Disease Control and Prevention (CDC)
    www.cdc.gov
Federal Emergency Management Agency (FEMA)
    www.fema.gov
Office of the Assistant Secretary for Preparedness and Response, Department of Health and Human Services
    www.phe.gov
Agency for Healthcare Research and Quality (AHRQ)
    www.ahrq.gov
National Association of County and City Health Officials (NACCHO)
    www.naccho.org
Council of State and Territorial Epidemiologists (CSTE)
    www.cste.org
Center for Public Health Preparedness and Disaster Response, American Medical Association
    www.ama-assn.org/ama/pub/physician-resources/public-health/center-public-health-preparedness-disaster-response.page
Center for Infectious Disease Research and Policy, University of Minnesota
    www.cidrap.umn.edu
Center for Biosecurity, University of Pittsburgh
    www. upmc-biosecurity.org

Commentary 7-2: Lessons Learned from Experience in Financial Management and Oversight

Melvin D. Shipp

I have learned important lessons in helping organizations navigate through periods of financial difficulty. Whether the organization is nonprofit, public, or academic, there are several procedures that can be designed and implemented to overcome the problems and move the organization back to financial stability.

An organization may need to address several types of financial or planning issues. Some of these are directly related to the organization's internal practices, while others are influenced by the external environment.

An internal problem may be due to causes such as:

- The lack of training for key staff members working in the finance/accounting department
- A recordkeeping system that is out of date or difficult to use
- Introduction of a new recordkeeping system
- Management difficulties, such as inadequate executive or board oversight or poor relationships among managers and staff members

An external problem may be due to causes such as:

- A sudden and/or significant change in the economy, which may decrease investment revenue
- A reduction in available grant funding
- Decreased income from registration fees or membership dues

Any of these challenges may require you to redesign the financial plan or business model of your organization.

Several of the nonprofit organizations with which I've worked have experienced financial and planning challenges. Based on my experiences, I offer the following ways to address these challenges:

1. RECOGNIZE AND DESCRIBE THE SCOPE OF THE PROBLEM

To do this, you will likely need to have open discussions with key leaders of the organization and perhaps a lending institution. You will need to acknowledge difficulties that contributed to the current situation. Your short-run priority will be to get the organization's financial status into an acceptable mode. Once a stable fiscal position is achieved, long-term fiscal planning can begin. It will likely be necessary to set new goals for the organization, ensuring that there is clear alignment between these goals and the organization's strategic plan.

2. FOSTER A GOOD RELATIONSHIP AMONG ORGANIZATION LEADERS AND LENDERS, FUNDERS, AND KEY SUPPORTERS

Frankly describe the problem to these important stakeholders and decision-makers. You may need to evaluate and change your organization's financial operations, such as by improving board oversight with creation of a finance committee that meets regularly to review and address financial issues. You may need to do the following:

- Arrange a retreat to discuss issues in a broad context.
- Mandate a balanced operating budget.
- Match funding priorities with the effectiveness of programs—in the context of the organization's overall strategic plan.

In sum, you and other organization leaders may need to make changes that provide better management of financial resources and also focus activities of the organization to maximize its value to members and those it serves.

3. ESTABLISHED NECESSARY CONTROL MECHANISMS AND ENSURE AVAILABILITY OF ADEQUATE EXPERTISE TO ADDRESS FUTURE CHALLENGES

For example, you may need to introduce zero-based budgeting and link budgets with work plans of each division and unit in the organization. Budget managers may need to review their work plans and revise them as needed. All work plans may need to be reviewed for outcomes and measured against the objectives of the organization's strategic plan. You and other leaders will need to ensure alignment between (a) the vision, mission, and goals of the organization, and (b) the work to be performed.

To ensure realization of the strategic plan, you may need to strengthen service functions of the organization in such areas as continuing education, communication, information technology, and grassroots advocacy. Others will need to ensure that budget requests are developed in concert with approved work plans, and that the budget is jointly finalized by budget managers, other senior managers and fiscal officers, and the executive director. Unfunded budget requests can be placed on a list for future consideration.

4. MAKE STRUCTURAL CHANGES AS NECESSARY

For example, to improve cash flow, your organization may need to change its fiscal year so that most revenues are received in the first part of the fiscal year.

Conclusion

By carefully stating the type and scope of the financial problems that your organization may face, you can begin a plan of action to make corrections that will result in a more sustainable, better-operating organization. You can help create a new financial environment for your organization that will enable it to achieve its goals and realize its mission.

8

Improving and Maintaining Quality

Ron Bialek and John W. Moran

Public health organizations serve as the first line of defense in keeping the public healthy and safe. This duty is best met by combining public health science with the highly reliable techniques of quality improvement (QI). By eliminating ineffi- ciency, error, and unnecessary redundancy, public health organizations can con- tinually challenge and improve core processes and functions, thereby reducing costs associated with poor quality. QI requires purposeful leadership in all levels of an organization, starting with a strong, unwavering commitment from the leadership team.[1]

Quality improvement in public health has matured from the exploration phase to the implementation phase, with many health departments implement- ing QI projects. The Multi-State Learning Collaborative (MLC) projects, the Robert Wood Johnson Foundation Evaluation grants, and the Public Health Accreditation, Turning Point, and other programs have enabled many health departments to apply QI concepts. There are now many success stories of how QI concepts, tools, and techniques have improved the effectiveness and efficiency of public health services.

A Case Study of QI in Public Health

An H1N1 immunization clinic designed by the Northern Kentucky Independent Health District Department has demonstrated how using QI tools and techniques to plan and deliver services can achieve a smooth process flow and high levels of customer satisfaction.[2] The Department built QI into the process while develop- ing its plan for H1N1 immunization clinics. It was able to perform a trial process by scheduling clinics for first responders. The first three clinics, in which 1,035 first responders were immunized, provided tests of the system and opportunities to gather, from staff members and those immunized, suggestions on where improvements could be made. As the Department acquired more vaccine, it vaccinated up to 10,000 people a day, including students at local schools.

A customer satisfaction survey was distributed to every 30th person attending a clinic. The results of the first five clinics showed that 90% of those immunized were extremely satisfied. Careful planning for the clinics and the follow-up survey corrected process flaws for subsequent clinics and brought a high level of satisfaction to those immunized.

The Department involved all staff members in the continuous QI process by using a Stop-Start-Continue Matrix (Fig. 8-1). This matrix can be used for a quick analysis to see which practices or actions should be stopped, which should be started, and which should be continued. In the staff break room, the Department had a flip chart for staff members to indicate what practices or actions they should stop, start, or continue doing. Within a few days, H1N1 management team members (the "Swine Flu Crew") then performed a wrap-up assessment to determine areas needing improvement and how to make changes for the next clinic. These Stop-Start-Continue suggestions were evaluated by staff members, who listed their planned actions next to each suggestion.

As with any other public health emergency, preparedness for an H1N1 outbreak will be strengthened if the public health system is tested in a comprehensive, systematic, and rigorous manner to find areas that can be improved, resulting in better outcomes and improved satisfaction of those immunized. The Department's critical analysis of its first three immunization clinics revealed areas of performance where change was needed in its immunization process.

For public health departments to reach their full potential in improving the health of the people and communities that they serve, high-quality performance, efficiency, and evidence-based practice are critical. Broad implementation of a QI management approach can enable an organization to perform at a high level. For this to happen, public health leaders must make a long-term commitment to eliminate inefficiency and to develop processes that yield improved results. Large-scale change is seldom quick or easy. It requires the commitment and personal

Start Doing	Stop Doing	Continue Doing
Aha	Learnings	Best Practices
What should we put in place to improve our next clinic?	What are we doing in our current clinic that is not working?	What is working well in our current clinic and should be continued in future clinics?

Figure 8-1 Applying a Stop-Start-Continue Matrix to make immunization clinics more successful. (Source: Katkowsky S, Kent L, Divine S, et al. *Using QI Tools to Make a Difference in H1N1 Flu Immunization Clinics: A Local Health Department's Experience,* January 2010. Available at: http://www.phf.org/pmqi/Using_QI_Tools_for_H1N1_ Clinic.pdf. Accessed on July 7, 2010.)

stewardship of public health leaders. These leaders must publicly declare their intention to make QI a reality and to develop visions for their organizations, build QI infrastructure, and implement basic QI methods, concepts, and principles.[1]

The Continuum of Quality

QI in public health is a never-ending process that pervades an organization when it is fully implemented. As shown in Figure 8-2, organizational leaders at the top address the quality of the system at a macro level (Big QI). In the middle, professional staff members work on problems in programs or service areas by improving specific processes (Little qi). At the individual level, staff members look for ways to improve their own behaviors and environments (Individual qi).[3]

When starting to use QI, public health organizations tend to embrace "Little qi"—striving for quality in a limited or specific QI project or area. This is accomplished by using an integrated set of QI methods and techniques to create a *flow chart*, which identifies each process step and key quality characteristics, analyzes process performance, re-engineers the process if necessary, and "locks in" improvements. "Little qi" can be viewed as a tactical or systems approach to implementing quality and beginning to generate a "culture of QI" within an organization.[1]

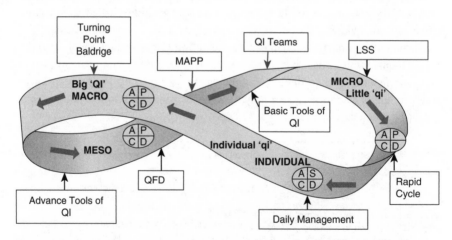

Figure 8-2 Continuous quality improvement system in public health. MAPP, Mobilizing for Action through Planning and Partnerships; LSS, Lean Six Sigma; QFD, Quality Function Deployment. (Source: Duffy GL, Moran JW, Riley WJ. *Quality Function Deployment and Lean Six Sigma Applications in Public Health*. Milwaukee, WI: Quality Press, 2010, p. 15.) Reproduced by permission of Grace L. Duffy, John W. Moran, and William J. Riley, *Quality Function Deployment and Lean Six Sigma Applications in Public Health* (Milwaukee: ASQ Quality Press, 2010). To order this book, visit ASQ at http://www.asq.org/quality-press.

The voluntary accreditation program of the Public Health Accreditation Board (PHAB) emphasizes the importance of QI for health departments in its accreditation standards (Box 8-1). As increasingly more public health departments embraced QI, a workgroup of the Public Health Accreditation Coalition, which comprises national public health organizations supporting implementation of voluntary accreditation of health departments, developed the following definition of QI in public health:

> Quality improvement in public health is the use of a deliberate and defined improvement process, which is focused on activities that are responsive to community needs and improving population health.
>
> It refers to a continuous and ongoing effort to achieve measurable improvements in the efficiency, effectiveness, performance, accountability, outcomes, and other indicators of quality in services or processes which achieve equity and improve the health of the community.[4]

Box 8-1: **Quality Improvement and Public Health Accreditation**

The goal of national public health accreditation is to protect and improve the health of the public by advancing the quality and performance of all health departments in the country—local, state, territorial, and tribal. Accreditation will drive public health departments to continuously improve the quality, efficiency, and effectiveness of their services and help make all our communities healthier places to live, work, learn, and play. Accreditation of health departments is a critical part of the future of public health, and as the national conversation around implementing health-care reform progresses, accreditation will be an integral part of that dialogue.

Why Does Accreditation Matter to Public Health?
For public health departments, accreditation means demonstrated accountability and improved quality. Nationally, public health accreditation means that people across the country can expect the same quality of public health programs and services no matter where they live. Accreditation is expected to strengthen public health departments and the services they provide, which will contribute to improve health outcomes in communities. Local public health departments already participating in state accreditation programs report a variety of benefits, including:

- *Performance feedback and quality improvement*: The accreditation process provides valuable feedback to health departments about their strengths

and areas for improvement, laying the foundation for improved protection, promotion, and preservation of their community's health.

- *Accountability and credibility*: Accreditation is also a way for health departments to show how effectively they are allocating often-scarce state and
  local resources. Achieving accreditation demonstrates accountability to
  elected officials and communities, resulting in increased credibility for
  public health departments.
- *Staff morale and visibility*: The recognition of excellence that comes with
  meeting accreditation standards has improved staff morale and enhanced
  the visibility of the health departments in their communities, enabling
  them to compete successfully for additional resources.

National accreditation addresses important priorities supporting all
public health departments in developing core capacities and improving their
performance. Since the accreditation process is focused on building and continuously improving upon performance, it will help ensure that everyone has
access to essential public health services and that all communities become
healthier, safer, and more resilient.

The Public Health Accreditation Board (PHAB) was created to serve as the
national public health accrediting body, and is jointly funded by the Centers
for Disease Control and Prevention and the Robert Wood Johnson
Foundation. The development of national public health accreditation has
involved, and is supported by, public health leaders and practitioners at the
national, state, local, and tribal level. To receive updates on national public
health accreditation, learn more about PHAB, or sign up for the PHAB
e-newsletter, visit http://www.phaboard.org.

(Source: Public Health Accreditation Board. Courtesy of Kaye Bender.)

How to Start to Use QI in Your Agency or Organization

Once the leadership of a public health organization decides to use QI to improve
the way it delivers services, it needs guidance on how to start, build, and maintain
a QI organizational culture. The following is a 10-step process to accomplish this:

Step 1: Prioritizing areas needing improvement
Step 2: Developing a team charter
Step 3: Providing adequate training
Step 4: Using the Plan-Do-Check-Act (PDCA) cycle improvement process
Step 5: Using QI tools and techniques

Step 6: Determining root causes
Step 7: Developing solutions
Step 8: Implementing solutions
Step 9: Monitoring changes
Step 10: Maintaining ongoing QI

STEP 1: PRIORITIZING AREAS NEEDING IMPROVEMENT

As an organizational leader, you choose those areas needing the most improvement. These improvement areas can be prioritized from Mobilizing for Action through Planning and Partnerships (MAPP), a community-driven strategic planning process for improving community health (MAPP assessment); a SWOT (Strengths, Weaknesses, Opportunities, and Threats) analysis; Community Health Assessment; the strategic plan; or other indicators of areas needing improvement (see Chapter 7). You should align the areas selected to be improved with the future strategic direction of the organization. Staff members should recognize these areas as high-priority areas that are worthy of the investment of time and energy to improve them. Selection of improvement areas must be done with a focus on areas that:

- Are high profile
- Are causing much pain in the agency or organization
- Will have a major impact on improving the way work is done by streamlining and improving efficiency
- Will reduce unnecessary steps in the work process
- Will improve services to the community

All leaders of the organization must be involved in the QI process from start to finish by selecting areas of improvement and by providing necessary direction, guidance, training, and support. Continuous involvement of leaders helps ensure that QI becomes part of the culture of the agency or organization.

STEP 2: DEVELOPING A TEAM CHARTER

Once you have chosen the areas needing improvement, you and other leaders of the organization need to develop a team charter for each improvement initiative. Drafting a team charter provides the initial direction for team focus and gives team members the opportunity to develop its details and final AIM statement (what you are trying to accomplish), with leadership approval.

The team charter is an official work contract that delineates the strategic goals, boundaries, measures of success, constraints and limits, and available resources.[5] It provides a framework for ongoing discussions among team members and the team's sponsor concerning the team's direction and progress.

The team charter is developed in an iterative process until the team and the sponsor establish baseline acceptance. The sponsor is a senior organizational leader who supports a team's plans, activities, and outcomes. The team charter must be reviewed on a regular basis by the sponsor, the team leader, the facilitator, and team members to ensure that it reflects what the team is doing or will be doing.

The team charter does not tell team members how to solve a problem or what a solution should look like. Rather, it sets the process in motion and establishes key milestones and desired outcomes. But it does not suggest a path to a solution. Team members must use available tools to figure out how to analyze and solve the problem they have been commissioned to solve. The team charter starts the team in the right direction and provides the process for negotiating changes in direction, if necessary.

QI problem-solving teams often flounder from the lack of initial clear and concise directions on what they are supposed to do, inadequate training and technical assistance, and a problem statement that is too broad and not focused. Once teams narrow their problem statement to a discrete issue, they are able to focus on and effectively apply QI tools. When teams lack focus on the real issue, they lose valuable problem-solving time and become disenfranchised from the process since they seem to be going in circles without making any progress.[6]

The team charter can save much time and reduce confusion for team members since it defines clear goals, expressed duties, and desired outcomes. Omitting this step in planning reduces the team's overall effectiveness and the sponsor's ultimate goals.

After the team charter is developed and agreed upon, the next step the team undertakes is to develop a statement. When doing so, the team needs to think in terms of concentric circles (Fig. 8-3). These circles represent layers of decreasing control from the center, where the problem-solving team is in complete control, to the outermost circle, where it has little or no control over events or resources. The outer circles represent global, rather than discrete, issues. The farther one moves from the center, the more difficult it becomes to directly influence outcomes. When the problem-solving team starts at the innermost circle, it can develop issues that are discrete, measurable, and bound by time. As the team gains experience and confidence, it will probably want to tackle issues in the outer circles, where the potential for benefits to community health improvement is larger.

With resources being limited, everyone in public health should use QI tools to maximize return on resources. The team charter and a well-designed AIM statement can save much startup time and reduce confusion for a team since they help define clear goals, expressed duties, and desired outcomes. To omit this step in planning for a successful team process is to reduce the overall effectiveness of the team and the ultimate goals of the sponsor and leaders.

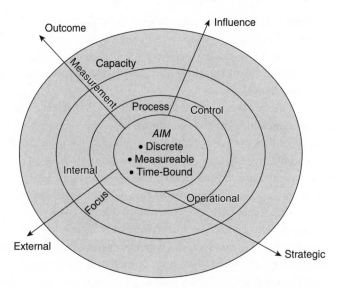

Figure 8-3   Developing AIM Statements. (Source: Beitsch L, Duffy G, Moran J. Ready, AIM, problem solve. *Quality Texas Newsletter*, October 2009;14–19. Available at: http://www.texasquality.org/SiteImages/125/Newsletter/October%202009%20% 20Newsletter.pdf. Accessed on July 8, 2010.)

STEP 3: PROVIDING ADEQUATE TRAINING

You and other leaders must provide adequate training for the QI teams you charter. You should present an overview of the QI process to staff members at all levels of the organization to help them understand what the QI teams are expected to accomplish. You should design QI training to help the organization and its members be on the cutting edge of quality and innovation—to assist in identifying and developing improvement objectives and aligning them to the organization's strategies. QI training should also:

- Develop skills to analyze root causes of problems—not treat symptoms
- Develop and use metrics and data collection to improve analytical capabilities
- Understand how to control costs, improve efficiency, increase morale, and engage those served to find out what services they want and need

Training should constantly emphasize how to develop and sustain, within a public health organization, a "culture of QI" that encourages all staff members to continuously improve the quality of services and programs. Ongoing and refresher training programs are needed to maintain the QI process.

Training usually involves the following three phases, each with learning objectives:

1. *Basic training* is for those exploring QI or just getting started in it. Its objective is to help participants to:
   - Describe the Plan-Do-Check-Act approach to QI and distinguish it from other planning and management approaches
   - Understand how to use basic QI tools to identify areas needing improvement
   - Understand why and how to identify root causes of problems
   - Observe public health applications of basic QI tools, such as Brainstorming, the Cause-and-Effect Diagram, Flow Charts, the Five Whys, Pareto Charts, and Graphical Displays of Data (described later in this chapter)
2. *Intermediate training* focuses on developing leadership skills necessary for those ready to expand the QI program throughout their organizations. Its objective is to help participants to:
   - Understand the support and leadership skills and support that are required to develop a "culture of QI" within an organization
   - Understand how to build a change management plan
   - Understand and articulate what the cost of quality is within an organization
   - Understand QI in the larger context of Performance Management
   - Define and describe key concepts and the four components of Performance Management in the Turning Point model (standards, measures, reporting of progress, and QI)
   - Describe potential roles to assist teams or individuals with QI projects
   - Increase confidence to support QI efforts of public health teams
   - Identify strategies to engage all leaders and staff members in QI
   These approaches are described in more detail later in this chapter.
3. *Advanced training* focuses on helping QI leaders to move their organizations to more advanced QI positions, to institute and sustain a "culture of QI," and to help move their organizations to the cutting edge of quality and innovation. Its objective is to help participants to:
   - Understand, develop, and articulate a strategic agency-wide or organization-wide QI plan
   - Begin involving their total communities in QI
   - Develop Balanced Scorecards to track and measure QI
   - Understand how to use the seven Advanced Quality Tools in a decision-making cycle to focus on organization-wide issues
   - Understand and articulate the benefits of a Total Quality Environment
   - Understand Core Process Redesign and Six Sigma methodologies to tackle larger projects of Business Process Redesign (rather than quality QI)

- Understand how to incorporate the "Voice of the Customer" into redesign and improvement projects

STEP 4: USING THE PLAN-DO-CHECK-ACT (PDCA) CYCLE IMPROVEMENT PROCESS

QI teams should use deliberate, defined, and evidence-based improvement processes. The Public Health Foundation recommends the PDCA cycle to guide team problem-solving (Figs. 8-4 and 8-5).[7]

PDCA should be repeatedly implemented in spirals of increasing knowledge of the system that converge on the ultimate goal—each cycle closer than the previous. Rapid Cycle PDCA applies a recurring sequence of PDCA in a brief period of time to solve a problem or address an issue facing a team or organization. It is designed to achieve a breakthrough or continuous improvement results quickly (Fig. 8-6).[8]

Launching a PDCA cycle can be accomplished in a short period of time—3 days or even 3 hours! QI teams can waste too much time and energy by not solving a problem quickly or by failing to hold onto gains so that they can move onto the next organizational challenge. Not doing Rapid Cycle PDCA causes team members to lose interest, become bored, fail to gain experience and knowledge in applying QI, and, for a long time, fail to see the impact of their work.

STEP 5: USING QI TOOLS AND TECHNIQUES

QI teams must use the basic QI tools to augment the PDCA cycle to develop a robust problem-solving process. The basic tools of QI and a general approach to use them in solving problems is shown in Figure 8-7.[9]

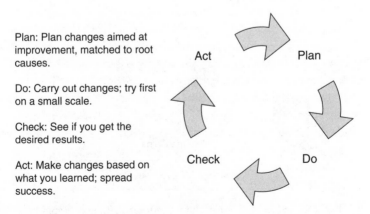

Plan: Plan changes aimed at improvement, matched to root causes.

Do: Carry out changes; try first on a small scale.

Check: See if you get the desired results.

Act: Make changes based on what you learned; spread success.

Figure 8-4 The Plan-Do-Check-Act (PDCA) Cycle. (Source: Deming WE. *Out of Crises.* Cambridge, MA: MIT Press, 1986, p. 88.)

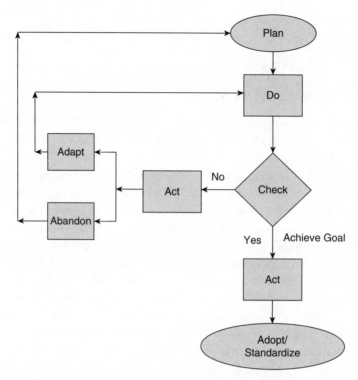

Figure 8-5 Flow chart of PDCA Cycle. (Source: Guest essay: The elements of the PDCA cycle. *ASQ Healthcare Update Newsletter*, June 22, 2010. Available at: http://www.asq. org/healthcare-use/docs/201006-guest-essay.pdf?WT.mc_id=EM5210C&WT. dcsvid=1506047082. Accessed on October 4, 2010.)

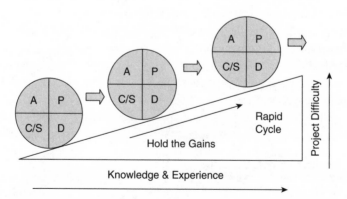

Figure 8-6 Rapid Cycle PDCA. (Source: Duffy G, Moran J, Riley W. Rapid cycle PDCA. *Texas Quality Newsletter*, August 2009; 2–4. Available at: http://www.texas-quality.org/ SiteImages/125/Newsletter/August%202009%20%20Newsletter.pdf. Accessed on July 8, 2010.)

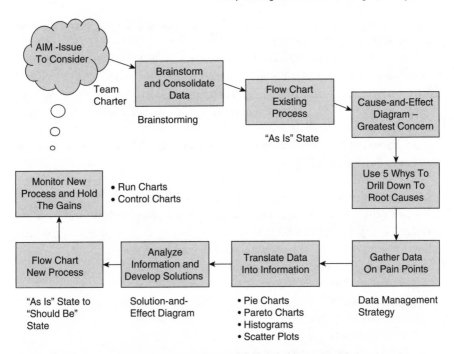

Figure 8-7 General approach on how to use the basic tools of quality improvement. (Source: Bialek R, Duffy G, Moran J, eds. *The Public Health Quality Improvement Handbook*. Milwaukee, WI: Quality Press, 2009, p. 160.)

1. Once the AIM statement is finalized, a QI team usually starts by flow-charting the current state of the process to understand how it is operating.
2. A flow chart is an organized combination of shapes, lines, and text. From this graphic picture, one can see a process and its elements. A flow chart can:
   - Demonstrate how "hand-offs" and "interactions" occur
   - Demonstrate where there are bottlenecks, barriers, and obstacles
   - Identify wasteful steps
   - Uncover variations
3. A flow chart provides a visual illustration—a picture—of the steps taken to complete an assigned task.
4. Flow-charting is the first step taken in understanding (a) how a process is functioning, (b) what the steps are that make up the process, (c) how the process is performing—by measuring key attributes of the process, and (d) how well it is satisfying the needs of those who benefit from it.

When a QI team flow-charts a process, it needs to ensure that it includes members who are experienced with the process. Alternatively, team members can go to where the process is operating—observe it in action, walk through each step, and speak with those performing the process to see if there are steps they are overlooking. Then, they can find out if there are any similar processes else-where that they can benchmark.

Spending the time to understand the process can enable you to (a) gather information on how the process flows from start to finish—to establish a baseline, (b) to clearly define each step in the process, and (c) to ensure that you have charted an accurate and honest portrayal of the current state of the process. Such a portrayal has a few baseline measurements to indicate how the process is performing over time. (These baseline performance data are relevant to analyzing changes as described in Step 9, below.)

Too often, many steps of a process are overlooked without walking through a trial process in real time to determine (a) what work is being done that adds no value to clients, (b) where rework (correcting defects) is built into the process, (c) where inefficiencies are built into the process, and (d) where workarounds (alternative methods) have been developed that add no value.

Some key questions to ask in documenting a process are:

• Who are the clients?
• Who are the suppliers?
• What is the first thing that happens?
• What is the next thing that happens?
• Where do the inputs to the process come from?
• How do the inputs get to the process?
• Where do the outputs of the process go?
• What are the measurement indicators that are being used to monitor performance?
• Is there anything else that must be done at this point?

STEP 6: DETERMINING ROOT CAUSES

Once the flow chart of the current state of the process is completed, the QI team begins the analysis phase, looking for potential problem areas and evidence to confirm that these indeed are problem areas. This is accomplished by examining the current-state flow chart and looking at each of the following:

• Activity symbol: What is the value? What is the cost?
• Decision point: Is it necessary or redundant?
• Rework loop: How much time is needed? What is the cost?
• Handoff: Is it seamless?
• Document or data point: Is it useful?
• Wait or delay symbol: Should it be reduced or eliminated?
• Transport symbol: How much time is needed? What is the cost? What is the location?
• Data input symbol: Is it in the right format and timely?

- Document/form symbol: Is it needed? What is the cost? What is the value?
- Current process measurement indicators: Is the process under control?

Once the analysis is complete and the potential problem areas have been listed, the QI team then prioritizes these areas and narrows the list to the top two or three to focus upon. Each of the potential problem areas is analyzed with the Cause-and-Effect Diagram (Fig. 8-8).

Each problem area being analyzed is written as a problem statement on the right-hand side of the page and a box is drawn around it with an arrow running to it. This problem statement is now the effect for which you want to find the root cause or causes. The QI team needs to perform an in-depth causal analysis. Usually when confronted with a problem, most people like to address the obvious symptom and eliminate it, but this often results in more problems. Using a systematic cause-and-effect approach to analyze a problem and finding the root cause is more efficient and effective in developing a solution that will provide a permanent fix.

The QI team then suggests main causes of the effect and labels these with main branch headers, such as People, Policies, Process, Material, Community, Environment, or Funding. Then, each of these main headers needs to be analyzed into its sub-causes by asking, "Why?" at least five times—the Five Whys—to peel away layers of symptoms, identify the root cause of a problem, and develop evidence to support its being the root cause through measurement.

When the Cause-and-Effect Diagram is completed, team members must decide what few areas to focus on to solve the problem. The obvious areas—"low-hanging fruit"—can be fixed easily. Others require some research by the QI team using the other QI tools, such as Pareto Diagrams, Run Charts, Surveys, and Histograms, to determine if it is the real root cause (Fig. 8-9).

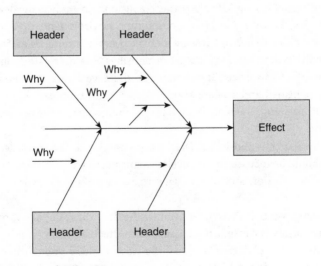

Figure 8-8 Cause-and-Effect Diagram.

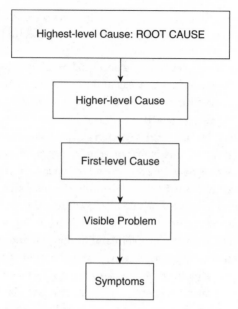

Figure 8-9 Root Cause Analysis.

STEP 7: DEVELOPING SOLUTIONS

Once the QI team has agreed upon the root cause, it begins to develop potential solutions for the problem. One way to address the root cause is by using a Solution-and-Effect Diagram (Fig. 8-10).

The root cause is made into a positive statement and placed in the box on the far right of the diagram. Then the QI team generates ideas as to what the Main Solutions of the effect are. It labels these as the main branch headers, such as People, Policies, Process, Material, Community, Environment, or Funding. The team then subdivides each of these headers into sub-solutions by asking, "How?" For each main solution category, the team identifies possible related sub-solutions that might affect the issue. The team uses the Five Hows technique when a solution is identified and repeats asking "How?" until no other solutions can be identified. In so doing, the team lists the sub-solutions using the arrows shown in Figure 8-10.

When the Solution-and-Effect Diagram is completed, the team decides what few areas should be focused on to develop solutions to solve the effect.

In using the Solution-and-Effect Diagram, beware of the following:

- Do not jump too quickly to a Solution-and-Effect Diagram; use it only after a detailed analysis of cause using a Cause-and-Effect Diagram.
- If you are still listing causes, you have not provided enough detail on the Cause-and-Effect Diagram.

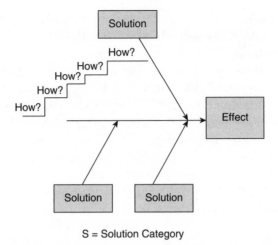

Figure 8-10 Solution-and-Effect Diagram.

- Ask if the proposed solutions will improve the effect or actually cause more problems.
- Note that the reverse of the cause is not always the solution.

STEP 8: IMPLEMENTING SOLUTIONS

Implementing potential solutions usually requires the QI team to develop the Should Be flow-chart state so everyone can see what will be affected or changed in the current state before moving to the future state. The Should Be flow chart will serve as a road map for the implementation of the proposed solutions developed in Step 7.

To correctly implement the potential solutions, you need to test the new process in such a way that you can control it and measure the impact of the change. The QI team needs to develop measurement indicators and plan for data collection for each change to be made to ensure that the evidence is in place to support that the desired change was achieved. These indicators and data-collection plans will provide the QI team with the necessary information to help determine if improvement is actually occurring, by a comparison with the baseline data obtained in Step 5. Before a QI team starts collecting data, it must answer the following questions:

- What is the purpose for collecting these data?
- What types of data will be collected?
- Where will the data be collected?
- Who will collect the data?
- When will they collect the data?
- How will they be trained to collect the data?

- What will be done with the data after they are collected?
- How will the data be summarized and presented?

The answers to these questions will help the QI team to develop a plan to collect data that are reliable and suitable for making decisions. QI tools such as a Pareto Chart, Run Chart, Histogram, and Pie Chart can be used along with some basic descriptive statistical measures (mean, median, mode, and standard deviation) to summarize the data obtained and to draw conclusions that can guide decision-makers.

In addition, the QI team develops a communication plan to inform everyone involved about the change of the timing, proposed changes, who is involved, and when the analysis of results will be available.

STEP 9: MONITORING CHANGES

The QI team tracks and measures the implementation to understand and document it and determine if the goals for improvements set forth in the AIM statement are being achieved. To determine if improvements have made a difference, comparisons are made to the baseline measures that were documented during the development of the current-state flow chart. The QI team documents any problems encountered, unexpected observations, lessons learned, and knowledge gained during the trial implementation, and communicates this information to all those involved.

The QI team then decides what action to take based on the trial implementation. If the pilot improvement is successful, the QI team must standardize the improvement by testing it on a wider scale in every area where the new process will be used. The QI team develops training for those affected so they can perform the new process and hold the gains made in the trial. In addition, the QI team continues to monitor the new process to ensure that, as it is expanded throughout the organization, it is still achieving the goals achieved in the trial period.

If the trial is not successful, the QI team members need to decide if they should modify the changes implemented and retest or if they should abandon the change and start the process again.

The QI team needs to make sure that it communicates all decisions made and their implications.

STEP 10: MAINTAINING ONGOING QI

QI is a continuous process. It never ends. So when a QI team ends its work, it is usually time to restart the PDCA cycle by repeating Steps 1 through 9—and by launching new QI teams to work on other organizational issues.

Continuous QI helps ingrain the principles of QI into the culture of an organization. It builds on existing efforts to improve how the organization functions, reinforcing leaders' commitment to the process, so that the organization can constantly improve its delivery of services to the community.

Why QI Projects Fail

Quality projects fail for the following reasons:

- Intuition is used, rather than data-driven management.
- Many policies, processes, and procedures are undocumented.
- QI teams receive insufficient training and guidance.
- Senior managers are inadequately involved.
- QI teams take on projects that are too complex.
- No Rapid Cycle PDCA is used—and therefore QI projects take too long to complete.
- QI teams do not involve clients or partners.
- QI teams use tools one at a time—not in an integrated process.
- QI teams do not update their tools as they gather new data.[10]

Conclusion

By following the 10 steps outlined in this chapter, your organization can successfully implement a sustainable QI process.

Acknowledgment

The Accreditation Coalition Workgroup, cited in this chapter, comprised Les Beitsch, Ron Bialek, Abby Cofsky, Liza Corso, Jack Moran, William Riley, and Pamela Russo.

References

1. Riley WJ, Moran JW, Corso LC, et al. Defining quality improvement in public health. *J Public Health Management Practice* 2010; 16:5–7.
2. Katkowsky SR, Kent LA, Divine S, et al. Using QI Tools to Make a Difference in H1N1 Flu Immunization Clinics: A Local Health Department's Experience. Available at: http://www.phf.org/pmqi/Using_QI_Tools_for_H1N1_Clinic.pdf. Accessed on July 7, 2010.
3. Duffy G, McCoy K, Moran J, Riley W. The continuum of quality improvement in public health. *Quality Management Forum* 2010; 35:1–9.
4. Riley WJ, Moran JW, Corso LC, et al. Defining quality improvement in public health. *J Public Health Management Practice* 2010; 16:5–7.

5. Moran JW, Duffy GL. Team chartering. *Quality Texas Newsletter*, April 2010, pp. 14–21. Available at: http://www.texas-quality.org/SiteImages/125/Newsletter/April%202010%20Newsletter.pdf. Accessed on July 8, 2010.

6. Beitsch L, Duffy G, Moran J. Ready, AIM, problem solve. *Quality Texas Newsletter*, October 2009, pp. 14–19. Available at: http://www.texas-quality.org/SiteImages/125/Newsletter/October%202009%20%20Newsletter.pdf. Accessed on July 8, 2010.

7. Gorenflo G, Moran J. The ABCs of PDCA. Available at: http://www.phf.org/pmqi/resources.htm#ABCs_of_PDCA. Accessed on July 8, 2010.

8. Duffy G, Moran J, Riley W. Rapid cycle PDCA. *Texas Quality Newsletter*, August 2009, pp. 2–4. Available at: http://www.texas-quality.org/SiteImages/125/Newsletter/August%202009%20%20Newsletter.pdf. Accessed on July 8, 2010.

9. Bialek R, Duffy G, Moran J (eds.). *The Public Health Quality Improvement Handbook*. Milwaukee, WI: Quality Press, 2009, p. 160.

10. Bialek R, Carden J, Duffy G. Supporting public health departments' quality improvement initiatives: Lessons learned from the public health foundation. *J Public Health Management Practice* 2010; 16:14.

RESOURCES

Books and Documents

Bialek R, Duffy G, Moran J (eds.). *The Public Health Quality Improvement Handbook*. Milwaukee, WI: Quality Press, 2009.

> *In this book, subject-matter experts in public health describe quality improvement tools and techniques that they are using to meet client needs more effectively.*

Duffy G, Moran J, Riley W. *Quality Function Deployment and Lean Six Sigma Applications in Public Health*. Milwaukee, WI: Quality Press, 2010.

> *This book introduces concepts to assist public health workers implement quality improvement within their agencies and other organizations.*

Gorenflo G, Moran J. The ABCs of PDCA. Available at: http://www.phf.org/resourcestools/Documents/ABCs_of_PDCA.pdf. Accessed on July 8, 2010.

> *This document describes the basics of the Plan-Do-Check-Act (PDCA) cycle.*

Sholtes PR, Joiner, BL, Streibel BJ. *The Team Handbook (3rd. ed.)*. Edison, NJ: Oriel STAT A MATRIX, 2003.

> *This book offers tools and strategies to help teams work well together in a quality improvement environment.*

Articles

Beitsch L, Duffy G, Moran J. Ready, AIM, problem solve. *Quality Texas Newsletter, October* 2009, *pp.* 14–19. *Available at:* http://www.texas-quality.org/SiteImages/125/Newsletter/October%20 2009%20%20Newsletter.pdf. *Accessed on July 8,* 2010.

Duffy G, McCoy K, Moran J, Riley W. The continuum of quality improvement in public health. *Quality Management Forum*, Winter 2010. Available at: http://www.phf.org/pmqi/ASQ_QM_Forum_Winter_2010.pdf. Accessed on October 4, 2010.

Duffy G, Moran J, Riley W. Rapid cycle PDCA. *Texas Quality Newsletter*, August 2009, pp. 2–4. Available at: http://www.texas-quality.org/SiteImages/125/Newsletter/August%202009%20%20Newsletter.pdf. Accessed on July 8, 2010.

Riley WJ, Moran JW, Corso LC, et al. Defining quality improvement in public health. *J Public Health Management Practice*. January/February 2010;16:5–7. (For additional QI training information, visit http://www.phf.org.)

> *These four articles provide more detailed information on the approaches to quality improvement described in this chapter.*

Web Site

GOAL/QPC

www.goalqpc.com.

GOAL/QPC offers practical tools in continuous improvement, quality, and organizational transformation. It is best known for its Memory Jogger series of organizational improvement pocket guides. GOAL/QPC also provides public and in-house training courses.

Commentary 8-1: Improving Quality in Your Organization

Paul Halverson

When considering how to implement quality improvement in your organization, remember that the concept of quality improvement must become part of the culture. It has to define the way that you do your work.

I counsel my managers to think in terms of *continuous quality improvement* (CQI). My philosophy is that we work to become an excellent organization at all times—not just when we're trying to assess those things that are not succeeding. For example, during the course of an employee's day, what are those job responsibilities that can be refined and made better? Can something as mundane as organizing e-mail allow an employee to be more efficient? Would an agenda for a staff meeting result in better time management and less "free-for-all" discussion? Even systems that are working well can be improved.

Make sure that your organization doesn't fall into the trap of creating situations laden with guilt or accusation. The focus should not be on who is to blame, but rather on finding ways that we can make things even better. William Deming, the "father" of the quality improvement movement, described the principle of "driving out fear." As a leader, you must ensure an environment in which fear doesn't rule.

Here are two scenarios for organizations practicing CQI:

1. Organization X does not practice CQI as part of its culture. This organization is currently doing well, and it tends to remain successful, despite the impact of difficult economic times on other organizations, because of its past success and geographic position in the region. Despite the fact that its success is not guaranteed, it resists changing to a CQI orientation because at present it seems to be doing well. Because of its apparent success, it joins with a few other organizations that don't currently see the imperative to make change.

2. Organization Y is teetering on the brink of disaster. There are major problems and a looming danger in its environment. There may be a compelling need to change. If Organization Y doesn't start practicing CQI, it may not survive. In this situation, its leaders should find it relatively easy to convince employees that change is needed to make an impact on the organization. There is shared pain. And CQI properly done may be seen as a way to help rescue the organization. The difficulty in this situation will be that this high-risk organization may have waited too long to implement change and may need a more immediate intervention than what a systematic approach to quality improvement might bring ordinarily. However, even in this situation, a CQI approach adopted after restructuring or more radical organizational transformation may help sustain needed change and attention.

The challenge that Organization X faces, when it encounters the financial and organizational pressures that ultimately impact every organization at some point, is gaining an understanding for change. Even when an organization starts to recognize that it is in the midst of a downward spiral, many of its members or employees often want to hang onto the past. Much like a marriage that is "on the rocks" and headed for divorce, they try to maintain a sense of normalcy and are averse to any meaningful change. The organization's culture is embedded in the belief that "It's good enough."

In some public clinics, for example, waiting time may be an indicator of staff efficiency and how it coordinates the flow of patients. Some public clinics operate on the principle that "We'll get to you when we can" and patients may wait for hours. Staff members may believe that the patients have less urgency with their time than patients who see physicians in private practice. Some employees of public clinics may even think, "They are lucky that we are here to serve them." This attitude can become institutionalized. Therefore, a challenge for this clinic is to create a sense of urgency about acceptable standards of care and service delivery.

As a leader of an organization, you should know that most employees are "tuned in" to the figurative radio station WIIFM—"What's in it for me?" How can you change your message so that they see a benefit to change? How can you engage and motivate them towards organizational goals and simultaneously provide personal benefit and satisfaction for them?

Look for opportunities to get employees excited about change. Give them permission to change. Give them enough time to learn about new concepts. Sometimes employees feel paralyzed. Empower employees to suggest changes—without fear of being punished. Show them that you are willing to "drive out fear." This can be especially challenging in a government organization because work is done in the public's eye. There are limitations as to how much "reasonable or calculated risk" employees can take. To counter this, give people explicit permission to make suggestions for change.

In our organization, we systematically review policies and procedures to look for opportunities for improvements. We also encourage supervisors to engage in discussions with workers who are involved in process improvements. By engaging employees at this level, a supervisor can heighten their sense of importance—a powerful personal and organizational motivator.

When I participate in the orientation of new employees to our health department, I encourage them to look to see how work is done, to make suggestions, and to ask questions. They have "fresh eyes," which can benefit everyone. New employees aren't jaded by an agency's historical successes and failures. They can point out what adds value or seems to make sense.

I'm reminded of the parable of a baker who after baking cakes always cut them in half. When someone asked him why, he said he didn't have a pan that was small enough, so he did this to have cakes that were just the right size. I wondered why he didn't just use the right-sized pan in the first place.

Many organizations also lack a spirit of innovation and creativity. Organizational leaders would like to see more creative thinking, which is difficult to find in today's frenetic work environment. Crisis management is often the norm, and creativity is missing. Part of an organization's CQI culture must include the belief that innovation and creativity are important and complementary to the CQI environment.

In government agencies, the organizational culture generally doesn't support innovation and creativity because work is done in the public eye. In these agencies, there are typically so many policies that govern all actions by employees that many feel unable to make any changes. There is little to no tolerance for "taking a risk" with—or for—the public's good. In these settings, there should be established parameters that enable employees to be innovative without creating a public perception that unmanaged risk is acceptable. It is important to recognize this distinction between work in the public sector and work in the more innovative and creative private sector.

There are tangible benefits for you and other organizational leaders to implement a culture of CQI. As you implement CQI, focus on measurement. What gets measured gets done. When employees start to focus on improvement, they need to identify the critical measurements for their own work. By doing so, they can recognize improvement—or lack of improvement—when it occurs. If employees have things that they are willing to measure, they have the will to improve.

During the initial implementation of CQI, celebrate important gains—even if they are small. Update employees on the progress that you are making together. They need to see results that use real numbers with real meaning so that they can measure their progress. Although much work in public health results in long-term improvements seen in the future, you and your employees need to have results that can be measured in the short term.

I often think of establishing CQI in our organization as creating a furious small fire. Keep fanning the flame of those goals and objectives that employees know they can achieve. Celebrate successes. And focus on things that are going right.

9

Obtaining Funding

Fern Percheski and Robyn Powers

This chapter provides practical information and tools to help you identify and obtain funding for your projects and programs: an overview of different types of funding, ways to identify and develop appropriate funding sources, a guide on how to write an effective grant proposal, and other helpful resources.

Understanding Funding Sources

There are two main categories of funding: (a) public funding, including grants, cooperative agreements, and contracts from local, state, or federal governmental entities; and (b) private funding from foundations, corporations, and individuals. This chapter focuses on public funding as well as private funding from foundations. Commentary 9-1 focuses on contributions from individuals and corporations.

There are similarities between public and private grants. Both require that you understand the grantor's funding priorities, application process, and method of evaluation. Distinctions between public and private grants include the regulatory requirements for governmental agencies and foundations, the process for grant solicitation and evaluation, and accountability and reporting requirements for funded grants.

FUNDING PRIORITIES

Priorities of public agencies are guided by legislation, agency directives, and public need. Priorities of foundations are usually set by their boards and are general or highly focused on a specific area.

You should understand that funding priorities of agencies and foundations are updated regularly. Once you have identified relevant agencies and foundations with priorities that match those of your organization, visit their Web sites to learn the beginning of their funding cycles and abstract relevant information for future reference.

APPLICATION PROCESS

The application, or solicitation, process for foundation grants varies among foundations. Many require online submission with standardized applications. Some foundations require a letter of intent before they "invite" submission of a complete application. Others encourage contact to discuss a potential project to ensure there is a fit with their priorities. Making this contact can save you much time and stress. When permitted, discuss your potential project with a foundation staff member—it begins building a relationship, which increases your chance of having your project funded.

Federal agencies are increasingly requiring electronic submission through Grants.gov, with standard application and budget forms. However, federal agencies differ in their formats and requirements for applications and budgets.

Early in your research, review submission requirements included in grant announcements. These requirements will affect your timeline for proposal development, internal resources needed for submission, and possibly the organization of your proposal narrative. When a contact is named in the announcement of a funding opportunity, discuss your proposed project with that person to better understand the interests, goals, and objectives of the funder. Ask potential funders about their goals and objectives to determine if there is a good match between your proposed project and funding opportunities.

REGULATORY REQUIREMENTS

Public funding agencies are bound by legislation, annual budgetary appropriations, and many governmental and agency-specific regulations that affect potential grant recipients.

Grant announcements will generally list all regulatory requirements for grantees. Review these before submitting an application and confirm that you are willing to comply. This advice can also apply to foundation expectations and reporting requirements.

TYPES OF FUNDING BY FEDERAL AGENCIES

Federal government agencies offer various types of grants. For example, the Department of Health and Human Services (DHHS) provides two categories of grants, which it defines as the following:

- "Mandatory grants are those that a federal agency is required by statute to award if the recipient, usually a state, submits an acceptable State Plan or application and meets the eligibility and compliance requirements of the statutory and regulatory provisions of the grant program."

- "Discretionary grants permit the federal government, according to specific authorizing legislation, to exercise judgment, or 'discretion,' in selecting the applicant/recipient organization through a competitive grant process."[1]

Individual agencies within DHHS have subcategories of grants. For example, the National Institutes of Health (NIH) uses "mechanisms of support" to distinguish between various types of grant programs. The mechanism for each opportunity is identified in the funding opportunity announcement (FOA). When you choose whether or not to pursue a specific NIH grant, understand what these mechanisms are and the subtle differences among them. (See the NIH Web site at: http://grants2.nih.gov/grants/funding/funding_program.htm.)

Cooperative agreements generally are used by federal funding agencies when a greater level of their involvement is required. Cooperative agreements are managed and treated like grants but generally have more deliverables and accountability, as well as substantial input from the funding agency. Always read the FOA carefully to identify expectations and involvement of the funding agency.

TYPES OF FUNDING BY FOUNDATIONS

Each foundation determines the parameters, funding cycles, reporting requirements, and other aspects of its grants. The Internal Revenue Service (IRS) requires each private foundation to distribute a specific percentage of its funds to maintain its status as a 501(c)3 not-for-profit organization. Foundations are usually established by individuals. Their board members aim to fulfill the desires of the founders. If the foundation is a family foundation, a donor-advised fund through a local community foundation, or a foundation affiliated with a for-profit organization, its funding distribution goals are determined internally. Therefore, a guiding philosophy of foundations is using donors' money to meet the donors' interests.

Fundraising through foundations requires research. The Internet is often the best resource for information—on the foundation's history, its mission, its application process, members of its board, and previous recipients and amounts of its grants. After you have obtained this information, add details about each foundation to the reference document you created earlier in the process. Even if you do not think there is a match for your current project, save this information for future opportunities that may arise.

KEY SKILLS FOR FUNDRAISING

Planning is the most important skill required for fundraising or development. Create a funding plan that includes establishing funding priorities that match your organization's mission and strategic goals. This plan can help you identify appropriate funding sources and relationships to cultivate, and to determine when personnel and other resources will be needed. It can also help you learn about gaps in levels of expertise in your organization that need to be improved. This plan can help you become proactive in seeking funding, rather than reactive to grant announcements as they are issued.

Research tools, evaluative questions, and professional networks and tracking systems can help you locate potential funding resources.

Tools for effective research include searches of databases, such as the Foundation Center, Grantstation, and Grants.gov; and listservs and newsletters, including the *Philanthropy News Digest* and those of the Foundation Center and specific foundations matching your interests.

Questions you should ask to determine the best match of a funding source to your project include the following:

- Is the mission of the funding agency or foundation compatible with our proposal?
- What are our chances for getting funded? (For example, if the funding agency or foundation is only funding one grant and its geographic focus is not in your area, you probably will not be funded.)
- Who are our likely competitors?
- Can we produce better results than our competitors?
- Is there a partnership opportunity with competing organizations?
- Can we develop collaborative partnerships in time for the application?
- If there is merit in partnering, should we write a joint application in this or the next grant cycle?
- What other programs or projects has the granting agency previously funded? (Check its Web site for a list of funded grants, or its annual report may include them. Its IRS 990 Form may also show a list of donations and grants.)
- Do we have the resources to complete the application and meet the grantor's deadline?
- Will we have the organizational capacity to manage the grant financially and programmatically, or do we need more time to develop this capacity?

Use your own personal networks. If you are a member of a professional association, ask colleagues about their success in working with different funding sources. What insights can they provide? Is there a particularly helpful staff member? Are the reporting requirements overly burdensome? Develop relationships with those agencies and foundations that seem most relevant to your organization's objectives. Your time spent in doing this is a valuable investment.

In your relationships with grantors, build their trust and confidence. They need to trust that your organization will be responsible and ethical in administering the funds they are providing.

Develop strategies in your relationship-building. Who in your organization is the best person to make the initial contact and to start building the relationship? Who tells your organization's mission and story the best? When should you bring your organization's leaders into the process?

Note and track details of each interaction with grantors, program managers, and foundation representatives. People like to be remembered on their birthdays or asked about subjects discussed in previous conversations. Even if you have a great memory for details, have a tracking system, such as a spreadsheet, that allows others in your organization to have access to this information, should the need arise.

Maintain open lines of communication. This will vary by funding source and is sometimes dictated by reporting requirements of a grant. Beyond required communications, share stories with grantors that affirm that the funds they have provided made a difference in people's lives. A phone call, e-mail, or letter could ensure success in your next grant request.

There are important things you should avoid. Your relationship with a grantor will deteriorate if you believe that the funds your organization has received are yours to do with as you please—that you can change the agreed-upon use of those funds. Your organization has a fiduciary responsibility to administer the funds in the ways described in the grant proposal. If you see a need to change program or project plans, first contact a representative of the granting agency or foundation. You must maintain trust.

Keep your commitments to fulfill reporting requirements—on time. If you cannot make a deadline, renegotiate a new one before the due date—not after you have missed the deadline.

Understand funding cycles so you can appropriately plan your applications. A funder's cycle usually is based on its fiscal year, which can be identified from its annual report or its IRS 990 form. Funds become available at the beginning of its fiscal year and may need to be obligated by the end of that fiscal year. When application deadlines are nonspecific or continuous, you may benefit by applying at the start of the funder's fiscal year—rather than at the end, when the organization may have only limited funds remaining for the year.

The federal government's fiscal year begins on October 1. Once the federal budget is approved, some agencies provide an overview of the anticipated funding. Learn what funds will be released over the next year for what goals, purposes, or projects. If your needs are targeted towards a specific agency or foundation, you might check its Web site to see if it has a funding portal or preview of its grant opportunities. The Health Resources and Services Administration (HRSA) has a "public portal" (the HRSA Preview) that provides a listing and description of current and planned funding announcements. (See https://grants.hrsa.gov/WEBEXTERNAL/fundingOpp.asp.) If you are interested in a broader view of upcoming opportunities, DHHS offers the HHS Grants Forecast for planned grant opportunities for all HHS agencies for the current fiscal year. (See http://www.acf.hhs.gov/hhsgrantsforecast/ .)

Writing an Effective Grant Proposal

There are five stages in the process of developing a grant proposal. Ideally, you will have a team to develop the proposal. But if you do not, you likely will be performing many of the following tasks by yourself. If you have limited time, you may not be able to complete all of the tasks described below.

ASSESSMENT

Before you expend resources on the application process, thoroughly review the funding announcement. Sometimes details that were not apparent in initial grant program summaries will reveal a different objective or additional unanticipated requirements.

Ask these questions to help determine whether to pursue this funding opportunity:

- Does this fit within and advance our mission?
- Is the funding sufficient to cover the costs of the project? (If not, will we be able to acquire the difference through other sources?)
- Are there likely to be other local or national competitors? (If so, would collaboration make the application stronger and also reduce competition?)
- Would other community collaborators or outside experts strengthen the application? (Community collaboration can often leverage each organization's resources.)
- Do we have the capacity to complete the application within the allotted timeframe? (Or should we hire a grant consultant to assist?)
- Do we have the capacity to manage the grant programmatically and financially if it is awarded? (Be careful what you ask for. If you are a small agency and are applying for a multimillion-dollar grant, make sure you are able to increase your administrative and programmatic capacities.)

If necessary, submit technical questions and a letter of intent.

Sign up for automatic notifications of amendments to the FOA, including posting of Frequently Asked Questions. (Instructions will be included in the FOA.)

EARLY PROPOSAL DEVELOPMENT

Set the stage for the proposal. Put together a team to create a shared vision for the end result of the funding project, set the timeline, and distribute tasks.

The proposal development team should include a lead person; other content matter experts, as needed; a research assistant; an administrative support person; and someone to develop the budget. One individual may fill multiple roles. Include team members from collaborating organizations, if appropriate.

Convene an initial proposal meeting with all team members and partners as soon as possible to accomplish the following tasks:

- Review the Request for Proposal (RFP) and its requirements.
- Identify the principal investigator or project director. Ideally, this person should be the lead person on your proposal team, and a significant contributor to the content.
- In a multi-partner application (consortium), identify the applicant organization.
- Discuss the overall goals, objectives, and high-level project design, including strengths you want to highlight and weaknesses that need to be addressed. Consider involving new people in this discussion.
- Create a shared vision of the final project and how it will be administered if the project is funded. You don't want to change direction once you start writing the proposal — unless the funder changes its requirements.
- Prepare a proposal development timeline.
- Determine the time and location for future team meetings. Schedule at least one or two meetings a week to keep people on task and to work through any issues. It's much easier to cancel an unneeded meeting than to schedule a new one.

Assign people to the following tasks, as applicable:

1. Prepare the proposal template, an outline based on the format suggested in the FOA, with requirements for each section. This gives the writers a framework for adding detail.
2. Prepare the requirements grid, to be used as a tool to ensure the proposal meets the needs of the funder.
3. Create a summary of the project proposal—no more than two pages long—for potential partners. This should be a concise document with enough information to solicit support or participation.
4. Write specific sections of the proposal. (See Box 9-1 for tips on writing grant proposals.)
5. Identify key project personnel, including those from partner organizations. You will likely need résumés, curriculum vitae, or "NIH Biosketches" and descriptions of roles for the project management section of the proposal.
6. Perform literature searches and other assessments of prior work on the subject to supplement the work of the principal investigator or project director and other key staff members.
7. Solicit and obtain letters of support. Although a template may be used for the letters, it should allow for very specific information from each supporter so that each letter will be distinct.
8. Engage additional partners.
9. Collect all necessary documents from partners.
10. Fill out application forms.
11. Develop appendices and attachments.
12. Perform other tasks specific to the proposal.

Box 9-1: **Tips for Writing Grant Proposals**

Remember the intended audience for your grant application: the funding agency's reviewers. They will probably not have the time to search through your application looking for the various required components listed in their evaluation criteria. So, as you prepare your proposal, do the following:

- Use captions to identify important sections.
- Use textboxes to highlight important messages.
- Use graphics to simplify a complex model or description.
- Use tables, when appropriate, to simplify a lengthy narrative description, depict a comparison, or display demographic information.

All of these tools will break up the text and make your proposal easier and more enjoyable to read.

Understand the objectives of the funding agency. If necessary, contact the funding agency to ask questions. This can help build your relationship with a representative of the funding agency, and it can give each of you an understanding of the other's objectives and how they relate.

Storytelling can be used to help the reader understand the impact of your current and proposed work (see Chapters 1, 3, and 4). Providing real examples of the problem you are trying to solve with grant funds can evoke empathy in a reviewer who may strongly support your project.

Write with clarity and purpose. Keep it simple and concise. Avoid jargon. Do not assume that reviewers will understand jargon. They may or may not be experts in the specific area on which you are writing.

Use the evaluation criteria to help guide what you need to include in your proposal. Reviewers will be asked to evaluate your proposal based on these criteria. Missing a single element can reduce your score or may even dismiss your application from further consideration.

Use graphics when they will add to your discussion. Sometimes it is easier to understand a complex description with a diagram, such as a project organization chart, a theoretical model, or a flow chart.

Use tables, when possible, to simplify a description of a large amount of information.

Describe your definition of success and how your program or project will be evaluated.

Identify how you will acknowledge and recognize the granting organization. This is especially important when making a funding request to a foundation or an individual.

MID PROPOSAL DEVELOPMENT

In this phase, you define details, refine, review, and obtain community support.

All team members write their sections and send them to a person charged with updating and maintaining the "master document." The "master document" should either be stored in a "shared" network location that is visible to all team members, or be updated daily and e-mailed to all team members. Version control can be difficult to manage if there is more than one person editing the document simultaneously. Tools such as MS Word's "track changes" or collaborative software make it easier to share and review documents.

During this phase, team meetings focus on:

- *The need for this project*: Build a compelling reason for the proposed work. Base your need statement on documented facts and use storytelling, when appropriate, to demonstrate impact.
- *How objectives will be met*: Make sure that you base your methods on sound science or practice. Back up your statements with facts and references to support them. Create a solid project design, with detailed project management components, including how multiple partners will coordinate their efforts. Identify potential barriers to show that you have addressed them.
- *How progress will be measured*: A strong evaluation is essential to any grant. When possible, include an analyst on your team. If you don't have one on staff, consider a graduate student or researcher from a local academic institution.
- *Why your team should be selected*: Articulate your team's experience, background, and capacity to do the proposed work. Give the funder a solid reason why it should select your team to implement this project.

Outside of team meetings, you will be soliciting support from the community. Obtain letters of support from individuals and organizations that will be affected by the work, such as members of an advisory board, those advocating for your shared concern, elected officials, and all partners named in your proposal. While letters of support may not be a requirement, including them demonstrates the community's confidence in your team's ability to address the needs. Make sure that each letter is somewhat distinct and written from the perspective of its writer.

A *mock review* is an extremely useful tool to improve your final product. This should be built into the original timeline to allow for completion of a full draft, and enough time for revision after the mock review.

Invite two to four people who have not been involved in the development of the proposal to be your reviewers. Provide them with the proposal draft, the FOA, and a reviewer's evaluation form with instructions. The form should include the review criteria, as specified in the FOA, with a place for comments. Instructions should direct reviewers to include comments on strengths, weaknesses, and suggestions for improvement. (Some reviewers may prefer to write their comments directly on their copies of the draft proposal.)

Schedule a review meeting with the proposal team and the reviewers. The meeting should begin with an overview of the proposal (given by someone on the proposal team). All reviewers should provide overviews of their reviews, followed by more detailed observations. The face-to-face meeting allows for clarification and discussion on how to improve the draft proposal.

FINAL DEVELOPMENT

In this phase, all items are finalized and the application is compiled and submitted in accordance with the funder's process. The following activities occur during this phase:

- A combined program and budget meeting to clarify budget needs. The project's overall lead person and lead budget person meet to discuss the final budget and its justification. The budget must be aligned with the project narrative.
- A compliance review, using the requirements grid created earlier in the process. One detail-oriented individual should be asked to review the proposal along with the grid and indicate those items that are not apparent in the proposal. The project's lead person should then determine whether—and, if so, how—to address any missing components that have been identified.
- Final proofreading. A last review for typographical and formatting errors should be done as the last step prior to compilation.
- All items should have been submitted by the partners, and all résumés and appendix items should be available in final format.
- Administrative staff members should review the terms and conditions of the grant to identify and mitigate any potential problems.

When development of the proposal is complete, assemble and deliver it according to requirements. Allow enough time, even if you are submitting it electronically; it takes time to enter information, and electronic glitches can arise. Always leave at least one day for compilation, one day for submission, and at least two extra days for the unexpected.

AFTER THE GRANT IS AWARDED

After a grant is awarded, you need to make the project operational. Meet with operations and administrative staff members to discuss the internal transition process and needs, clarify grant management issues and requirements, and redeploy or hire appropriate staff members. Identify programmatic and financial deliverables and establish a management tracking database. Shortly after you are notified of the award, send funding agency representatives letters of appreciation for the award with contact information for your program and financial leaders, and any other necessary information.

If you are not awarded the grant, send the funding agency a letter thanking it for the opportunity to apply, and request feedback so that you can learn how your proposal can be improved. In doing so, you will reinforce your organization's desire to develop a relationship with the funder and leave the door open for future opportunities.

Some funding agencies allow you to resubmit a revised proposal for potential reconsideration if additional funds become available. Track your success rate and feedback so you can improve with each additional proposal. Maintain files with copies of all of your final proposals, whether you are successful in receiving an award or not. These documents will serve as useful references for future proposals.

Development Through Foundations

Much of this chapter thus far also applies to funding from foundations. Some foundations have extensive requirements in their application processes. To facilitate your application process, follow the same timeline and activities for proposal writing for government agencies described above. Make sure your funding request fits within the guidelines and mission of the foundation—or in the case of an individual funder, the person's philanthropic interests. Search foundations' Web sites to identify their missions and funding interests. Determine if the goals of your organization are compatible with those of the foundation. The Foundation Center (http://www.foundationcenter.org/) is an excellent resource for obtaining information on specific foundations, such as their funding interests and regional preferences. For a fee, it enables subscribers to search for and access extensive information on its Web site.

Be prepared to address why a private foundation or individual funder should financially support public health: Isn't "public health" paid for by the public? Answer this question for your own organization. Demonstrate that your program is worthy of private financial support. Have data and illustrative examples readily available on how your organization has benefited its target population.

Your organization's Web site should represent your organization in the most positive way possible. Foundations to which you are applying for support will likely check it and other available sources to determine if your organization is reputable.

As a representative of an organization seeking funding support, you have a public identity that is not only your own, but also that of the organization you represent. Your public identity fosters the trust that you seek in building relationships with funders. Guard these perceptions carefully and respectfully.

A reference document summarizing foundation or individual funder information is a very useful tool. This tool helps identify progress made by various team members who are contacting multiple foundations or individual funders during the research, cultivation, and solicitation process. This document should be updated at each team meeting to track progress in moving forward with discussions and activities with prospects.

INCREASING YOUR LIKELIHOOD FOR SUCCESS

Build Relationships

Build relationships with potential funders, government agencies, foundations, and individual funders. Open communications and strong relationships can help build a dialogue that will give you important insight into what actions will lead to receiving funding.

Acknowledge Assistance

When working with a proposal team, celebrate your accomplishments—whether or not you receive funding. Share your praise for team members' efforts with their supervisors—even if they work in other organizations. Place supportive memos in the personnel files of people you supervise.

Handle Rejection

No matter how large and well-funded a government agency, foundation, or individual funder may be, there is not enough money available to fund all projects and programs that request support, so be prepared for the possibility that your proposal may be rejected. If it is rejected, meet with your team for a debriefing session. Review what you learned through the process. Review how team members collaborated. Determine what worked well and what you could have done better. Was everyone committed to the shared vision? Did you adhere to your timeline? Were there problems that you can address before writing the next proposal? Learn from your successes and challenges. Summarize the findings of your debriefing session so you can apply the lessons learned in developing the next proposal.

Build Your Organization's Funding Capacity by Developing Professional Expertise in Grant Writing and Fundraising

Courses are available through local colleges, the United Way, and professional associations. Online webinars are provided by various professional organizations. Join a national professional association to access free resources, and join the local chapter of that association to network with and learn from your peers in your area. Professional associations include:

- Association of Fundraising Professionals (http://www.afpnet.org)
- Grant Professionals Association (http://grantprofessionals.org)
- CharityChannel (http://www.charitychannel.com)
- Alliance for Nonprofit Management (http://www.allianceonline.org/)

Hiring a grant or fundraising consultant is another option for building your capacity. Respect professional protocols and negotiate a fee with the consultant based on a rate that reflects the amount of work involved. Contingency payments and commissions are considered unethical. Most funders will not allow their funds to be used to recoup proposal-development expenses. When interviewing consultants, look for a professional credential, such as Grant Professional Certification (GPC) or Certified Fundraising Executive (CFRE). Find an individual who relates well to your mission and has a demonstrated track record of success.

Reference

1.   U.S. Department of Health and Human Services, Office of the Assistant Secretary for Financial Resources, Office of Grants and Acquisition Policy and Accountability, Division of Grants. *Grant Information for Current and Prospective HHS Grantees*. Available at: http://dhhs.gov/asfr/ogapa/aboutog/grantsnet.html. Accessed on November 17, 2010.

RESOURCES

Journal and Books

Chronicle of Philanthropy: http://philanthropy.com/section/Todays-News/284/
> *This journal is a great news source for nonprofit organizations. It includes news and trends on management and philanthropy as well as grant announcements. Eighteen newspapers are issued yearly. Subscribers have access to research and data on nonprofit organizations and philanthropy.*

Coley SM, Scheinberg CA. *Proposal Writing: Effective Grantmanship*. Thousand Oaks, CA: Sage Publications, Inc., 2007.
> *This book provides a solid foundation for writing an effective grant proposal.*

The Foundation Center. Proposal Writing Short Course (online at http://foundationcenter.org/getstarted/tutorials/shortcourse/index.html)
> *This book provides a condensed version of* The Foundation Center's Guide to Proposal Writing.

Geever J. *The Foundation Center's Guide to Proposal Writing (5th edition)*. New York: The Foundation Center, 2007.
> *This guide provides detailed instructions on preparing successful grant proposals for foundation grants. Its table of contents can be viewed at: http://foundationcenter.org/marketplace/catalog/product_monograph.jhtml?id=prod10047.*

Gitlin LN, Lyons KJ. *Successful Grant Writing Strategies for Health and Human Services Professionals (2nd ed.)*. New York: Springer Publishing, 2004.
> *This is a basic instructional guide to grant writing for health and human services workers.*

Lysakowski L. *The Development Plan*. Hoboken, NJ: John Wiley & Sons, 2007.
> *This is a practical guide to developing a comprehensive fundraising plan.*

Ogden TE, Goldberg IA. *Research Proposals: A Guide to Success (3rd ed.)*. Salt Lake City, UT: Academic Press, 2002.
> *This is a helpful guide for writing sections of NIH grant proposals. However, it was written before the era of electronic submissions.*

Grant-Seeking Databases

Foundation Directory Online (http://fconline.foundationcenter.org/)
> *This is an online database of grantmakers and other resources.*

Grantsmanship Center: Catalog of Federal Domestic Assistance
(https://www.cfda.gov/?s=generalinfo&mode=list&tab=list&tabmode=list)
> *This is the prime source of information on federal funding. Also available is "How to Use the Catalog of Federal Domestic Assistance," which is a step-by-step approach to using this catalog. Available at: https://www.tgci.com/publications.php*

Grants.gov (http://www.grants.gov)
> *This is the source for all federal grants, providing tools, resources, and robust search features for the grant-seeker.*

Grantstation (http://www.grantstation.com/)
> *This is an online database of grant-makers and research tools.*

HHS Grants Forecast (http://www.acf.hhs.gov/hhsgrantsforecast/)
> *This is a database of all "planned" grants for the current fiscal year.*

Educational and Other Resources

Association of Fundraising Professionals
> www.afpnet.org/
> *This is a professional association providing resources and tools for fundraisers.*

The CharityChannel
> www.charitychannel.com/
> *The CharityChannel provides education and resources for the nonprofit organization community.*

The Foundation Center
> foundationcenter.org/
> *This national nonprofit service organization, which is an authority on organized philanthropy, provides resources and tools to nonprofits.*

Grant Professionals Association
> grantprofessionals.org/
> *This is a professional association that provides resources and tools for grant professionals.*

The Grantsmanship Center
> www.tgci.com/publications.php
> *The Grantsmanship Center publishes a variety of books, including* Program Planning & Proposal Writing *(in both introductory and expanded versions) and* Proposal Checklist & Evaluation Forms.

Guidestar
> http://www2.guidestar.org/
> *Guidestar provides free resources for nonprofit organizations and gathers and publicizes information about nonprofit organizations. It is a good resource for locating the IRS 990 forms of foundations.*

Kaiser Family Foundation
> http://www.kff.org/
> *This is a good resource for health statistics and demographic information.*

Subscription Services

Federal Register
> listserv.access.gpo.gov/
> *This is a daily list of Federal Register releases.*

Grants.gov
> www.grants.gov/applicants/email_subscription.jsp
> *As a subscription service or RSS feed, this provides information on federal grant releases.*

National Institutes of Health (NIH)
> grants.nih.gov/grants/guide/listserv.htm
> *This is a daily list of NIH Guide announcements (also published on Grants.gov).*

Philanthropy News Digest
> foundationcenter.org/newsletters/
> *This is a weekly news digest.*

RFP Bulletin
> foundationcenter.org/newsletters/
> *A weekly summary of recently announced Requests for Proposals (RFPs) from private, corporate, and government funding sources.*

Robert Wood Johnson Foundation
> http://www.rwjf.org/grants/
> *The Foundation provides program-specific alerts via e-mail or RSS feed.*

W. K. Kellogg Foundation Evaluation Handbook
> wkkf.org/knowledge-center/resources/2010/W-K-Kellogg-Foundation-Evaluation-Handbook.aspx
> *This is a free guide that provides a framework for evaluation. Written for W.K. Kellogg grantees, it is also relevant to others.*

Commentary 9-1: Fundraising from Individuals and Corporations

Lyndon Haviland

Fundraising from individuals and corporations can offer new sources of funding, partnership, or much-needed assets, including technical assistance. To build partnerships and raise funds from these sources, you need to be entrepreneurial and strategic.

First, condense your organization's missions and goals into a simple statement that identifies the unique and critical role your organization plays and specifies its anticipated impacts. Think of this as your *elevator speech*, a statement on why your organization matters is essential as you seek funding from individuals and corporations. The first step in developing a fundraising pitch is making the language simple and accessible—and eliminating jargon.

Individual Donors

For many nonprofit organizations in public health, individual donors are the primary source of income. Individual donors can be either individuals of high net worth who give large sums, or individuals who give small amounts. Both types of donors are valuable. It can be challenging to develop and maintain a strong base of individual donors. Traditionally, many organizations contact donors once a year and ask for contributions—during an "annual appeal," often targeted around an event or the end of the fiscal year. Some donors may be willing to contribute on a regular basis, such as monthly, as part of their ongoing financial contribution to the organization. Payment may be facilitated by automatically debiting donor's checking accounts or charging their credit cards. Regular donors to your organization may be also interested in making in-kind contributions, including volunteering their time and making non-monetary contributions, such as contributing a vehicle or items for an online or special-event auction. Individual donations are often unrestricted, which can be an advantage. However, some individuals may prefer to contribute to a specific program or activity.

Understanding donor motivation is the second step in fundraising. Cultivate your relationships with donors and potential donors, and understand what your organization can offer them. Donors may be attracted to your cause, may live in your community or your state, or may have a personal connection to a staff member or client. Many times, small donations lead to deeper engagement in the mission of an organization and can result in larger funds later. Key to donor relations is personal interaction and ongoing engagement over time.

You need to explain what the funds will be used for—and then report back on how the funds were actually used. You need to demonstrate your passion and your excitement for the organization and its vision and mission. Donors react with their heads and their hearts—but their hearts often motivate their checkbooks. A compelling story told in an upbeat and positive way is a critical tool in your fundraising.

All fundraising is personal. Donor relations mean that you must be accessible to donors and potential donors and return communications promptly—both before and after a gift is made. To be successful at donor relations, you must allocate human and financial resources to identify and vet new donors, maintain relations with existing donors, and build a sustained commitment to your organization's mission, vision, and values. Just as you develop and recruit staff for other positions in your organization, you should carefully select the right people with the right skills to manage your donor relationships. You should develop an appropriate performance plan that will help guide them and allow for feedback on how well they achieve their goals.

When you identify potential donors, consider both individuals who are willing to make large contributions as well as those who may be able to make only small contributions. Also consider what skills and non-cash contributions would be useful for your organization (consider donated airtime, software, personnel, or space). Past donors can be a critical source for information as well as funding. Don't be afraid to ask past donors why they gave in the past, what would motivate them to support your organization now, and who else they might suggest that you approach. In addition, cultivating individual donors may also be important for a strategy on planned giving—soliciting bequests to support your organization.

Funding from Corporations

Corporations are often an important source of financial support for nonprofit organizations. There is always a variety of motivations for corporations to make charitable contributions, ranging from positive publicity to improving their market share. Corporations may be especially interested in new or special initiatives that relate to their missions, staff members, or customers.

To begin the process of soliciting corporate support, you need to learn a basic corporate vocabulary. For example, you will need to develop a *value proposition*— an offer to an individual or corporation that describes the quantifiable benefits your organization promises to deliver. Thoroughly evaluate potential funders and consider any disadvantages of potential funding relationships; for example, taking funds from a tobacco company for an anti-smoking program makes little sense and could adversely affect your organization's—and your—reputation.

If your work is unique and essential, ask yourself which corporations might fund it and how you can acquire short-term and long-term funding from them. Find out what they have already funded. Ask the following questions:

- Have similar programs been funded by them?
- If yes, what programs were funded and for how much?
- Why were these programs funded?
- What were the outcomes?
- Is the corporation interested in funding other similar projects?

If the corporation is interested, your next step is to identify the people who make its funding decisions and how you can contact them. Request an informational meeting, and ask for guidance on submitting a funding proposal. Like individual donors, corporations want to feel valued, and informational meetings can provide strategic guidance on the size, shape, and cost structure of your proposal.

Special Events

Planning and holding special events can be an important part of your fundraising and communications plan. Special events are often designed to highlight your organization's mission and offer an important opportunity to recognize individual and corporate sponsors. Although special events can be designed to bring in additional revenue, initially the event—even with contributions of work by volunteer staff members—may cost more than the revenue brought in at the time of the event. However, even if a special event does not generate net revenue immediately, it provides a number of other important opportunities, such as acknowledging sponsors and volunteers, building relationships with existing or potential donors, engaging volunteers and other supporters of the organization, and creating positive publicity about your organization—its mission and its activities. Often special events are venues where your organization can give awards, such as for the corporation, volunteer, or legislator of the year. Awardees and their corporations may help bring in additional revenue through ticket sales or generate "buzz" for your organization or cause.

For a special event, your organization may need more than money. Consider requesting the following:

- Free advertising space in newspapers or on TV, radio, or the Internet
- Use of a facility
- Free transportation for participants to come to your event
- Donated time from people with specific expertise

- Free entertainment (Is there a celebrity who has a personal stake in your orga-nization or cause?)
- Access to distribution channels, such as a flyer enclosed in the Sunday newspa-per or free advertising on a carton of milk

Fundraising and program implementation focus on building unexpected rela-tionships. Who are your organization's allies and partners? What do they need and want from a relationship with your organization?

In an ideal world, individual donors and corporations might make decisions about funding and partnerships based entirely on merit. But in the real world, these decisions are made in a more complex manner, relying on the multiple rela-tionships among all the key players—funders, partners, community members, and the public at large.

Relationships take time to develop. Sponsors and partners want to feel person-ally valued—not only for their financial contributions. Successful sponsorships and partnerships are based on trust and a shared understanding of what the value of the sponsorship or partnership is to each partner. Identifying what each part-ner brings to—and needs from—the partnership can help you to develop long-term, sustained relationships. Consider how your program can highlight the work of partners while improving public health. In fundraising, you will need to describe how the partnership or funding will be reported or highlighted, from print publi-cations to acknowledgement on a Web site or "co-branding." Each option must be considered carefully and priced accordingly.

Communications

Good fundraising is based on good storytelling—a critical skill for building sus-tained financial support (see Chapters 1, 3, and 4). To be successful, your organi-zation must identify its most valuable stories and identify the key storytellers and key audiences. Think about how funds are raised for disaster relief.

Sustainable funding requires a communications plan to engage all partners and potential supporters. You need to answer the following questions:

- Who are the targets of communications?
- What does success look like?
- Which people speak for the campaign and to whom do they speak?
- Who addresses problems as they arise?
- Through what media are messages communicated?
- Is the language culturally appropriate? And is it free of jargon?
- What is the most succinct way that you can communicate the essentials of your program—how it will improve the health of the public?

Conclusion

Fundraising from individuals and corporations may be a critical way of funding your organization's programs and projects. Keys to success include cultivating relationships with donors and potential donors, understanding their motivations for contributing, and effectively communicating the mission and activities of your organization and how funds will be used. A well-developed communications plan, including effective storytelling, is an integral part of a successful fundraising program.

10

Recruiting and Developing Employees

Donna R. Dinkin, Sylvester Taylor, and
Joyce R. Gaufin

As a manager, you need to attract and hire high-performing employees to your team, and support their growth and development for current and future roles in your organization. This chapter provides tools, techniques, and advice to help you and your organization in recruiting and developing employees.

Hiring and Managing Talented Employees

Talent management is a set of integrated systems and processes designed to enhance the success of recruitment, retention, development, and planning related to human resources in organizations. To successfully perform talent management, you need to:

- Identify talent needs and gaps
- Recruit talented employees to meet strategic competencies
- Evaluate and manage the performance of employees
- Identify the leadership potential of employees
- Develop the talent of employees for current and future needs
- Move talented employees throughout the organization, as needed

Decisions concerning talent management are often driven by both organizational core competencies and position-specific competencies. A set of competencies includes knowledge, skills, experience, and, sometimes, personal traits demonstrated through defined behaviors.

As a "best practice," your organization needs to clearly describe what constitutes effectiveness for each employee. These descriptions are often in the form of detailed competency models, which specify the competencies that contribute to each employee's effectiveness—often delineating low, moderate, and high levels of a competency at various levels in an organization.

As a manager or leader, you may find that already developed lists of competencies can help you in identifying the skills and abilities needed by members of your team.[1,2] You should know what competencies your organization needs for high performance, both now and in the future. You and other managers in your organization can use this information in creating a job description for each position and a development plan for each employee.

All employees should understand for which tasks and functions they are responsible and what work conditions and supervision they can expect. You should include this information in each job description for every position of your team. Typical job descriptions have the following six sections:

- *Job title*, as well as pay grade or range, supervisor's title, and employment status
- *Job summary*, as well as the major responsibilities of the employee in the position
- *Major tasks and duties*: an extensive list
- *Knowledge, skills, and abilities* required to perform the job
- *Education and experience* required
- *Special assignments or requirements* related to the position

SELECTING THE RIGHT PERSON

Once you have determined the types of talent and skills required in an employee in a position, you need to find the appropriate person. Strategies to do this include:

- Developing relationships with placement offices, recruiters, and search firms
- Advertising on Web sites of professional associations and in professional journals and magazines
- Encouraging current staff members, as they participate in professional meetings and conferences, to actively recruit potential candidates
- Monitoring online job boards for potential candidates and their résumés
- Using Twitter, LinkedIn, and other social media—especially if you need to recruit staff members who are technologically savvy
- Offering meaningful paid and unpaid internship opportunities, which may lead to regular employment
- Conducting formal recruitment at job fairs and professional conferences and meetings, such as the Annual Meeting of the American Public Health Association

Ease of recruiting is affected by many factors, including salary, personnel policies and procedures, the job market, and your skills. If pre-approved by your organization's human resources department, special strategies, such as providing signing bonuses and moving expenses, can often help you recruit for positions that are difficult to fill.

You should ensure that processes used for selecting and hiring new employees are organized, fair, and compliant with applicable laws and standards. You need to review résumés and applications, check references, and interview the leading candidates. By working closely with human resources personnel, your staff members, and, if appropriate, key stakeholders, you can increase the likelihood that you will choose the right person for the job.

You can reduce the pool of applicants by reviewing résumés, although résumés do not predict how well an applicant will perform in a position. Interview the best applicants in a way that allows them to share their interests, previous work, and behaviors related to past work experiences. (Box 10-1 lists common interviewer mistakes.) You may choose to perform a behavior-based interview, which focuses on job-related competencies and work habits; if you do so, ask questions that focus on examples of behavior from previous work experience—not only what the applicant did, but also how and why (Box 10-2).

CREATING AN ORGANIZATIONAL CULTURE

To retain high-performing employees you need to establish a culture for talent management in your organization. To do this, you need to recognize and value diversity—the various needs, interests, and cultures of both employees and constituents. To promote a dynamic and innovative work environment, you can draw on the diversity of staff members—in terms of age, gender, race, ethnic and cultural background, sexual orientation, religion, personality, educational level, job function, and physical and mental capabilities (see Chapter 5).

As a manager in an organization that supports and manages talent, you need to provide honest feedback to employees frequently, evaluate them through a formal performance-management process, and develop and implement plans to support their performance and development. However, employees need to take the initiative in managing their careers and professional development. Senior managers need to evaluate line managers on how they build and manage the talent of the employees whom they supervise. You can create a work environment that motivates employees by appreciating their diversity, providing them with feedback, and helping them develop their talent.

Box 10-1: **Common Interviewer Mistakes**

- Failing to articulate job expectations clearly
- Talking more than the applicant does
- Asking hypothetical or leading questions
- Allowing applicants to generalize answers or speak about theories
- Evaluating applicants based on similarities with or differences from yourself or other employees

---

Box 10-2: **Sample Behavior-Based Interview Questions and Requests**

- Describe a situation in which you were able to use persuasion to enact a change in your organization. What did you do? Why did you choose that approach?
- Tell me about a time when you overcame serious objections of a key change stakeholder and the person became a supporter. How did you accomplish this?
- Tell me about a time you when you led a team where one member was not performing as expected. What did you do?
- Describe a time when you had to work in a very ambiguous situation. What was it? How did you handle it? How did you cope with it? What was the outcome? What did you learn?
- Tell me about a time where you made an unpopular decision. How did you know it was unpopular? What did you do to influence others and gain their cooperation?
- Describe a time that you improved a specific work process. Why did you take on the challenge? What did you do?

Performance Management: Systems, Tools, and Personal Needs

To be effective as a manager, you need to recruit, retain, and manage employees in ways that improve organizational outcomes. Performance management systems and tools can help you achieve these goals. *Performance management* is a systematic approach for making organizations effective and productive. It is a "strategic and integrated approach to increasing the effectiveness of organizations by improving the performance of the people who work in them and by developing the capabilities of teams and individual contributors."[3]

Performance management can also be viewed as a cycle in which you do the following:

- Identify organizational performance requirements
- Develop measurable individual performance objectives
- Track progress towards these objectives
- Provide feedback for improvement
- Evaluate performance
- Offer incentives for achieving expected results

All large organizations have established specific requirements for performance management and compensation practices. Governmental agencies are generally governed by merit systems that use "educational and occupational qualifications, testing, and job performance as criteria for selecting, hiring, and promoting civil servants."[4] You should become familiar with the policies, guidelines, or rules within your own organization for performance management. Union employees may have additional requirements.

Each unit within an organization must have a plan that defines its specific performance goals to help the organization be productive and effective. As a manager, you should ensure that all employees understand both their individual performance goals as well as the organization's goals. Employees who feel that their work supports a larger purpose tend to be more engaged. If they sense their increased value to the organization, they may increase their willingness to be actively engaged with the work of the team.

As you create individual performance goals for all employees, include them in the process. Learn their perspectives on priorities, processes, and productivity. If your organization does not have a specific process for creating performance goals, you may wish to follow the outline for creating SMART Performance Goals, which are specific, measurable, attainable (but aggressive), results-oriented (and future-oriented), and time-based.[5]

Some goals emphasize quantitative measures, such as the number of immunizations to be given during each flu clinic or the number of restaurant inspections to be completed per week. To determine if a goal is attainable, you may consider existing standards for a given profession or you may create a standard that is based on historical performance data. You should consider external factors that may influence standards over time, such as the introduction of a new technology or the addition or loss of staff members. And don't expect that every employee will perform at the same level.

You should become familiar with performance-management systems. Performance reviews usually consist of written assessments of employees' performance, including to what extent they achieved previously established performance goals. An assessment may include a qualitative rating system—with ratings such as exceptional, good, average, below average, and unacceptable—or a pass/fail rating system. Often, compensation increases are linked to these ratings. These systems often specify a required frequency for performance reviews—most often once or twice a year. Feedback may need to be more frequent if an employee is new to a position, requires corrective action, or simply prefers more frequent feedback. If your organization adopts a performance-management system, it should provide training to all supervisors before the process is begun.

Performance reviews can be made more useful if:

- Employees perform self-assessments.
- Supervisors and employees meet face-to-face to enable supervisors to acknowledge employees' accomplishments and to address any necessary changes in their work.
- Supervisors and employees develop plans for continued training and education.

How do you adapt to the needs of all employees? Ask them! Set aside time for private meetings with all employees you supervise and ask them how often they would like to receive feedback on their performance.

All feedback should be done in an atmosphere that ensures confidentiality and encourages openness of communication between supervisors and employees. You should also ask employees how they would like to receive feedback if they have done something that deserves special recognition or if there is something that they should be doing differently or better.

In addition to formal performance reviews, all employees want and need positive feedback and encouragement—not limited to financial incentives. You should find out how each employee likes to be acknowledged and for what, such as demonstrating innovation; starting a new project; or showing attention to detail, a willingness to take risks, or excellent writing skills. Customizing feedback for each employee helps you to ensure that recognition and encouragement will satisfy each employee's individual needs.

When an employee needs to be coached to improve performance, plan a private conversation with adequate time. Consider how the employee has asked for feedback. Don't delay the conversation until the behavior or task becomes routine for the employee. Don't wait until the employee requires formal corrective action. Be prepared to accurately describe both the problem and what needs to be done differently. Ask employees to recommend solutions to problems, and then agree on plans that include their commitment to follow these plans. For example, if employees repeatedly come to work late, ask them for their solutions on how they can regularly arrive on time, then ask them to commit to implement these solutions.

Arrange for follow-up. If performance has improved, acknowledge this and have the employee commit to continued improvement. If problems persist, implement your organization's process to address persistent performance issues in a step-by-step manner.

Your organization may have a specific process for creating individual development plans that focus on long-range goals and training opportunities. These goals are often part of the formal process of planning and reviewing performance. If your organization does not have such a process, you should schedule time at least once a year to meet with each employee in a confidential setting for this purpose.

To start a performance-review process, encourage employees to think about personal goals for development and advancement—before meeting with you. Ask them what they would like to be doing 2, 5, and 10 years in the future. Ask them what they will need to do, have, and be to achieve these long-range goals:

- Does your development and advancement require job-related training that our organization can provide?
- Do you need to return to school for more education?
- Can you achieve some of these goals by being given new responsibilities and performing new tasks in your current job?

As a manager, you should ensure that some of these goals relate to the needs of the unit or the organization, which might pay for some necessary training or education.

Some employee contracts specify educational benefits. While employees should develop their own development and advancement plans, the human resources department of your organization can offer counseling and assistance to help them develop these plans.

Organizational policies and budgets affect the performance management system that is used for ensuring that your organization performs efficiently and effectively. Managers should receive formal training to ensure that they understand the requirements for performance management in your organization.

Even if your organization's policies and procedures do not require anything more than a formal performance assessment, as a supervisor you should ensure that all employees regularly receive relevant personal recognition and encouragement. You should address performance issues or problems as soon as they are noticed by coaching and supporting employees in making necessary changes.

Developmental Assessment: Systems, Tools, and Instruments

As a manager, you should provide employees with opportunities to develop early and throughout their careers. You can use personal assessment instruments to help employees identify areas for development. *Learning-management systems—* which are software applications used to manage and administer training records and content—can help you match employees with available training and learning opportunities. You should use work assignments to support their developing and applying newly acquired knowledge and skills.

PERSONAL DEVELOPMENT INSTRUMENTS

Assessment tools help employees understand and assess their strengths and their needs for development so they can improve their performance. (Table 10-1 gives a sample of these assessment tools.) These tools can also support an organizational culture that facilitates individual growth. Some of these instruments are completed only by the person being assessed, while others seek input from additional "respondents" or "observers." Instruments that allow for feedback from multiple perspectives, such as from supervisors, subordinates, and peers, are called *360-degree assessment instruments.* Feedback from multiple perspectives can enable employees to see more clearly their strengths and developmental needs as well as how they affect others. As a manager, you can use assessment tools to complement other sources of information for the growth and development of employees.

Table 10-1: **Sample of Assessment Tools Used in Talent Management Processes**

	Fundamental Interpersonal Relations Orientation-Behavior (FIRO-B)	Emotional Competency Inventory 2.0 (ECI)	BENCHMARKS	Myers-Briggs Type Indicator (MBTI)	Discovery Learning Leadership Profile for Public Health
Assessment Name					
Publisher	Consulting Psychologists Press, Inc. (CPP)	Hay Group	Center for Creative Leadership	Consulting Psychologists Press, Inc. (CPP)	Discovery Learning, Inc.
Purpose	To measure three interpersonal needs: inclusion, control, and affection	To assess emotional competency	For 360-degree assessment of key leadership lessons, skills, behaviors, perspectives, and career derailment potential	For training and development, such as one-on-one coaching, team-building initiatives, and communication workshops	For 360-degree assessment of leadership skills for public health leaders
Audience	All levels of management	Individuals and teams at all levels	Middle- and upper-middle-level managers	Individuals and teams at all levels	Middle- and upper-middle-level managers
Cost	$11.50 per manager	$150 per manager	$275 per manager, unlimited number of raters	$11.60 per manager	$135 per manager, up to 17 raters

When choosing an assessment tool, answer the following questions:

1. Has the instrument been validated, refined, and researched?
2. What behaviors, skills, or competencies does it measure?
3. Are results communicated by interaction with a qualified facilitator?
4. Is the assessment tool supported by good resources for both respondents and facilitators?

Outside facilitators, such as consultants, coaches, or trainers, often administer assessment instruments in workplace settings. Even those who are qualified by their education to purchase these assessment instruments should study the materials that have been specifically designed for instrument facilitators. This enables them to offer comprehensive background and guidance to employees being assessed and to those administering these instruments.

When administering assessment instruments to employees, you should first describe the purpose of taking the assessment and how the results will be used. If possible, offer employees the option not to participate. Ensure that the results of developmental assessments will never be used to label, evaluate, or limit employees in any way. Ensure that assessment tools are used in compliance with authors' and publishers' guidelines, including confidentiality standards and procedures for scoring and reporting. The following are some strategies for sharing results of assessment instruments:

- Give results directly to the employee in an active discussion with a qualified facilitator. Avoid delivering results in impersonal ways, such as by e-mail.
- Make it clear that the employee is the expert—the only person who can know the complete context. For example, employees may be the only people who know that the input for their 360-degree assessments came only from supervisors or co-workers with whom they have worked for less than 6 months—and, therefore, the results represent only early impressions.
- Don't counsel an employee toward—or away—from a specific career, relationship, or activity based solely on information obtained from a single assessment.
- Since employees change with time and experience, recognize that the accuracy of a report will decrease as time passes, as circumstances change, and as the employee engages in development processes.

PUBLIC HEALTH LEARNING-MANAGEMENT SYSTEMS

While assessment tools help identify strengths and gaps in employees' knowledge and skills, learning-management systems can help fill these gaps by linking employees with available training programs and courses. Courses and other training opportunities can help employees develop and grow in the areas identified through the performance-management process or from results of personal assessment instruments. To support the continuous development of employees, learn about available educational opportunities.

Online learning-management systems can help you identify and access assessment and training opportunities for employees. These systems provide information and links to training programs, including e-learning opportunities, conferences, discussion sites, and classes. Learners can find opportunities related to specific public health competencies or specific discipline-related requirements.

As an example, the Public Health Foundation administers and supports the TrainingFinder Real-time Affiliated Integrated Network (TRAIN), a system that lists over 14,000 onsite and distance-based training opportunities that are offered by approximately 3,000 academic and governmental programs. TRAIN is also linked to 23 affiliated systems, which offer additional resources to state and local public health workers (see https://www.TRAIN.org).

States not affiliated with TRAIN may have their own online learning-management systems that offer similar support to public health workers. Three such systems are New York Learns Public Health, Public Health Learning (Illinois), and the North Carolina Center for Public Health Preparedness Training System.

Developmental Experiences

Decreased funding for public health services may limit access to external training programs and conferences for public health workers. Budget restrictions may force some organizations to cut back on travel to events not related to a direct or essential public health service. Web-based courses or other distance-based training programs can provide public health workers access to educational opportunities.

While distance-based training programs can provide public health managers with access to both new information and to other managers who are working on similar challenges elsewhere, they are more valuable for personal growth if they are accompanied by on-the-job developmental experiences. People learn by doing. On-the-job assignments—sometimes called development in place—represent the most effective way to develop new skills and new competencies. This approach is less expensive than sending employees to external courses or programs. And it can be more effective for building individual and organizational talent.

CREATING AN ENVIRONMENT TO SUPPORT LEARNING IN YOUR ORGANIZATION

A *learning organization* is one in which employees are enabled to learn, grow, and develop and, as a result, are more engaged in their work, more adept at meeting work demands, and better able to seize opportunities. Individual employees and teams of workers may acquire new knowledge or skills unintentionally as they work. However, in a learning organization, they need to be strategic and deliberate in pursuing novel and creative ways of working.

While the benefits of creating a learning organization may be obvious, the ways to establish one may be less apparent. To create a learning organization, as a manager, you need to:

- Establish a safe environment for risk-taking and failure
- Ask probing questions that allow employees to see and challenge their own mental models or beliefs about how things are—or should be
- Encourage and support employees as they explore the unknown
- Establish organizational structures for sharing various points of view, for obtaining new insights, and for sharing them with others
- Establish communities of practice or peer learning circles (see below)
- Create audio podcasts or CDs that highlight lessons learned from work

Appreciate diversity. Teams of workers, who have diverse points of view, plan and perform the work of your organization. They draw on concepts and experiences from diverse sources and disciplines. In a learning organization, employees can rise to meet new and complex challenges—which, in turn, can provide them with opportunities for additional development. (See Chapters 5 and 8.)

While developing an organizational culture for ongoing learning, expect and prepare for an increase in "organizational noise." Employees with a strong commitment to the organization and with increased skills feel empowered to question why and how things are being done in your organization. This questioning can create uncertainty or confusion. Anticipate this increase in energy, acknowledge it, and direct it in ways that help employees understand the mission and strategies of their work in a new and more meaningful way.

DEVELOPMENT IN PLACE

Sending employees to courses and training programs is a common strategy for developing their talent. While these experiences are helpful in providing employees with new information or in helping them develop new relationships, their attendance at an onsite educational event does not always translate into learning. Learning can be enhanced when new knowledge or skills are applied immediately to relevant, real challenges. Four strategies for helping employees continue their development while they work are:

- Developing a mentoring program
- Providing executive coaching
- Using action learning teams and peer learning circles
- Creating developmental experiences

Each of the strategies is described in more detail below.

Developing a Mentoring Program

Creating or encouraging formal relationships between younger or less experienced employees and senior or more experienced employees can help transfer knowledge throughout your organization. Mentors can share their experiences and their understanding of the system in which they are working, and in response they can gain new perspectives on old problems from their younger or less experienced co-workers.

If you choose to establish a mentoring program, answer the following questions:

- How will mentoring relationships help our organization achieve its mission?
- What, if any, incentives will there be for participating in the program?
- Will the focus of mentoring relationships be career development, system navigation, business outcomes, or something else?
- How will we select mentors and mentees?
- How will we train mentors?
- What are the expectations for successful pairings of mentors and mentees?
- What are the options for terminating unsuccessful pairings?
- Will mentoring be done in person or at a distance, and for how long?
- How will the program be monitored and evaluated?

Establish ways to monitor and support mentors and mentees. Ensure that they discuss needs, interests, goals, and ground rules for their work together. Provide them with samples of mentoring agreements and action plans. Provide mentors with training programs and guidebooks with sample questions and suggestions for mentoring activities. Advise mentees on how to "own" their learning, seek feedback from others, and ask probing questions to maximize learning.

Develop evaluation strategies during the planning phase of the mentoring program. Use quantitative and qualitative methods to identify successes and problem areas of your mentoring program. Evaluation measures can include promotions or departures in your organization, accomplishments of individual workers, achievement of organizational goals, and personal levels of satisfaction.

Providing Executive Coaching

Pairing employees with a personal coach can provide them with "just-in-time" feedback as they use new skills or experience problems at work. Executive coaches can help employees assess their personal style, preferences, and behaviors in various situations. As a manager, you can also serve as a coach, asking employees questions that help them address challenges from various perspectives and allowing them to identify alternate solutions. If you become a coach or learning facilitator, you need to put your ego aside and learn to ask transformative questions, strengthen your listening skills, take advantage of teachable moments, and provide constructive feedback. Becoming a "manager coach" can be a rewarding experience for you, your employees, and your organization.

Using Action Learning Teams and Peer Learning Circles

Since much public health work is collaborative, use team project experiences for employee development. *Action learning teams* are groups working on projects whose members agree to use their experiences to learn and grow. These teams are typically supported by learning coaches and/or subject-matter experts. Team members commit to achieving learning goals and action goals. Members of teams that use an action learning approach spend much time learning about problems they are about to address and potential solutions—and learning about other team members and themselves. Knowledge gained from this investment in learning improves how the team works and the outcomes of its work.

Peer learning circles (or communities of practice) are structured groups in which workers meet to learn from the successes and challenges of others who are working on similar projects or who share a common work-related interest. They can also provide structure for collaborative or shared learning.

To create a successful group learning experience, ensure that:

- Teams or groups each have five to seven members.
- Team members have diverse backgrounds and prior experiences.
- Discussions focus on actual challenges that are related to the mission of your organization.
- Action goals as well as individual and team learning goals are established.
- A skilled learning coach, who is not an employee of the organization, supports the group.
- An organizational sponsor holds the group accountable for its achievements.

Creating Developmental Experiences

Work assignments that provide employees with new and varied experiences can be used to promote learning and development without moving people into new positions. Temporary assignments, such as starting a new project or resolving a problem situation, can provide employees with opportunities for developing key skills or competencies needed for current or future jobs. Support is essential for maximizing the learning and development from various assignments. As a manager, you should help employees understand what they are learning as they work and provide support as they have new experiences.

The Center for Creative Leadership has identified developmental assignments that can stimulate learning. These include the following:

- Starting new projects or changing the direction of projects
- Taking on projects with inherited problems
- Taking on projects with major increases in scope and complexity

- Addressing problems with employees
- Assuming unfamiliar responsibilities
- Taking on high-stakes assignments with tight deadlines
- Taking on assignments with external pressure from important stakeholders
- Influencing decisions, even without authority
- Working among multiple cultures
- Leading a diverse workgroup[6]

Providing employees with various work-related projects can help them develop a well-rounded set of skills and experiences. As you work with employees to identify (a) specific skill sets that they would like to strengthen and (b) specific projects or "stretch assignments" for them to build these skills, make sure that they have adequate support to deal with discomfort that arises from learning and risk-taking. With appropriate support and encouragement, these projects and assignments can be extremely effective ways of developing talent.

If your organization is committed to providing opportunities for continuous learning, it will recruit and retain employees who are committed to continuous improvement of their abilities—and your organization will be better positioned to respond to complex challenges.

Workforce Trends

Several trends influence your recruitment and development of public health workers, including workforce shortages, generational diversity, and use of technology.

WORKFORCE SHORTAGES

Major universities and national organizations have developed estimates of current and future workforce shortages. These reports highlight worker shortages in specific public health occupations and specific parts of the United States. With increased ethnic and cultural diversity in many areas, there are shortages of bilingual and multicultural public health workers. In addition, state and local public health agencies are concerned about possible shortages of managers and leaders.

Budget constraints represent the main barrier to adequate staffing of governmental public health agencies. Noncompetitive salaries and lengthy processing time for new employees are also barriers. Many public health leaders who are nearing retirement believe that younger workers have not been adequately prepared to assume leadership roles. All of this makes training and development more important—to help retain and motivate superior employees, ensure a competent "pipeline" of new leaders, and help create an attractive workplace for recruitment of new employees.

GENERATIONAL DIVERSITY

There are four generations of public health workers:

- *Traditionalists* born before 1945
- *Baby boomers* born between 1946 and 1962
- *Gen X'ers* born between 1963 and 1985
- *Gen Y'ers* born since 1985

With traditionalists re-entering the workforce after retirement and baby boomers resisting retirement, many administrators are finding that they are now supervising and managing diverse teams that include employees from each of these generations. Employees from these different generations often bring different needs, interests, and perspectives to the workplace. This generational diversity can be valuable to your organization, but it can also lead to challenges. As a manager, you need to understand how employees from each of these generations view work and where differences among employees of different generations may lead to conflict. While it is important to avoid stereotyping, describing common characteristics of public health workers in each of these four generations makes it easier to understand each group. Few workers have the typical characteristics of only one generation.

Traditionalists are typically hard workers and loyal to their organizations. They prefer to interact with others in person rather than communicating by e-mail or other technological tools.

Baby boomers are also loyal to their employers and are generally willing to work long hours. They accept authority figures and value "working their way up the ladder."

Gen X'ers tend not to believe that they will work for one organization throughout their lives; they are more comfortable than people from older generations in changing jobs. They tend to prefer an informal work atmosphere and want more balance between their work and other parts of their lives. They also tend to think globally and embrace diversity.

Younger Gen X'ers as well as Gen Y'ers have grown up with technology and tend to be very comfortable using it for all aspects of life. Gen Y'ers tend to be very self-confident and outspoken. These characteristics may make them appear arrogant and disrespectful. They can be very entrepreneurial and creative, and they tend to enjoy continuous learning and development.

While these characteristics are helpful in your understanding of how people of various generations work together, as a manager you need to recognize that each employee is unique and may or may not share the same characteristics, values, and perspectives of other employees of the same generation.

Potential areas of conflict between workers from different generations include:

- Work ethic
- Loyalty to the organization

- Organizational hierarchy
- How they deal with change
- How they use technology
- Level of formality

As a manager, you need to recognize and embrace generational differences among employees. To maximize the value of this diversity, host discussions about the diversity of viewpoints among workers of different generations; build on the talents of various workers, such as the political savvy of baby boomers and the technological capabilities of Gen Y'ers; and use multiple training methodologies for development. Employees of all generations want to continue to learn, and they all value using technology for at least some aspects of learning.

USE OF TECHNOLOGY

As a manager, you need to learn about new and more efficient uses of technology. Advances in technology have improved surveillance and monitoring, sharing and analysis of information, education and training, and networking of stakeholders. Technology has also changed or expanded the ways in which employees are recruited and trained. These advances, however, have their limitations and challenges. For example, new technologies have contributed to information overload for many employees, and they have created the need for new technology-related positions in public health organizations.

Conclusion

The tools, systems, and advice described in this chapter will help you to recruit and develop employees. An effective performance and development system will help your organization to achieve higher levels of performance and will result in a more supportive working environment.

References

1. Public Health Foundation. *Core Competencies for Public Health Professionals*. Available at: http://www.phf.org/resourcestools/Pages/Core_Public_Health_Competencies.aspx Accessed on May 27, 2011.
2. *Public Health Leadership Competency Framework*. Developed by the National Public Health Leadership Development Network. Available at: http://www.heartlandcenters.slu.edu/nln/about/framework.pdf . Accessed on November 11, 2010.
3. Wikipedia. *Performance Management*. Available at: http://en.wikipedia.org/wiki/Performance_Management. Accessed on September 21, 2010.
4. The Free Dictionary. *Merit System*. Available at: http://www.thefreedictionary.com/merit+system. Accessed on September 21, 2010.

5. Wikipedia. *SMART Criteria*. Available at: http://en.wikipedia.org/wiki/SMART_criteria. Accessed on December 30, 2010.
6. McCauley CD. *Developmental Assignments: Creating Learning Experiences Without Changing Jobs*. Greensboro, NC: Center for Creative Leadership (CCL) Press, 2006.

RESOURCES

Books, Reports, and Documents

Association of State and Territorial Health Officials. *State Public Health Worker Shortage Report: A Civil Service Recruitment and Retention Crisis*. Washington, DC: ASTHO, 2004.

> *This report highlights public health workforce shortages in public health nursing, epidemiology, laboratory science, and environmental health, and provides strategies to recruit and retain workers.*

Core Competencies for Public Health Professionals. Council on Linkages between Academia and Public Health Practice, Public Health Foundation website. https://www.train.org/Competencies/corecompetencies.aspx?tabid=94 Accessed on February 15, 2011.

> *This document provides a list of the skills, knowledge, and abilities needed by public health workers.*

Deal JJ. *Retiring the Generation Gap: How Employees Young and Old Can Find Common Ground*. San Francisco: Jossey-Bass, 2007.

> *This book summarizes research on the generational differences and similarities of leaders, and provides practical advice for managing the talents of workers from different generations.*

Health Resources and Services Administration (HRSA). *Public Health Workforce Study*. Rockville, MD: HRSA, 2005.

> *This report summarizes a study of the public health workforce that focused on recruitment and retention of physicians, nurses, and dentists.*

Lombardo MM, Eichinger RW. *For Your Improvement: A Guide for Development and Coaching* (5th ed.). Minneapolis, MN: Lominger Limited, Inc., 2009.

> *This book provides tips that can be used to improve performance of individual public health workers.*

McCauley CD. *Developmental Assignments: Creating Learning Experiences Without Changing Jobs*. Greensboro, NC: CCL Press, 2006.

> *This guide provides examples of how to help employees develop leadership skills through challenging assignments at work.*

Public Health Leadership Competency Framework. National Public Health Leadership Development Network. Available at: http://www.heartlandcenters.slu.edu/nln/about/framework.pdf

> *This list of core leadership competencies for public health leaders identifies transformational, political, trans-organizational, and team-building competencies.*

Senge PM, Kleiner A, Roberts C, et al. *The Fifth Discipline Fieldbook: Strategies and Tools for Building a Learning Organization*. New York: Crown Business, Random House, 1994.

> *This book teaches skills for creating a learning organization, including systems thinking, vision, strategic planning, team building, and executive involvement in change management.*

Article

Gaufin JR, Kennedy KI, Struthers ED. Practical and affordable ways to cultivate leadership in your organization. *Journal of Public Health Management and Practice* 2010; 16: 156–161.

> *A useful article on developing leadership.*

Commentary 10-1: Hiring and Retaining the Right Workers in the Right Jobs

Kristine M. Gebbie

Critical to your achieving this goal are the following four elements:

- Clear position descriptions, written in behavioral terms
- Thoughtful interviews and careful hiring decisions
- Effective use of the probationary period to guide new employees and decide on their long-term employment
- Annual performance appraisals as part of ongoing performance improvement

Your partnership with human resources (HR) personnel can help you, as a manager, ensure that effective workers are recruited, retained (or not), and developed to realize your organization's mission and achieve its goals.

Defining the Position

The position description for any job is the foundational document for any personnel action that may be taken. Therefore, it must be carefully developed before you recruit prospective employees. Most civil-service agencies and many nongovernmental organizations have templates for positions in any one job class or level of employment, often with standardized language on (a) knowledge, skills, and attitudes necessary for the job; (b) required level of education or way of demonstrating an alternative achievement based on work experience; and (c) requirements for computer literacy for some office support positions.

There are usually methods for updating these requirements, or for clarifying specific requirements for a specific position—especially important when the system uses nonspecific job titles (such as Supervisor 1, 2, or 3). There are usually ways to add specific prior experience or necessary occupational credentials, such as licensure as a nurse or physician for the position of supervisor of a primary care clinical team. If you are defining the position, the demand on you is to think through what is really essential for success—possibly moving away from habit and history concerning the position.

One of my more painful decisions as a state health director was a critical appraisal of the position requirements for the director of the state's oral health program, which included holding a license to practice dentistry. The program was entirely preventive in nature—primarily a school-based topical fluoride program, which was familiarly known as "Swish-Swash." There was no real need for a licensed dentist to direct the program. The position involved maintaining and building relationships with school districts and local health departments to maintain and increase participation of students. After we revised the position description, applications increased. The position was filled by a dental hygienist with a Master of Public Health degree who excelled in the role.

The HR manager (or designated HR staff person) should be your partner throughout the hiring process. You might otherwise believe erroneously that your expertise concerning the vacant position is the only relevant issue and that the personnel system requirements are only "bureaucratic red tape" created to frustrate action. But executing personnel actions correctly is a legal and ethical requirement that must be met, and few individuals who have not worked in an HR office have the full range of information to ensure that all standards are met.

You may feel that meeting requirements can be done only one way—with a very fixed set of forms, steps, and timelines. There are usually ways to adapt the standard forms, steps, and timelines to meet a specific situation, and your partnership with HR personnel can facilitate the process. For example, your collaboration with the personnel in determining what education and work experience is required for a position—and what is preferred—can save much time and reduce much distress.

Making the Hiring Decision

If you will be making hiring decisions, you must become familiar with the personnel processing requirements of your organization. These requirements might include:

- The length of time an announcement must be "open"
- The range of advertising expected to ensure access by candidates from under-represented groups
- "Automatic" candidates who must be considered as they are on pre-established promotional or applicant lists
- Composition of interviewer panels
- Steps prior to the job offer

If you are overly eager to identify a preferred candidate without taking all necessary steps, you may well be stymied when the final hiring paperwork needs to be processed—leading to embarrassment, an extended period of position vacancy, and loss of organizational capacity.

Assuming all of the required processing criteria are being met, there are three main stages of a hiring decision:

- The interview, for which you should involve more than one interviewer and use questions or assessment exercises that are planned in advance

- Reference checking, which you should do after the interview but before you make a final decision
- Your assessment of the "fit" of the individual into the existing work group

It is often too easy for you, as a hiring manager, to have a preferred candidate—or to quickly become attached to an individual applicant—without listening to the voices of others who have interviewed all of the candidates or to the voices of those who have previously worked with each of the candidates. Everyone wants to like the people with whom they work and often like best those people who are similar to them. But successful teams usually include a range of skills and approaches to work. Having everyone thinking alike may mean that critical alternatives are not considered and that "group think" minimizes the flexibility and creativity in the work group. Your careful interviews of candidates, reference checks on them, and thoughtful consideration about what skills and work habits are needed by the work unit will increase the likelihood of a successful hiring process.

Using a panel and a planned exercise, such as "sorting an inbox" to identify priorities, will often help identify the candidate who knows the subject area well but misses key organizational priorities or handles communication poorly. Questions about how a problem situation might be handled can reveal much about priority identification and communication.

When I was being interviewed for possible appointment as a state public health director, the key interviewer used two fairly recent cases in which policy and public communications had become a challenge, and asked me what I would have done. I apparently answered correctly, as I got the job! And I was impressed by the technique and used it in several interviews that I later conducted. (See Box 10-2.)

Probationary Period

Every employment process includes provision for a 3- or 6-month probationary period, during which the newly hired individual can be removed with a minimum of procedure, based on evidence that there is not a workable match between the job requirements and the individual's abilities. What happens all too often, however, is that the supervisor is (a) pushing to catch up on work that may have been left undone during the period the position was vacant, (b) pleased that there is someone on board to begin assignments, and (c) not scheduling regular review meetings with the new employee. As the end of the probationary period nears, there is tension because a decision to terminate the new employee would recreate a position vacancy, causing further delay.

If the new employee was an internal candidate for the position, there may also be tensions about the employee's right to return to a prior position or criticism from others in the organization. Remember that internal promotions or transfers should not be seen as the way to get rid of an unsatisfactory employee with an extremely positive—but inaccurate—reference.

In a recent case in which I was involved, the supervisor of a newly hired employee quickly identified a mismatch, and the employee was quickly informed that her prior position was still available, and that she could return to it. We reached a three-way mutual agreement—described publicly as, "She found that the prior job was a better match for her interests and skills." The supervisor thought, "That was the easiest firing I ever did." This was a poor choice of words because the employee was in a probationary period to see if there was a good match between her and the job.

Three or six months is almost never sufficient time for a newcomer to fully master all of the nuances of any job, so there may also be hesitation to decide at the end of the probationary period that the hiring was not successful. On the other hand, "20-20" hindsight 9 or 12 months later often suggests that problems were evident during the probationary period and could have been acted upon then. Any supervisor working with a probationary employee should have a clear idea of a minimum, realistic level of successful performance at 1, 3, 6, and 12 months. These milestones should be conveyed to the new employee and regularly reviewed, with gaps documented. Failure to meet the milestones for the probationary period then validates the decision to terminate at that point.

Annual Performance Appraisal

The annual performance appraisal, for employees who have passed from probationary to regular employment, is often treated as a bureaucratic irritant—to be completed at the last possible date or after multiple reminders, and considered irrelevant to the actual work performed. It is often at this time that the myth of durability of public employment is cited, often in the form of the question, "Why do it, since no one ever loses a job?" But, sometimes, the time of the annual performance appraisal is when an exasperated manager decides that an employee who is not performing must be fired, and asks the HR office for assistance in the termination process. Unfortunately, the personnel file may contain a series of prior annual appraisals that indicate satisfactory or superior performance, often signed by the same exasperated manager. There may be no evidence of feedback to the employee on what is lacking in performance and no indication that specific guidance on how to improve has been given. In fact, there are often commendations of various types!

Modern personnel management rightly requires that all employees be given sufficient feedback so that they know what is expected and have opportunities to perform at the expected level. Feedback must be based on the job description. Therefore, if the description does not match the supervisor's requested performance, either expectations must be adjusted or the job description rewritten.

Feedback should be clear and include measurable items, such as "Must respond to public requests for information within 3 working days" or "The report of a community outreach meeting must be submitted within 2 working days of the meeting." If the failure to perform involves not only information communicated but also the style or attitude of the employee, specific descriptions of failure to perform should be documented and the preferred approach described.

As a supervisor, your partnership with the HR office will provide you with guidance and support throughout the process. Without adequate documentation, it will be impossible to fire the employee. For example, I once lost a court case on terminating an executive-level employee for cause because in the termination letter my discussion with the employee was referred to as a "meeting"—rather than an "opportunity for a hearing." In a termination done well, there may be mutual agreement that there was not a good match between the employee and the job, leading to collaboration to find the employee a better job. As a supervisor, you must be able to critically assess both your employees' performance and your own, to give and document feedback, and, with the help of the HR office, to terminate employees when necessary.

Part Three

LEADERSHIP

11

Creating a Vision and Inspiring Others

Robert S. Lawrence and Barry S. Levy

Close your eyes for a moment. Think of a time when you were moved or inspired to take action by another person's vision. Recall what you thought. Recall how you felt. Recall what inspired you. What did you think about the person who inspired you? What commitment did you make? What actions did you take? How did that person's vision change your life?

At first, it may seem difficult to analyze a prior experience in which you were moved or inspired to take action as a result of another person's vision—or to identify specific elements and factors that can enable you to create a vision and inspire others. This chapter aims to explore these subjects and to enable you to identify these elements and factors so that you may be able to use them to create visions, inspire others, and motivate them to find new purpose or direction in their professional work.

Be clear on what your values are. Be grounded in them. And be passionate about them. Values that underlie work in public health include, among others, integrity, respect for human dignity, social justice, community responsibility, cooperation, the pursuit of truth, prevention, harm reduction, and caring about the well-being of those you supervise.

Every public health worker and every public health agency or organization needs to have a vision. Your vision is shaped not only by your values, but also by your previous work and educational experiences, your beliefs, your commitments, and ongoing input and feedback from other people. To inspire others with your vision, you must believe deeply in that vision. You must believe that (a) the effort to translate your vision into reality is worthwhile, (b) doing so will make a positive difference in other people's lives, and (c) you have taken the necessary steps to reduce the risk of unintended negative consequences of your actions.

To translate your vision into reality you need a framework—an organization or a movement—with a mission, goals, objectives, and activities to achieve these goals and objectives.

One definition of a vision is "a thought, concept, or object born by the imagination." Developing a vision is a creative process that requires imagination. A bold vision that transcends limits imposed by traditional thinking inspires others.

Many of the greatest achievements in public health were initiated by people who had a vision. The eradication of smallpox, chlorination of public water supplies, removal of lead from paint and gasoline, mandatory use of child safety seats in automobiles, and prohibition of smoking in public places were all seemingly impossible until a person or group of people created and articulated a vision.

One definition of inspire is "to exert an animating, enlivening, or exalting influence on." To inspire others, you must be inspired by your own vision. And, since inspiration is infectious, you must lead by example to inspire others in your vision. Directly participate in activities and share in frontline responsibilities. By doing so, you demonstrate your commitment to the vision. And you gain valuable experience with issues and challenges to realizing your vision (Box 11-1).

If you want to inspire others, you must demonstrate the values that underlie your vision in both your professional and personal life. Your behaviors are critical, such as the respect and empathy you demonstrate when you interact with colleagues, patients, and those in the communities you serve.

For example, if you are concerned that greenhouse gases contribute to climate change, demonstrate your values with your behavior: Commute to work or school by riding a bicycle, driving a hybrid vehicle, or walking. A colleague who directs an environmental nongovernmental organization personifies his vision in the way he lives his life. He helps mitigate greenhouse gas emissions by refusing to travel

(Text continues on page 245.)

Box 11-1: **Community Health Services in North Carolina: Walking the Talk**

Robert Lawrence

I did not initiate my first opportunity for creating a vision and inspiring others—it was thrust upon me by circumstances. In 1970, I joined the faculty of the University of North Carolina at Chapel Hill (UNC) to participate in the new Community Health Services Project. The federal government had just given a grant to a community group to establish three health centers to serve 65,000 people living in a 1,000-square mile area without primary care practitioners. The community group was to contract with UNC to provide professional services, while it employed non-professional staff members, arranged for construction of the centers, provided transportation, and managed the budget.

I was attracted to this opportunity by the prospect of working for—and learning from—a distinguished senior community health physician, who, at the last moment, chose not to work on the project. When that happened, the dean appointed me as project director—and an opportunity to create a vision and inspire others was suddenly thrust upon me.

The population to be served was 60% white and 40% black. Almost all of these people were tenant farmers or cotton mill workers. The black community was highly suspicious of the overwhelmingly white university, which was suddenly expressing interest in community engagement. The black project director, who had been hired by the community group, regarded me as an opportunistic outsider hired by some UNC faculty members and with much suspicion.

While initially stumbling through tasks for which I felt unprepared, I sustained myself with my vision of providing high-quality, comprehensive primary health care to an underserved population—and my commitment to realizing this vision.

Since North Carolina then had an inadequate number of primary care physicians, many people had to travel long distances for medical care at hospital emergency rooms. I was energized by the compelling need and my vision of developing this program with a multi-racial staff serving a multi-racial patient population.

A small group of dedicated people coalesced to share our commitment to the project. We benefited greatly from our mutual support and understanding—which ultimately made it easier to recruit exceptional health professionals and staff members for three health centers.

My new leadership role was to negotiate with UNC physicians to provide service, recruit additional physicians, help develop and implement a curriculum for training nurse practitioners, and perform administrative tasks. And my responsibilities also included practicing as a primary care internist.

I soon learned that it was critical for me to be engaged in the hands-on nature of the enterprise—providing medical care to patients. I led by example—taking my share of night and weekend call, filling in for colleagues with schedule conflicts, and working directly to resolve the problems in providing services. My demonstrating empathy for patients, phoning patients to ensure they were responding to treatment, and respecting the input of nurse practitioners and community health workers were more important contributors to my leadership than any exhortations at staff meetings.

My direct involvement also gave me valuable information on which to base management—and leadership—decisions. When leaders devote time to hands-on work, they can see and experience problems, fix or reduce them, and communicate solutions to others—from the perspective of people who have "walked the walk."

The greatest challenge to my leadership was the need to reconcile the profound differences in perspective of what the core purpose of the project was all about. For the academic leadership of the university, the lure of "doing well while doing good" was powerful. Here was a new source of federal funding through the Office of Economic Opportunity (OEO)—which directed the "War on Poverty," established during the Johnson administration; a new opportunity to rationalize clinical services and expand the referral base for specialty services, teaching, and research; and the chance to build bridges to a community that was feeling empowered to make demands for more inclusion in university hiring, student and faculty composition, and other aspects of community-university relationships. The clinical staff was committed to providing high-quality care in an efficiently organized and administered setting. The project director and his community board emphasized the opportunities for entry-level employment for the poor. Rarely were these differences overtly expressed, but their disruptive influence was pervasive.

Matters finally came to a head when I scheduled a meeting with the project director to communicate the growing frustration that clinicians were experiencing with errors and inefficiency in the appointment system at the health centers and with the limited skills of support staff members. After laying out my concerns about the potential erosion of quality in our clinical care and the morale problems among the physicians and nurse practitioners, I suggested that we needed to do more in-service training for staff members and be more rigorous in our hiring of new staff members. The project director glowered and said, "You think this is a *medical program*, don't you? Well, it isn't! It's a *jobs program* and the sooner you understand that, the better off we'll be."

At first I was stunned. But, after discussions with a few of my trusted colleagues and further reflection, I recognized that I had failed to investigate fully the goals and values of the other stakeholders. I had assumed that we were all on the same page without having bothered to check the validity of my assumptions. I had not been attentive to the input from others about developing a truly shared vision for the project.

It was now time for me to focus on the challenge of reconciling these different visions to develop together a shared vision of our mission. On several long evening drives to meet with community groups, the project director and I spoke about our personal motivations. He shared childhood stories of walking to his segregated school and watching a school bus pass filled with white children on their way to a better-equipped and better-staffed school. I told him of my original plans to work in international health and of my change in course after the assassinations of Martin Luther King and Robert Kennedy. Slowly, we established the level of personal trust that allowed us to do the hard work of reconciling our different visions for the project.

Coming to terms with the university represented a different challenge. Community board members, filled with suspicion about the motivation of the university, insisted that no students be allowed in the health centers and that no research be conducted there. These terms had been accepted during the contract negotiations that preceded my move to North Carolina. And I soon learned that people at the highest level in the university believed that the community would "come around soon enough" to recognize the importance of teaching and research to the university.

As I argued for maintaining a focus on service, I also agreed to develop a "Medicine and Society" course for first-year medical students—a phenomenon of the times as medical schools across the country were swept up in the focus on social change during the late 1960s and early 1970s. By agreeing to develop and do much of the teaching in this new course, I was able to share my vision with the medical students and demonstrate to community board members that the values of the project were influencing the curriculum at the university.

by air. He even travels across the Atlantic by freighter—using the longer travel time to read and write. Not all of us can follow his example, but each of us can demonstrate through our personal actions and behaviors the values that are foundational to our leadership.

Like your behaviors, your attitudes are vital in inspiring others, such as your attitude when you deal with difficult situations or crises or when outcomes are not to your liking. As a colleague recently said in celebrating the lifelong accomplishments of a faculty member assuming emerita status, "She is someone who brings out the best in the people working for her and stands by them when they are not at their best." The late Carl Rogers coined the term unconditional positive regard for valuing others regardless of their faults or failings.

This concept—and the behaviors needed to communicate it—can help to build teams and can help inspire trust in those we lead.

Translating Vision into Action

Translating a vision into the mission, goals, objectives, and activities of an organization or a movement is challenging. As you do so, remember Margaret Mead's words: "Never doubt that a small group of thoughtful, committed citizens can change the world. Indeed it is the only thing that ever has."

Consider the following suggestions:

1. ARTICULATE YOUR VISION AND HOW IT CAN BE ACHIEVED

Communicate your vision in a manner that others can clearly understand. Make it real for them. Enable people to see how their values—and yours—relate to the vision. Describe the challenges of the vision and opportunities for helping to achieve it. Describe broad sets of actions that will be needed. (See Box 11-2.)

2. LEARN ALL YOU CAN

Immerse yourself in the subject. Read whatever you can. Listen to others. Seek out differing perspectives. Be open to new ideas. Show respect for the ideas and opinions of those reluctant to join in the effort while presenting your vision. An element of healthy skepticism—and even a designated naysayer on the team— helps avoid the pitfalls of a vision being hampered by "groupthink."

3. ENGAGE OTHERS

Being an inspiring leader is not a solo act; get others involved. Engage your colleagues in your vision by sharing it at every appropriate opportunity. Enable them to see the benefits to be gained by achieving the vision. Engage others, even those whom you might not initially think would be supportive of your vision or ways of

(Text continues on page 248.)

Box 11-2: **Creating the Future of Public Health: Values, Vision, and Leadership***

Barry S. Levy

Public health is what we, as a society, do collectively to assure the conditions in which people can be healthy." [That's the Institute of Medicine definition from *The Future of Public Health* report of 1988.] It takes a society to practice public health . . . .

The future of public health is not in a crystal ball somewhere; it is not some predetermined fate that we live out. Instead, as APHA Past President Dr. Bill Foege often says, we create the future of public health together . . . .To accomplish this, we must engage the public in public health . . . .

What We Need to Do
We need to listen to people in the communities we serve; we need to listen to what they believe is needed and wanted. We need to understand their perceptions of health and public health and what they see as their roles in public health.

---

* Excerpted from Levy BS. Creating the future of public health: Values, vision, and leadership (1997 Presidential Address). *American Journal of Public Health* 1998; 88: 188–192.

We need to educate and inform the public in many different ways. We need to educate and inform people directly, where they work, where they live, where they play—in their communities and in their homes. We also need to work more effectively with the media and to take advantage of "teachable moments."

We need to advocate for strong public health policies and programs and to teach ourselves and others how to advocate more effectively . . . .We need to advocate not only for specific public health policies and programs, but also for support of the overall infrastructure of public health—the research institutions, the educational institutions, and the public health agencies, particularly at the state and local levels . . . .And our advocacy needs to be based on sound public health science.

We need to develop partnerships, which are so critical to the work that we do—not only partnerships made with like-minded public health and health-related organizations, but also partnerships established by reaching out to all groups in society. . . .Whatever are our differences with other groups, we can always find some common ground for the good of society. It takes a society to practice public health, and we cannot write off any person or any group.

Who We Need to Be
[Our values, our vision, and our leadership define who we need to be.]

Values define us as a group of public health professionals; values drew many of us into public health in the first place. Ultimately, we often feel most passionate about values. General values include respect for human dignity, health and well-being, and quality of life. They include social justice and community responsibility . . . .

We need to have visions, visions of healthy and safe lives in healthy and safe communities—even visions that seem impossible. Robert Kennedy used to say often, "Some people see things as they are and ask, 'Why?' I dream things that never were and ask, 'Why not?'" We need to dream things that never were and ask, "Why not?" . . .

The philosopher Sören Kierkegaard once said, "Life can only be understood backward, but it must be lived forwards." To do so effectively, we must have visions—even seemingly impossible visions—and the courage and persistence to see those visions come to reality.

Finally, we need to have leadership—leadership that translates these values and visions into actual policies and programs. We need to call forth leadership, not only in ourselves, but also in others. We need to be leaders who not only do things right but also choose to do the right things. We need to demonstrate what public health is all about—not only by what we say, but also by what we do. As Mahatma Gandhi said, "Be the change you want to see in the world."

We also need to have leaders who are not seeking credit for what they have accomplished but know that their acknowledgement is in seeing the fruition of their values, their visions, their leadership.

A wonderful poem from the Chinese tradition [by Lao Tzu] addresses these qualities of leadership:

Go to the people,
Learn from them,
Love them,
Start with what they know,
Build on what they have;
But of the best leaders,
When their task is accomplished,
Their work is done,
The people will remark,
"We have done it ourselves."

That's the kind of leadership we need to call forth . . . .

So, as we move forward and create the future of public health together, let us remember the values that brought us into public health in the first place and not be afraid to articulate them, even in unfavorable political climates—to articulate them with passion, with courage, and with persistence.

Let us remember our visions—even seemingly impossible visions—for healthy and safe lives in healthy and safe communities.

Let us be leaders of public health, leaders to shape the future of public health.

And let us not forget that it takes a society to practice public health, a society in which the public is in public health.

---

achieving it. When you communicate about your vision, be in the moment and share with passion. And actively listen to others and be willing to be inspired by them. Identify people and organizations that may promote and support your vision. You may find common ground with "strange bedfellows"—people or organizations who generally do not share your opinions but who share commitment to your vision (or a piece of it).

4. DEVELOP AND IMPLEMENT A STRATEGIC PLAN

Engage others who share your vision in strategic planning that enables everyone to help develop and refine a mission for your organization or movement—and to develop short- and long-term goals, measurable objectives, and activities to achieve these goals and objectives. But don't be over-invested in a particular outcome—what evolves in an inspired group of people develops organically. And don't get distracted; keep your eyes on "the prize."

5. CARE FOR THOSE YOU SUPERVISE

Managers have a profound influence on the job satisfaction of the people they supervise. Data suggest that people who think they work for managers who care about their well-being intend to remain with their current employers. Without satisfaction in the work required to translate a vision into reality, employees are less likely to be motivated to develop their skills and remain with the organization to fulfill its mission. Recognizing and rewarding your staff members for their achievements inspires their commitment to the vision of your organization.

6. LEARN TO DEAL WITH RESISTANCE AND DISAPPOINTMENT

Find ways to maintain your vision when you meet with resistance from those who do not share it or see it as a threat to the status quo. Do not get discouraged when things don't work out initially. Maintain your own morale and that of your colleagues. Managing change is a critical component of successful leadership (see Chapter 13).

7. TAKE INCREMENTAL STEPS

The Chinese philosopher Lao Tzu said, "A journey of a thousand miles begins with a single step." To get started, undertake small incremental steps to establish a track record and to enable more people to become familiar with your vision. Establish a pace that allows others to keep up with you, especially if joining in the achievement of your vision requires fundamental changes in existing priorities or activities. Be strategic in identifying critical opportunities to promote your vision and inspire others.

8. PERFORM SELF-EXAMINATION

Critically evaluate how you are creating a vision and inspiring others. Invite input from others. Learn what is succeeding and what isn't. Actively solicit feedback about your leadership. Consider formal mechanisms for evaluation of your performance, such as a *360-degree assessment* (see Chapter 10).

To build an organization or a movement, you may need to do all of this—and more (Box 11-3).

In addition to intensely interacting with others, visionary leadership requires periods of solitude for you to reflect. These periods allow you to analyze and reflect upon possible outcomes and consequences of alternative courses of action. They allow you to distinguish between your personal goals and those of the

(Text continues on page 252.)

Box 11-3: **Physicians for Human Rights: Engaging, Motivating, and Guiding Others**

Robert S. Lawrence

During my junior year in college I read Alan Paton's *Cry, the Beloved Country*, a wrenching novel about racial injustice in South Africa, and I was inspired to learn more about social injustice. As a history major, I wrote my senior honors thesis on apartheid. As a medical student, I followed news about South Africa and signed petitions for divestment of university funds that seemed to sustain apartheid, but I saw no path to getting directly involved. For me, human rights remained an abstraction. But a seed had been planted.

Almost a quarter-century later, I began writing letters to the Committee on Human Rights of the National Academy of Sciences calling attention to physicians and scientists who were prisoners of conscience in the Soviet Union and elsewhere. In 1983, a staff member for the Committee asked if I would be willing to travel to El Salvador to investigate the disappearances of 13 physicians and medical students in the civil war there. I went and examined political prisoners in the women's and men's prisons, documented physical and psychological signs of torture, met with members of a human rights investigating unit and family members of "the disappeared," and found evidence that only three were still alive. On my return, I testified before Congress on our findings and spoke to community groups that were concerned about events in Central America.

Several months later, a staff person from the Committee on Scientific Freedom and Integrity of the American Association for the Advancement of Science asked if I would be willing to investigate the murders of two physicians in the Philippines. When I pointed out that I had participated in only one previous similar investigation, she replied, "That's one more than most doctors have done."

With Jonathan Fine and Eric Stover, I visited detention centers, took testimony about torture from political prisoners, and met with officials from the Marcos government and the U.S. embassy. On our return, we testified before Congress and met with staff members of the Department of State. Soon after, as chief of medicine at Cambridge City Hospital, I worked with legal aid services to provide medical examinations for asylum-seekers who had been threatened with deportation back to Central America. I began to develop a vision of using the knowledge and skills of clinical medicine to document and expose human rights abuses.

Several months later, Jonathan Fine told me he was resigning from his position as director of a community health center to direct a new organization, the American Committee for Human Rights (ACHR), and wanted me to join the board of directors. I agreed and began meeting regularly with Jonathan and fellow board members. Over the next year and after several investigations, we realized that our most effective work was using health professionals to investigate human rights violations. We changed the name of the organization to Physicians for Human Rights (PHR). Jonathan and I became founding board members along with four other physicians.

Our initial challenge with PHR was to engage, motivate, and guide other physicians and medical students to address the many cases of human rights abuse throughout the world. I participated in investigations in Chile, Egypt, Czechoslovakia, Guatemala, and South Africa, which enabled me to become a stronger advocate for human rights and social justice. Together with colleagues at Cambridge City Hospital and an attorney, we used our experience with asylum-seekers to develop a guidebook for health professionals to document torture and inhumane treatment and to provide therapy for their suffering.

Physicians for Human Rights grew and was able to hire a full-time professional staff. We engaged physicians, medical students, and other health professionals in advocacy. We solicited contributions to support the work of PHR. We spoke to groups of health professionals and students. We developed student chapters. We built interest in health and human rights, and we motivated physicians, students, and others to commit to creating a culture supportive of human rights.

After several years of serving as a major nongovernmental organization in the campaign to ban anti-personnel landmines, PHR shared the Nobel Peace Prize in 1997 with five other organizations and Jody Williams, campaign coordinator.

The initial group of leaders of PHR refined the vision in response to experiences gained in the field. By engaging other health professionals in the application of their professional knowledge and skills to advance human rights, we continued to learn and refine the mission.

The early work of PHR focused on gross violations of civil and political rights, many of which were perpetrated by repressive regimes supported by the United States in its Cold War struggle with the Soviet Union. With the end of the Cold War, PHR expanded its mission to include violations of social, economic, and cultural rights—the "aspirational" rights of international human rights law. We became increasingly uncomfortable devoting all our efforts to the gross violations of human rights occurring in other countries while ignoring the insidious violations of the social and economic rights at home. We were especially concerned about violations of the right to health.

Physicians for Human Rights adopted new programs in juvenile justice in the United States, advocacy for expanding prevention and treatment for

> HIV/AIDS patients in sub-Saharan Africa, and support for threats to the health and well-being of noncombatant civilians living in conflict zones. PHR recognized the need to expand and grow the vision while adhering to the original concept of applying medical knowledge and skills to advancing the cause of human rights.

organization—to ensure that you do not subordinate the mission of the organization to your needs for self-fulfillment. And they allow you to cultivate independence of mind—away from the day-to-day demands that intrude—to create new visions and ways to inspire others in these visions.

Finally, to be an inspiring leader you need to be open to being inspired by the people whom you serve—and, in turn, sharing that inspiration with others (Box 11-4).

Conclusion

Any public health worker can develop the necessary skills to become an inspiring leader. This chapter has described some of the essential elements for creating and articulating a vision and for engaging and inspiring others. Commentary 11-1 presents the spoken words of four public health leaders who have inspired us.

Box 11-4: **Working in a Camp for Cambodian Refugees***

Barry S. Levy

For six weeks in February and March 1980, I served as a physician at Khao-I-Dang, the largest of the camps for Cambodian refugees in Thailand [with a team from Cornell University Medical College and New York Hospital that was sponsored by the International Rescue Committee] . . . .

My experience and those of many other relief workers probably do not conform to most readers' expectations about what it must be like to work in a refugee camp. My overwhelming sense there was not of death, but of life; not of the Cambodians' ability merely to survive, but of their vitality; not of their grief for the past, but of their hope for the future; not of our superficial differences, but of our shared humanity; and not of the hopelessness of the situation, but of the difference we and they were making . . . .

---

* Excerpted from Levy BS. Special report: Working in a camp for Cambodian refugees. *New England Journal of Medicine* 1981; 304: 1440–1444. © Massachusetts Medical Society.

By the time we arrived in early February 1980, Khao-I-Dang's population had grown to over 120,000, and no more Cambodians were legally permitted entry. On this 5-km² former rice paddy was the second largest aggregation of Cambodians in the world and the second largest "city" in Thailand. Although the people lived crowded together in huts of bamboo and thatch, the overall organization of the camp was miraculous. It contained 10 sections, each of which was subdivided into about 100 groups; it had an organized political system with section and group leaders; and each section had facilities and services, including food and water distribution, an outpatient clinic, a sup-plementary-feeding center, a police station, and usually a school and an orphanage. The United Nations, the Thai government, the International Committee of the Red Cross, and two dozen private agencies and their vol-unteer workers deserved much credit for this organization and the relatively smooth functioning of the camp. But so did the Cambodian people . . . .

Many of the Cambodians at the camp worked long hours in the heat—not merely for the 50-cent daily wage, but largely out of pride and a desire to contribute to their community. Cambodian construction workers built huts and hospital wards and dug latrines. Cambodian public-health workers gave thousands of immunizations for polio, measles, and other diseases to children who were susceptible to them. Cambodian technicians performed microscopic examinations in the clinical laboratory. Cambodian craftsper-sons—including one woman who was almost blind—made bamboo baskets, mugs, and fish traps and sold them at the crafts center to relief workers for $1 or $2 each . . . .

Wind Song, the most remarkable Cambodian whom I met at Khao-I-Dang, reflects in many ways the strength and spirit of his people. During the Pol Pot years, he was sentenced to death four times, but he miraculously sur-vived "by acts of God." [During those years,] he usually worked 18 hours a day moving dirt with his hands. He secretly supplemented his daily ration of two spoonfuls of rice and a thin porridge with roots, insects, and snakes, but his weight steadily dropped to 72 pounds, and he was left for dead . . . .At Khao-I-Dang . . . , he worked as an assistant by day and a translator by night in the camp hospital; he taught an English class for adults hoping to emigrate to the West, translated for other courses, and recruited blood donors—over 300 by the time I left in mid-March. Why? He once explained to me, "I love so much helping people.". . .

A striking characteristic of the Cambodians at Khao-I-Dang was their spirit, most clearly manifested by the happiness of the children. By February 1980 only about 1 percent of the children were severely malnourished (down from 15 percent three months before), and there were few outward signs, as I walked through the camp, that they had lived through a holocaust.

When not in school, they were jumping rope, tossing Frisbees, kicking soccer balls, and most often playing makeshift games—pebbles and bottle caps served as checkers on a cross-hatched piece of cardboard—or dutifully toting pails of water hanging from bamboo poles balanced on their shoulders . . . .

[In our work in the emergency department of the 1,000-bed field hospital,] we were assisted by a dozen Cambodian translators, some of whom were among the most sincere, brightest, and most ingenious people I have met. They anticipated our questions to patients and often obtained much information before we began. We were also assisted by a dozen Cambodian "helpers," who escorted patients to other wards, brought specimens to the laboratory, and [helped] in other ways. In addition, Chu Pheng, one of 53 surviving Cambodian physicians of the 500 who were alive [in Cambodia] in 1975, worked with us. He was about to graduate from medical school when Pol Pot took over; he had forgotten much of what he had once known and was relearning medicine as he saw patients under our supervision . . . .

On four pediatric wards with about 80 patients each, mothers and sometimes other family members stayed with children to assist in their care and also to keep families intact lest the camp suddenly be dispersed . . . .In family medicine, physicians and nurses dealt largely with psychosocial problems and developed working relations with monks and shamans—folk doctors whose traditional practices, like rubbing or burning a coin on the skin, were sought by many Cambodians . . . .There was also an eye clinic, where many Cambodians put on glasses for the first time in five years; one old man cried when he donned his new glasses, saying that he had forgotten how beautiful the world was . . . .

Many of us participated in ongoing in-service training for Cambodian physicians, translators, and "helpers"; a three-month nursing program; and a course in communicable-disease control for 60 Cambodian public-health workers. We were continually amazed by the eagerness of the Cambodians to learn . . . .

In many ways, the Cambodian people contributed more to me during my six weeks at Khao-I-Dang, and since, than I did to them. They brought me much personal and professional gratification. They taught me to be even more grateful for all that I have, especially my freedom. By sharing themselves, they enabled me to see who I am and to realize how similar we are. Despite superficial differences of diet, language, and custom, [they] are motivated by the same things that motivate us: the desire to contribute to their communities and their nation, to love and be loved, and to create a better life for their children.

RESOURCES

Books

Denning S. *The Secret Language of Leadership: How Leaders Inspire Action Through Narrative.* San Francisco: Jossey-Bass, 2007.

This book provides explanations, examples, and practical tips on writing and speaking for inspiring leadership.

Dilenschneider RL. *A Briefing for Leaders: Communication as the Ultimate Exercise of Power.* New York: HarperCollins Publishers, 1992.

This book can help leaders listen more effectively, promote values, ensure integrity, and motivate others to undertake initiatives.

Garcia CP. *Leadership Lessons of the White House Fellows: Learn How to Inspire Others, Achieve Greatness and Find Success in Any Organization.* New York: McGraw-Hill, 2009.

This book distills leadership lessons from generations of inspiring individuals and provides excellent examples of what it takes to make a difference.

Kouzes JM, Posner BZ. *The Leadership Challenge* (4th ed.). San Francisco: Jossey-Bass, 2007.

This book describes the following skills that leaders must demonstrate for success: modeling the way, inspiring a shared vision, challenging the process, enabling others to act, and encouraging the "heart."

Kurtzman J. *Common Purpose: How Great Leaders Get Organizations to Achieve the Extraordinary.* San Francisco: Jossey-Bass, 2010.

This book provides insight into how great leaders achieve "common purpose" and success in their organizations. It sheds new light on the meaning of leadership, the necessary qualities of leaders, and how to lead.

Love A, Cugnon M. *The Purpose-Linked Corporation: How Passionate Leaders Inspire Winning Teams and Great Results.* New York: McGraw-Hill, 2009.

This book provides a concise framework and practical means to understand and unleash the passion of people at work.

Sinek S. *Start With Why: How Great Leaders Inspire Everyone to Take Action.* New York: Portfolio Hardcover, 2009.

This book enables readers to determine why their organizations exist and why that should be meaningful to others in society.

Sloane P. *The Innovative Leader: How to Inspire Your Team and Drive Creativity.* London: Kogan Page, 2007.

This book, filled with innovative techniques and tools, can help readers build innovative cultures in their organizations.

Commentary 11-1: People Who Have Inspired Us

Robert S. Lawrence and Barry S. Levy

In this commentary, we present the spoken words of four public health leaders who have inspired us: James (Jim) Grant, Helene Gayle, Helen Rodriguez-Trias, and William (Bill) Foege. For each of them, key aspects of their successful leadership and calls to action involved their describing important public health problems in a compelling manner—often with stories that put a human face on a problem—and calling listeners to take action to bring about a better future.

James (Jim) Grant

What made Jim Grant so inspiring was his passion for improving the lives of children around the world and his relentless belief that he could recruit everyone as a partner in the work of making children healthier. A lawyer by training, he worked for many years for the United States Agency for International Development (USAID). In 1969, he established the Overseas Development Council and then served as its president and chief executive officer. From 1980 until shortly before his death in 1995, he served as Director of the United Nations Children's Fund (UNICEF). His leadership of UNICEF was inspired by his vision to confront and manage what he called "the silent emergency," embodied in the "daily tragedy of millions of children caught in the relentless downward spiral of poverty, population, and environmental degradation."[1]

During the 1980s, Jim Grant directed UNICEF staff to gain support among poor countries, multinational and bilateral donors, and sister United Nations (UN) agencies, such as the World Health Organization (WHO) and the United Nations Development Programme (UNDP), to develop and implement a "package of low-cost interventions and services called the Child Survival and Development Revolution."[1] The campaign, launched in 1983, emphasized four methods to improve the health and well-being of children. Two of them—breastfeeding and growth monitoring—focused on nutrition, while the other two—oral rehydration therapy (ORT) to prevent death from diarrhea-related dehydration and immunization—emphasized low-cost preventive measures.[1]

Jim Grant always carried a packet of ORT salts in his pocket and used it to persuade heads of state or potential donors from foundations or business to invest in a "pennies-per-treatment" method of decreasing the millions of childhood deaths from diarrheal disease that occur each year.[1] His campaign was successful in reducing the deaths of children under 5 years of age, despite the emergence of the HIV/AIDS epidemic.[2] In its first 15 years, the campaign saved the lives of an estimated 25 million children. And in 2007, UNICEF reported, "For the first time in modern history, the number of children dying before the age of five has fallen below 10 million per year."[3]

The adoption by the UN General Assembly of the Convention on the Rights of the Child in 1989 was a major milestone in Jim Grant's career. The Convention was initiated by him and developed by the Commission on Human Rights during almost 10 years of difficult negotiations. It included ideas put forward in earlier documents about the rights of the child, such as the Geneva Declaration on the Rights of the Child (1924), the Universal Declaration of Human Rights (1948), the UN Declaration of the Rights of the Child (1959); various international covenants; and documents of agencies and organizations concerned with the welfare of children.[4] It also included articles addressing civil, political, economic, social, and cultural rights. As a direct result of Jim Grant's vision and capacity to inspire others, the Convention provides a comprehensive framework for meeting the needs of poor children.

Another aspect of his visionary leadership was his ability to select the right people to senior positions in an organization and then give them freedom to pursue their dreams. He transformed UNICEF "from a supply-oriented organization to the center stage of social development."[5]

Jim Grant used his bully pulpit at UNICEF to bring people together to achieve a shared vision, whether their personal and official interests were in health, environmental protection, economic development, or population control. He was a great role model for all of us in finding those overlapping areas of interest and commitment that enable people to recognize their shared vision.

Addressing the tension between those concerned about reducing infant and under-5 mortality and those wanting to focus on population control, he said, "The reality, of course, is that neither group needs to abandon its own cause. They have only to make common cause, because achievement of either goal—increased child survival or slowed population growth—virtually presupposes and requires accomplishment of the other. Effective child survival strategies work in tandem with effective family planning services to significantly weaken the links among poverty, population growth and environmental deterioration."[6]

In addressing the International Development Conference in 1991, he said:

> Crafting a new world order begins with simple visions. . . . We seek a world which places the individual human being at the center of society and at the center of the responsibilities of [nations]. We seek a world in which each human being is assured his or her essential needs for nutrition, health and shelter; a world in which the role of the state is to foster and protect, and not abridge or neglect, the rights and dignity of each person.
>
> We seek a world in which the human community has found a sustainable balance of its needs with the carrying capacity of the earth. And we

seek a world in which nations have found a different way of inter-relating than marching across borders, carpet bombing, dueling their missiles in the sky, or starving civilians, the great majority of whom are children and their mothers.

In his statement to the Task Force for Child Survival and Development in 1994, he again asserted the power of vision:

> Looking back, we can sense what we have all accomplished together by having a shared vision, and by working together as developing countries . . . international organizations . . . bilateral donors . . . to achieve that vision of better health for children. It was a vision that seemed utopian to many in 1984, when we had our first gathering. A global recession had set in. In most countries, children were clearly the most neglected part of society. They had no legal rights—they were the property of their families. Even readily preventable and curable diseases like measles, tetanus and diarrhea were still taking the lives of more than 10 million children annually. Only a very small proportion of the world's children were being served by the new vaccines, or benefiting from the new knowledge of how to deal with diarrhea. Some 10 million children were dying needlessly each year—30,000 daily—from causes for which the life-saving knowledge was there and readily available. Millions, scores of millions of children—two thirds of them girls—were out of primary school. And everywhere in the early 1980s, health and education budgets were being cut under the impact of the global recession and debt crisis.
>
> . . . What we have been demonstrating in the last 10 years is that when we work together, we really can begin to change the face of global society, the face of the world.

Helene Gayle

Helene Gayle is president and chief executive officer of CARE, Inc. Previously she was chief of international HIV/AIDS activity at CDC; AIDS coordinator for USAID; Director of the National Center for HIV/AIDS, Sexually Transmitted Disease, and Tuberculosis Prevention at CDC; and Director of the HIV, TB and Reproductive Health Program at the Bill & Melinda Gates Foundation. The following are excerpts from the Johnnetta B. Cole Lecture that Dr. Gayle gave at Spelman College in Atlanta on January 30, 2008:[7]

> Holding a position of leadership—a high-powered title—doesn't make you a leader. More and more, people are talking about the concept of

"authentic leadership." . . . It means aligning your leadership with who you are as a person. So authentic leaders are able to demonstrate a passion for their mission, practice their values consistently, and lead with their hearts as well as their heads. . . .

The most important capability . . . is self-awareness. Before asking others to follow, a leader must begin by knowing who she or he is. So what does that mean for all of us? It means getting in touch with who [you] are. And how do you do that? Well, there is no one right way to do that either, but it can start by just asking yourself some simple questions. Which people had the greatest impact on your life? What are your values? What motivates you? What is your true passion? . . . My sense of passion and commitment has driven me and has been the most consistent factor in my career.

I have known for most of my life that what I wanted to do was contribute to bringing about positive social change and social justice. . . . I didn't set out to be a doctor. I grew up at a time when social change was in the air your breathed in this country. I grew up during the civil rights movement, the women's movement, [the] anti-Vietnam War protest period, [the] liberation struggles in Africa. . . . I saw the power of collective action causing change and grew up wanting to be part of something bigger than myself.

My commitment to social justice led me to medical school and, ultimately, into public health. Becoming a doctor seemed like a concrete way to contribute to society and to use a focus on health status as a way of addressing inequities between the haves and the have-notes. I decided on a career in public health, even though I trained in pediatrics, because public health is that marriage between society and medicine. . . .

The more I worked on HIV, the more the relationship to poverty and inequity became clear. Those who are most disproportionately impacted by HIV/AIDS are generally those most impacted by stigma, discrimination, marginalization, and inequality. This is especially the case for women whose risk for HIV is often linked to low status, low negotiating power in sexual relationships, and lack of economic options. . . .

Ending poverty is the ultimate way to save lives, and coming to CARE gave me a chance to focus in depth on the issues of inequity and social injustice that had led me to medicine and health to begin with . . . .

Our world is desperately in need of good leaders—in all parts of the world and in all parts of society. And we need more of these leaders to be women.

Our world is changing in that regard. In countries around the world, women are assuming leadership positions and shifting the leadership landscape. Currently, 10 countries have female presidents or prime ministers. . . . These are women who are opening the doors for others to follow. . . .

Looking at national parliaments or legislative bodies like our Congress, a global survey in 2005 found that 16% of members were women. As a comparison, in 2000, that figure was 11%. . . . Which country has the highest number of women in its parliament? . . . Rwanda, with 49%. Compare that with the United States, with 16% of members of Congress being women. Thirty percent representation is considered the threshold at which women legislators gain a critical mass to have an impact.

Now, Rwanda's [rank] is no accident. The current Rwandan constitution, adopted in 2003, states that 30 out of the 100 seats in parliament must be reserved for women. . . .

There have been many studies trying to [determine] how female leaders are different than male leaders . . . [with] two fairly consistent findings:

First, women tend toward a consensus style of leadership—bringing people together and trying to work toward a shared vision. Generally speaking, women establish themselves as leaders by gaining followers' trust and confidence. We are more natural mentors and prone to seek to empower others around us. Research has found that this style is much more well-suited for leading a modern organization and for solving our current-day problems than the more authoritarian style that is associated with male leadership. . . .

Second, women bring a different perspective to issues, and bring different issues to the table. So women approach issues like peace-building and traditional notions of power and structure differently and help to add balance to problem-solving. . . .

More than half the people on this planet live on less than $2 a day. Of them, 70% are women and girls. Consider these facts:

- Nearly two-thirds of children out of school are girls.
- One woman dies every minute of every day during pregnancy or in childbirth.
- Women work two-thirds of working hours, but earn only 10% of the world's income.

No matter how you measure it, women and girls bear the brunt of poverty. They are also our greatest hope for eradicating it. Improving women's lives can be the crucial first step toward creating lasting social change in poor countries.

Here are just a few examples why:

- Each extra year of primary education that a girl receives boosts her wages later in life by 10% to 20%.
- Children of mothers who attended at least 5 years of school are 40% more likely to survive past their fifth birthday.

- A study in Kenya found that crop yields could rise by more than 20% if female farmers had the same education and decision-making authority as men. . . .

CARE places a great emphasis on investing in girls and women. Educating girls, providing quality health care for pregnant women and new mothers, helping women gain access to financial resources—all of these efforts lift entire communities. . . .

Take time to know who you are. Find your passion. Develop your skills. Travel, but also practice being a leader right here, right now, every day. Leaders aren't born. They are made. You have a fantastic opportunity at this very moment to make yourself into a leader and, by so doing, to change our world.

Helen Rodriguez-Trias

Helene Rodriguez-Trias was a pediatrician, an educator, a human rights activist, and a consultant in health programming. She helped to increase public health services for women and children in low-income and minority populations in the United States, Central and South America, Africa, and elsewhere. She was the first Latina president of the American Public Health Association. The following are excerpts from her presidential address, presented at the APHA Annual Meeting in San Francisco on October 25, 1993.[8]

[We] sense a great urgency about the health of our environment. Aware that our and the earth's health are inseparable, we are deeply concerned about the effect environmental degradation will have on us all. We meet to resolve some controversies on causes and effects and to share public health strategies for the promotion and preservation of healthier neighborhoods, communities, nations, and planet. Among controversial issues, few arouse our passions as much as that of global population.

The most alarmist among us share the views voiced by population control proponents who call overpopulation our number one environmental problem, attributing to it much damage, "from global warning to rain forest destruction, famine, and air and water pollution."[9] The bumper sticker from one population group is a good example of their thinking: "#1 Pollution Solution: Birth Control."

Proponents of a more balanced view focus on poorly planned industrial expansion and rapacious harvesting of natural resources as principal causes of environmental damage. We need look no further than Montana to find rapacious harvesting! One lumber company has in one decade created and abandoned a wasteland.

Those holding a balanced view also point to poverty and the inequitable distribution of resources as posing the greatest threats to health, environment, and social and political stability. Again, we do not need to leave our cities or our poorer rural areas to find supporting evidence for that argument. For population stabilization at sustainable numbers throughout the world, proponents of balanced approaches argue that we must first alter consumption patterns and contribute to the economic development of all. As we in the United States are among the 22% of the world's population that consumes 70% of the resources,[10] we have little moral ground on which to counter their arguments.

My views are closest to the latter. I also hold a firm belief that women's participation and full partnership in discussions on population, development, and the environment are crucial, not just to achieving a clearer understanding of interrelationships, but to crafting policies and programs that will work.

Whether [a] dialogue on population—both in the United States and abroad—leads to new levels of understanding, empathy, and acknowledgment of common cause is up to us. Only we can bridge the chasms of class, gender, nationality, race, and ethnicity that threaten to entrap us in accusations, counter-arguments, and stalemates.

What must we do to gain the respect of all participants in this dialogue? How can we craft policies that will work? We need to start at home, guaranteeing reproductive and other health rights to all women. We need to care as much about providing women with the means to protect themselves from infection with the human immunodeficiency virus (HIV) as we do about helping them avoid pregnancy. We must show respect for our children by contributing to their future and lifting them out of poverty. We need to invest in the creation of a nonmilitarized society and in the resolution of problems of racism, all forms of discrimination, and violence. Our credibility abroad is only possible if we have credibility at home. The Hyde Amendment, which excludes coverage for abortion services and contains other restrictions on reproductive choice, cannot coexist with an external position that makes the issue of safe abortions a major point for other countries.

Why is all the preceding fundamental to us as public health workers? Simply because we cannot succeed in improving and saving the environment without a coherent vision. To succeed at home as well as abroad, we need to make commitments to reject all coercion in family planning and contraception, whether it is the punitive use of Norplant or its use without adequate informed consent. The full range of funded reproductive services in health care reform must include safe abortion services. We must defend the right and access to reproductive health services and meet the unmet demands for family planning and sex education. We must work toward family policies that empower families and women and reverse the feminization of poverty. Women who define reproductive rights as the right to have children and nurture and shelter them must be supported. We must support the right of children to safe childcare. Racism and class attitudes permeate our institutions, and we must work to eradicate them. Our insular, narrowly defined approach to our professional work must give way to a broader understanding of our role as collaborators with communities. We must unite with grassroots environmental movements and understand that, for communities of color, the main environmental issues may be violence in their neighborhoods, toxic dumpsites next to their homes, or uranium mining in their sacred grounds. For other nations, the issues may be our deployment of nuclear weapons or our use of their territory as sites for our most toxic and unregulated industries.

We must recognize that alliances between environmental and population groups must not build on the old elitist notion of the environment and must instead resuscitate the idea that "people pollute." The environment does not comprise only pristine forests, lakes, and rivers; it also includes workplaces, communities, schools, and homes. We must find new ways of integrating issues, methods that recognize the centrality of people and their empowerment in the decision-making process.

We need to learn from women—not just from the content of what they want, but from their processes, how they organize and communicate with each other, how they effectively bridge gaps and differences among themselves, and how they transcend the historical rifts that have impeded international cooperation. The women's agenda is based on integration and humanism. Women bring a holistic view that emphasizes how poverty undermines people's rights. Women bring a humanistic view that has at its core respect for the individual woman, man, and child. Women bring a view that quality of life is the ultimate measure of our success. The women's agenda is for all of humanity.

William (Bill) Foege

Bill Foege is a former Director of CDC, a Health Policy Fellow and former Executive Director of the Carter Center, a Senior Fellow of the Bill & Melinda Gates Foundation, and a Professor Emeritus of the Rollins School of Public Health. He is a past president of APHA. The following is from a speech entitled "Public Health Without the Barriers,"[11] which he presented at a conference on "Leadership in Public Health," sponsored by the Milbank Memorial Fund in 1994.

INTRODUCTION: WITHOUT A VISION, THE PEOPLE PERISH

Public health is grounded on the assumption that this is a cause-and-effect, non-fatalistic world. Actions can be taken that change risks and thereby outcomes. The vehicle for exploiting this cause-and-effect world is epidemiology. Epidemiology becomes the interface between science and public policy as it interprets the science, measures the problem, suggests interventions, assesses what could happen if the interventions were applied, and monitors their effects on the population.

Public health is grounded on a second foundation, that the truths of science will be used to benefit everyone. Therefore, the philosophical basis of public health is social justice. A look at "public health without barriers" is best viewed not as the result of a magic wand that could produce miracles, but rather as a look at what could happen if the usual barriers were removed at each step of the process, from discovery to application.

What if we had an environment that stressed the best science possible, the best interpretation of that science, the best policies based on those interpretations, the best application of interventions resulting from those policies, full participation of people in reducing their risks, and the best evaluation of results with ongoing corrective actions, all within the context of the best imaginable equity and ethics? To date, successes in public health have always been partial, always relative. With the exception of smallpox eradication, we have never met the potential suggested by science [or] the equity required by social justice. . . . What could happen if we pushed our science to the limits, thought globally, and developed policies that combined what we could do with what we should do?

WHAT IF WE COULD APPLY THE SCIENCE AVAILABLE?

. . . What if we revisited the concept of what could happen, both in the United States and the world, if we were suddenly free to apply what we know? What would we actually do?

Principles
We would first develop a set of principles to guide all future public health work. Just as health care delivery discussion has been organized around access, cost, and quality, public health workers would probably organize their new freedom to deliver public health around equity, quality, prevention, and outcomes.

Equity. Public health workers would promote the idea that the interrelationships between people, both throughout the world and through time, are such that all decisions must be based on what is best for the greatest number of people over a long period of time; that is, a horizon of centuries rather than years.
Quality. The best science, policy, and administration must be brought to bear on public health problems.

Prevention. Every condition would be evaluated to see if it could have been prevented, and to identify the steps to prevent similar occurrences in the future.

Outcomes. The tool for decision-making in public health should be outcome rather than access, which is only another process measure in the equation. The most important measures would be premature mortality, unnecessary morbidity, and life quality. The first two could be combined to form a measure of disability-adjusted life years (DALYs), and efforts would be required to quantify life quality and add it to the equation . . . .

Policies would be based on the possibilities offered by science, the interpretation of that science, evaluations of cost-effectiveness, and the best predictions of their impact. Programs would not be introduced just because there are no barriers to their delivery, but because they make sense, are prudent, and improve the quality of life at a reasonable cost. Interventions that have a positive benefit-cost ratio, such as vaccine prevention programs and tuberculosis treatment, would become entitlements. Programs that improve life quality would qualify based on the cost of recovering a "disability-adjusted life year.". . .

WHAT IF WE COULD SPEED UP WHAT WE KNOW?

. . . If there were fewer barriers, could research be made more rational? Could we improve on the tools available to public health?

One way to do this would be to imitate the *World Development Report* in its approach to the global burden of disease. First priority would go to studying prevention, measuring our disease problems, and improving the process of public health. For example, research support would be given to improving the efficiency and effectiveness of surveillance, methods of quantifying morbidity, approaches to improving the speed and quality of analysis, ways of improving communication and evaluation, and methods for automating response.

The entire process would then be used to develop both applied and basic research priorities. . . .

Funding decisions for global research could be based on the importance of the problem and the best judgment of the scientists regarding the possibility of a breakthrough.

Without the usual barriers, one can envision major breakthroughs in respiratory infections by means of vaccines, better detection, rapid field diagnostic techniques, appropriate therapy, and supervision. Likewise, a variety of vaccines could be available within decades for other infectious diseases if such a priority would be selected. Public health needs would be more adequately addressed by the research establishment, and, within public health, priorities would be established on a rational basis of need.

Within this scenario, violence would be a major recipient of research resources. Five separate areas of violence each account for more than 1% of the total burden of disease in the world (automobile injuries, falls, homicide, suicide, and war). When violence is aggregated, it represents the largest cause for the world's burden of disease. The rapid fall in automobile mortality in the United States, the strides made in injury control in the past decade, and the pervasiveness of this problem in all geographic areas of the world gives hope that basic and applied research is not only likely to be productive but that the reduction in DALYs could be substantial.

WHAT IF WE COULD SEE THE FUTURE?

. . . What if, on the basis of this experience, we agreed that all future public health activities would be based on the following:

1. Programs would be planned from a global viewpoint, with the goal of providing what is best for the largest number of people.
2. Programs would be planned with the longest time span possible. What would the impact of a program be on persons living hundreds of years in the future?
3. What is the level of impact? For example, an episode of diarrhea in an adult, while extremely annoying, may have no long-term impact, whereas such an occurrence in a young child may be the pivotal event leading to death; the child's illness thus would assume greater priority. . . . However, some problems have a "Humpty Dumpty" impact in the sense that they can never be repaired. Population growth, the destruction of rain forests, and depletion of ozone are examples of conditions that must be attended to no matter what the cost. . . .

It is possible to provide a new vision for public health, where truth and equity propel the decisions, and common sense frames the priorities. Health would be seen to involve all aspects of the world. Interventions would benefit this generation as well as those to follow. We could be ideal ancestors while making relatively few changes in the way we operate.

References

1. *UNICEF Director James P. Grant Dies at 72*. Unity News, April 1995. Available at: http://www. resultssf.org/media/unity199504grant.html. Accessed on August 10, 2010.
2. UNICEF. *The State of the World's Children 1996*. Available at: http://www.unicef.org/ sowc96/1980s.htm. Accessed on August 10, 2010.
3. UNICEF. *Young child survival and development*. Available at: http://www.unicef.org/childsurvival/ index_40850.html. Accessed on August 10, 2010.
4. Center for the Study of Human Rights. Preamble to the Convention on the Rights of the Child. In *Twenty-five Human Rights Documents*. New York: Columbia University, 1994.
5. Cassell M. *Unwind. The Crazy American: Jim Grant*. Available at: http://www.merrillc.typepad. com/unwind/2006/01/the_crazy_ameri.html. Accessed on October 20, 2010.

6. United Nations Population Information Network. 94-09-07: *Statement of UNICEF, Mr. James P. Grant.* Available at: http://www.un.org/popin/icpd/conference/una/940907130633.html. Accessed on October 19, 2010.

7. Gayle H. Johnnetta Cole Lecture, Spelman College, Atlanta, January 30, 2008. Available at: http://www.care.org/newsroom/articles/2008/01/20080130_speech_spelman.asp. Accessed on December 16, 2010.

8. Rodriguez-Trias H. Women are organizing: Environmental and population policies will never be the same (1993 Presidential Address). *Am J Public Health.* 1994; 84: 1379–1382.

9. Ehrlich P, Ehrlich A. *Healing the Planet.* New York: Simon & Schuster, 1993.

10. Wirth TE. *The United States and the International Conference on Population and Development.* Washington, DC: U.S. Department of State, 1994.

11. Foege WH. *Public Health Without the Barriers.* Conference on Leadership in Public Health. Milbank Memorial Fund, New York, 1994. ©Milbank Memorial Fund. Available at: http://www.milbank.org/mrlead.html. Accessed on December 27, 2010.

12

Transforming Organizations by Using Systems Thinking

Charlotte Roberts and Frankie Byrum

Systems Thinking, also known as *systemic thinking*, is the ability to holistically consider an entire entity at once and understand how its parts interact with one another to create an observable behavior or outcome. Systems Thinking requires the discipline to consider past, present, and future simultaneously rather than one event or one crisis at a time. In practice, you embrace the complexity of the situation and imaginative ways to address it. By mastering Systems Thinking, you can design your organization to fulfill its mission and strategize effectively to achieve your vision.

Systems Thinking is not the same as *systematic thinking*, which is a methodical, linear (step-by-step) analysis of an entity, such as your organization. Systems Thinking is messier than systematic thinking and integrates logical, holistic, and intuitive thinking.

As a public health leader, you can put Systems Thinking to good use. For example, if your organization provides services to a diverse population in a geographic area with political demands within state, national, and global economies, you need to comprehend all forces operating in any situation you're addressing. Systems Thinking enables you to deal with complexity—and to have the courage to move forward with incomplete information.

The health-care reform movement in the United States cannot measure all the shortcomings of the current system or quantify all the improvements of a reformed system—and cannot precisely delineate what is causing the system to fail or precisely predict the changes that will enable it to work for everyone. Well-intentioned people need to comprehend the complexity of the system, design a new one based on their innovative thinking, intuitively sense how to change the mindset of stakeholders, and logically create a strategic plan for change.

As you practice Systems Thinking over a period of time, you are likely to move through three phases:

1. Using a set of Systems Thinking tools for solving problems
2. Developing a valuable leadership competency
3. Living a personal philosophy

In the first phase, you develop facility with the tools of Systems Thinking. Like any management tool, such as performance reviews or monthly budget reports, you think about or listen to someone describe a difficult problem that triggers your memory of one of the Systems Thinking tools and begin thinking broader and deeper. With the right stimulus, you use the tools to make a qualitatively different decision.

In this phase, you use the tools for analyzing and addressing recurring problems. You see interdependencies "upstream and downstream," and apply leverage to create different outcomes, recognizing that there could be both intended and unintended consequences. Approaching problems from a systemic action perspective, you draw on personal courage to speak and act across functions, and learn from the effects rippling through systems.

After some time, you enter the second phase and naturally begin to not only see but also anticipate connections among driving forces and elements in the communities you serve. You use the tools of Systems Thinking with other people and take conversations out to a wider perspective. You are recognized by your peers and manager as someone with a valuable competency for not only current problems, but also strategic issues.

With practice and learning from using the tools, you can develop Systems Thinking as a personal competency of understanding the whole *and* the parts, and the dynamic interaction of these parts—all of which together create a behavior or outcome. When called upon, you can naturally engage a larger system to take effective action for a cause and simultaneously engage stakeholders. Not being intimidated by complexity and being willing to ask people to follow a courageous plan, you can become a humble and responsible leader.

Competence in Systems Thinking does not stop at the office door. In the third phase, you begin to live your life from a systems perspective and encourage others to see their reality differently. As you read the news or vote for candidates or serve on a nonprofit organization's board, you ensure the group asks the right questions and achieves a deeper understanding before making long-lasting decisions. Systems Thinking—and Systems Acting—becomes integrated into your personal philosophy.

You appreciate complexity in time, space, and energy. You acknowledge that everything is connected to everything else. You realize that there is always more to reality than is currently seen or understood. And you exhibit deep respect for those who came before and those who will come in the future. Others recognize your new style of leadership. When you adopt Systems Thinking as a personal approach to living, you are likely to be more tenacious, creative, and forgiving, with a bias for wholeness and integrity.

Systems Thinking is a discipline for lifelong study and practice. Your learning to think and act systemically engages several types of intelligence, involves changing some precious paradigms, alters the expression of power in relationships, and expands the ways you approach situations.

Great leaders approach their responsibilities from a systemic perspective. Rather than repeatedly fixing the same problems or "putting out fires" that frequently occur, you can begin creating the organization you imagine and have the impact you envision.

Why should you develop this capability?

- To understand the system you're leading from several perspectives, so you can take more effective action
- To engage people throughout your organization in meaningful conversations about what is possible and then working together to make improvements for employees, for individuals and populations that your organization serves, and for the general public
- To be a creative force in designing changes—in policies, practices, mindsets, and relationships—that will lead to significant positive change
- To achieve the vision of the organization

Why isn't this leadership capability embraced more widely? Perhaps the most frequently stated reason is: "They don't appreciate it and wouldn't tolerate the level of engagement that's needed." Notice *they* are the problem in this explanation. Many executives are just waiting for *you* to pick up your head and look beyond your scope of responsibility to see what is—and what is possible. In reality, the ways we address problems are limited by the way we think.

Some of the mental barriers to becoming an effective systems thinker include these thoughts:

- "The reality I experience is *the* reality. Therefore, if others have a different perspective, they are wrong."
- "Since I can separate myself from what I observe, my biases and prejudices don't really influence my experience or opinions."
- "Focusing on events and fixes is more practical than seeking to understand the dominant systemic forces. Don't just stand there. Do something now!"
- "A situation is best understood if broken into its parts and dealt with according to specific accountabilities. If we think systemically, then no one is responsible."
- "Enemies are out there. Focusing on beating *them* has the highest leverage. *They're* the cause of our misery."
- "Transformation will only occur with big initiatives, such as re-engineering the organization. We need to find a leader or a consulting group with a large reputation to save us with bold moves."
- "It is possible to control the reality that I experience."

- "Wisdom resides at the top of the system and comes from specific experience. We have to wait for people at the top to come up with the best ideas on how we should move forward."

Because we all have been taught principles that are counter to Systems Thinking, it is easy to surrender to these thoughts. To adopt Systems Thinking, you need to test and refine your paradigms.

Basic Tools

There are several disciplined approaches to thinking systemically, such as open systems, family or social systems, process engineering, living systems, and systems dynamics. Each of these approaches has a basic model and methodology to understand the forces at play in a system and to identify possible interventions to transform a system's performance.

Systems can be approximated in diagrams, which can be used as tools to show connections between and among the forces that are operating. In the next section, five tools for Systems Thinking are presented. The first three—The Iceberg, The Fishbone Diagram, and Systems Dynamics Loops—employ a method of picturing. The last two—Boundary Definition and Root Cause Analysis—are ways of reframing a situation.

A good basic tool for practicing Systems Thinking is The Iceberg (Fig. 12-1). It is a metaphor representing four levels of explanation of current reality: Events Thinking, Patterns (or Trends) Thinking, Systemic Structures, and Mental Models.

At the Events level, managers see only the circumstance in front of them, with little or no regard for history, interdependencies, time delays, or other factors. They believe only in what is measurable and urgent.

An Events explanation of what just happened tends to closely examine pressing symptoms—and then react. Any event is easy to address—just act against the last person who intervened or try to remediate the most recent action taken by someone else. For example, if the number of immunizations administered is less than expected and vaccine inventory is increasing, someone may say the cause must be the medical director's poor planning or the public's poor understanding of the benefits of immunization. The response would therefore be teaching the medical director to plan better or making public-service announcements to encourage people to be immunized. At the Events level of thinking, we generally employ a tool or technique to "fix" the situation quickly. We're asking, "What just happened?" and "What do we need to do to fix it now?"

Consider the agendas for the past several meetings of your management team. How many of the topics were dealing with "fixing" problems? Events Thinking is a frequent mode of dealing with issues because it seems quicker and easier; we feel like we're doing something constructive. The manager can take credit for

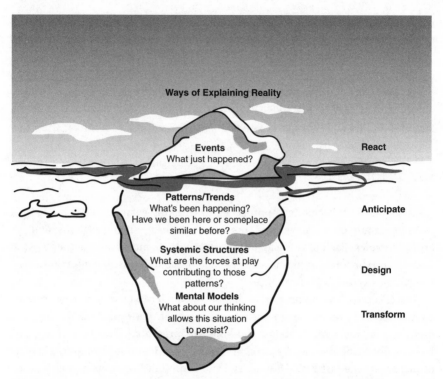

Figure 12-1 The Iceberg. ©2000, the Fifth Discipline Fieldbook Project; originally appeared in Peter Senge, Nelda Cambron-McCabe, Timothy Lucas, Bryan Smith, and Art Kleiner, *Schools That Learn, A Fifth Disciple Fieldbook for Educators, Parents, and Everyone Who Cares About Education* (2000, Doubleday), page 80; www.fieldbook.com.

resolving the problem. Good problem-solvers will get promoted. And it doesn't require another meeting or getting more people involved.

Early in the Quality Movement* in the United States, we applauded companies that could handle events well—such as solving a customer's technology problem in 24 hours or taking back merchandise from dissatisfied customers, no questions asked. That's Events Thinking. It addresses what is visible, urgent, and/or measurable—what's above the water line in The Iceberg.

In Patterns Thinking, we start by reviewing history. Is this the first time we've seen this? How long have we been monitoring these particular symptoms? Have

---

* In the early 1980s in the United States, the Quality Movement was a transformative management system designed to improve the performance of processes and the products produced in response to superior quality products from foreign countries. W. Edwards Deming, along with Joseph M. Juran and Philip B. Crosby, taught methods for improving employees' performance by building effective systems, learning from feedback, and innovating based on customer needs.

we seen something similar in the past? What other patterns surround this problem or crisis?

Patterns Thinking requires drawing on an organization's "institutional memory" that is stored in databases or in the minds of long-term employees. Facts are subject to interpretation, as we obtain a picture *over time*. Patterns Thinking uses charts and graphs as tools. Patterns Thinking is empowering because we have, before making a decision, a different quality of information than in Events Thinking.

Epidemiologists are trained to employ Patterns Thinking to discern patterns of time, place, and person from sets of data. For example, they look for geographic patterns, patterns of age or gender, and patterns of concomitant factors that precede disease.

Patterns Thinking is limited by a key assumption: The past is the best predictor of the future. If we rely on historical data to predict the future, we are assuming external forces will not change substantially. In public health, this can be a dangerous assumption. People migrate. Hazardous exposures evolve. Viruses mutate. Climate changes. New policies are developed.

At a later stage in the Quality Movement, companies began to observe patterns of customers' complaints and anticipate problems. Their responses frequently focused on inspecting problem products or service providers. Customers' experiences were more positive than before, but providers' costs were substantially increased, trying to identify problems before they were perceived by customers.

The purpose of Systems Thinking is to understand why patterns are occurring and how to design systems to achieve desired outcomes. But moving to thinking of Systemic Structures is usually a big shift. This level of thinking is deeper in the water, where there is little light and there are no directional signs. You're on your own to explore, map, understand, and act. You are trying to comprehend how the driving forces are reinforcing or canceling out each other over time.

The Fishbone Diagram can be a helpful start. The head of the fish represents the problem and the bones represent factors, such as financial pressure and quality of service. A limitation of this tool is that it doesn't show the interdependencies among factors. In Figure 12-2, financial pressure from reduced allocations is contributing to turnover of employees, which, in turn, is adversely affecting quality of service. These factors are dynamically connected—not independent as the diagram implies.

Another methodology uses Systems Dynamics Loops, or Causal Loops, which can highlight connections among factors (Fig. 12-3). Because everything is connected to everything else, identifying "the single cause" of a problem is more difficult.

Each diagram has assumptions embedded in the connections, which need to be tested. For example, in Systems Dynamics Loops, is financial support always necessary to test a new program? Will the public recognize its support role in the growth of a high-impact program? Time delays are often overlooked. How much

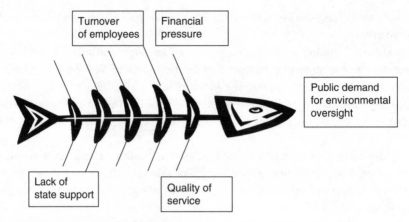

Figure 12-2 Fishbone Diagram.

time will pass before a quality program is implemented and the public recognizes the value enough to demand more financial support from government?

Systems Dynamics Loops have limitations. It's impossible to capture all the dynamic forces operating in a system. Some forces are visible and measurable—such as layers of management or units of time required in a budget cycle—while other forces are intangible—such as fear, trust, the political savvy of leaders, and the public's willingness to participate in a program. Acknowledging this limitation, you can still use Systems Dynamics Loops to engage in enhanced conversation and thinking with others to understand a part of the system and its performance—and what you want to do to improve it.

An essential question as you try to comprehend a system is: "Where are the boundaries of this issue?" Boundary Definition is an important concept. In general, boundaries should be set to ensure that your group's focus is wide enough to

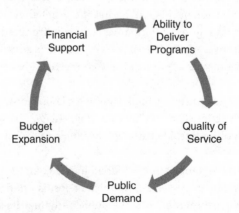

Figure 12-3 Systems Dynamics Loops.

include all factors that are relevant. Consider going beyond the boundaries that your group sets—literally "going outside the box"—and then looking for unexpected factors and interdependencies. For example, if your group believes that the boundaries of an issue are at specific dividing lines in your organization, move the boundaries further out to include the entire organization, and then look for causal factors or interdependent forces. Your answering the following three questions can help:

- Who belongs in this system?
- Do they know they belong in the conversation?
- If our strategy is successful, what are some possible unintended consequences throughout the system?

Yet another tool is Root Cause Analysis, which Systems Thinking uses to determine the underlying cause or causes of a problem. A *root cause* is a causal factor that is not in plain sight. Within a Root Cause Analysis, you can ask the Five Whys: Ask "Why do we have this situation?" and record the answers. In response to each answer, ask "Why is that?" until you've asked "Why?" five times—five levels down. Then begin to analyze the deepest responses to help you redesign the system—its policies, processes, procedures, and practices. (See Chapter 8.)

With Root Cause Analysis, you see well below the surface, discover symptoms, and see opportunities to intervene. Clear and precise "answers" do not await you. *You* must use your systemic, logical, and intuitive modes of thinking to identify the next action to take—to eliminate an old policy, to change the flow of monthly budget information to all managers, to design a system of patient advocacy, to publish program proposals for public response, or to initiate an educational program in local schools. The large impact of systemic decisions may intimidate some people so that they revert to Events Thinking for solutions that, at best, will make only short-term impacts.

You need to dive deep for the next level of thinking: Mental Models. At this level, you ask, "What about *our* way of perceiving and thinking allows this situation to persist?" The heart of transformation is a fundamental change of mind. Examples include (a) letting go of a long-held principle, such as "Employees must always be at their desks to ensure productivity," and (b) incorporating a new principle, such as "Electronic social networks within an organization can increase productivity and management effectiveness." When you engage in this level of thinking, you have to stop acting and begin reflecting. Even more, you need to have reflective conversations with others.

An example of a Mental Model is: "Public Health is a local and state business." Perhaps we should change the name of what we do to "Global Health" since the term has worldwide implications, compared to "Public Health," which implies local boundaries. If you included "Global Health" in the name of your organization, what questions would emerge? What conversations would be stimulated inside and outside your organization?

The best tools for engaging Mental Models are generative conversations and powerful questions. At this level of thinking, you are required to bring representatives from all levels and all functions of the system—and outside the system—into dialogue. This is why it is important for you to have enlightened and independent people on the board of your organization. You will need to gather the most complete picture of reality by asking strategic questions, without intimidating or excluding people or presuming answers. You will need good facilitation and relationship skills (see Chapter 14) as well as cultural competence (see Chapter 5). As the conversation evolves, it often stimulates a vision for a new reality.

Why don't we naturally test and refine our Mental Models? Well, have you ever tried to change another person's mind? It's difficult work, with no step-by-step process that guarantees a positive outcome. You have to uncover your own and key stakeholders' *current* beliefs and assumptions about how the system *currently* works to produce *current* outcomes—before you can address how the system should work *in the future*. As a result, a much bigger picture emerges. Sometimes it's hard to know what you should do next to move the thinking along. Leading reflective sessions requires you to have patience and persistence. Frequent barriers are insufficient time, inadequate facilitation skills, unavailability of the right stakeholders, and inadequate political permission or savvy.

At this level of thinking, you invest more time. But you are able to influence the system by expanding Mental Models throughout the organization. Here are two examples: Members of the sports team who change their self-image from a group of hopeless losers to one of hard-working winners before the season begins. The city health department that starts thinking of itself as a global health department and begins acknowledging—and responding to—its international and global influences.

Quality is a state of mind and everyone's job. When employees are given the tools to understand their processes and empowered to redesign their work and workflow for best outcomes, the model of power and responsibility for quality shifts from belonging with managers to being shared among all employees (see Chapter 8).

Once you "see" the system from a different and larger perspective, you cannot go back to acting narrowly. People are energized and want to take action. That's transformation. And changing Mental Models is at the heart of transformation.

A Case Study: Applying The Iceberg to a Specific Situation

A county councilwoman angrily enters your office. She says she has received several phone calls from constituents living in the same neighborhood, complaining that their well water is smelling bad. She's running for re-election, and she wants something done now.

If you approach this situation with Events Thinking, you would ask what the councilwoman wanted you to do. She's the person in front of you making demands, so you would focus on her. She might answer that she wants you to get someone to investigate the situation right away, take samples, and report the findings to her. With Events Thinking, you would do what she asked—and nothing more. Having kept your agreement, you would be done with the matter.

If you used Patterns Thinking instead, you would gather data from all the residents of this neighborhood and adjacent neighborhoods and from environmental records in the department. After a few days, you would find that there have been intermittent complaints for the past 4 years. When the water was tested in the past, there were only traces of chemicals, all within acceptable ranges. You would also find that there have been several cases of leukemia among young adults—an occurrence difficult to interpret with no cancer database for comparison. Your solution might be to carefully monitor these neighborhoods and close those wells with high levels of chemicals. You might also send letters to residents of these neighborhoods, suggesting that they buy bottled water. And you might encourage the councilwoman and residents to advocate for bringing municipal water to these neighborhoods. Your actions would focus on studying patterns and anticipating how the situation might evolve.

If you led the thinking to Systemic Structures or forces operating, you would find out what's behind the water issue. You would continually ask, "Why?" You would want to know what happened before that could have led to contamination of the well water—possibly something that happened 10 or 20 years before. You might also interview the leukemia patients to see if they might have had any common exposures. You might learn that an oil company's tanks 3 miles away, which were built 12 years before, were found to be leaking petrochemicals into the groundwater. You might seek help in rectifying this problem from the state department of natural resources or the U.S. Environmental Protection Agency.

If you performed with the community a Root Cause Analysis of the water contamination, you might determine how much well water in the area is contaminated and then supply regular deliveries of safe water to families in need. You might also work with the councilwoman to visit officials of the oil company. They might promise more testing onsite. But you might feel like you're at a dead end.

You could go the next level and use Mental Models to understand why this situation has persisted over several years. You would find that several families have moved into these neighborhoods in the past several years and couldn't afford to leave. The residents believe they "can't fight city hall" and feel powerless to force a change at the company. Given their low incomes, they say that they need to work—and retain their jobs in a tight economy—more than they need clean water. In the past several years, as upper-middle-class residents moved away, the city has become more dependent on the oil company for tax revenue. In fact, you discover that, after a previous investigation into the water contamination, two council members stopped further inquiry for fear that the oil company might leave.

With this information, you could choose to bring together neighborhood residents, council members, and company representatives to discuss the issues from several perspectives and find mutually acceptable solutions. As a result, you might uncover strategies that advance the community.

Systems Thinking doesn't try to find someone to blame and punish. Its purpose is to understand the complexity of a situation and design ways to move forward toward a shared positive outcome.

Social Systems

Another approach to Systems Thinking comes from the study of social systems. Organizations are comprised of people, working in hierarchical structures and making decisions throughout the workday. Human relationships are complex. And groups of people often perform in ways that individuals cannot. The structure of systems determines performance. Hierarchy powerfully produces predictable behaviors—no matter how hard individuals may try to overcome them, as Barry Oshry, a social systems expert, has observed.

It makes sense to design organizations in hierarchies, with three broad groups of employees, each with unique responsibilities. Executives (*Tops*) have ultimate responsibility for the current and future performance of an organization. Often seen as "the brains" of an organization, they spend their time thinking—and they often hire consultants to think with them. *Middles* hold the organization together by addressing "simple requests" and serving as conduits of communication within the organization. Middles are responsible for and to front-line managers. They meet to learn about situations, determine what needs to be done, and implement actions. They are the eyes and ears—and often the voices—in an organization. *Bottoms* ("hired hands") are frontline employees who are at the mercy of managers' decisions and often feel invisible. They are valued for their productivity—not their thinking.

The behavior patterns of these three groups are predictable. If the performance of the organization declines, Tops feel burdened and begin to act as if they are indispensable. They may start meddling in the work of the Middles, making the Middles feel that the Tops see them as incompetent and not trusted to implement corrective strategy. Because Middles, in this situation, are scrambling to hold everything together, they don't have time to meet with their colleagues and will likely feel isolated. Bottoms, who are often ignored when they offer ideas, feel unsupported if they have to integrate changes into their work while maintaining productivity. (See Chapter 13.)

When you initiate a systemic change, your organization will experience stress, so you can't avoid the kind of reactions just described. However, if you don't deal with the social issues created by a systemic change, a situation can get much worse. Tops will get protective of people in their divisions and territorial with each other.

Middles will become fragmented and lack a sense of purpose; some talented ones may leave. And Bottoms get tired of all the craziness and organize to save their work; they become "anti-Them" and shut out communication with most managers. If this happens, the situation will become much more difficult to address.

In dealing with social systems, you need to monitor your feelings and Mental Models as well as those of others to sense their level of frustration. Keep your Middles connected and frequently informed. Don't let them lose purpose or connection. Respect the interdependencies in your organization by holding focus groups, "brown-bag" lunches, or other types of small-group meetings to have employees and stakeholders discuss the changes, how their implementation of the change is progressing, and—most of all—the outcomes that you all envision. Your role is to facilitate—not dominate. Allow the social system to comprehend the change and work through social networks to achieve shared goals.

Albert Einstein said, "We shall require a substantially new manner of thinking if [human]kind is to survive." Systems Thinking is a discipline that has the power to change and transform your world as you know it. As a leader, you should develop your capabilities to think and act on deeper levels. And you should teach those who will come after you how to "see" the whole system and understand the interaction of its parts.

Lewis Thomas, a physician and author, wrote, "When you are confronted by any complex social system . . . whatever you propose to do, based on common sense, will almost inevitably make matters worse. If you want to fix something, you are first obliged to understand, in detail, the whole system."

You will be lost if you deal with each crisis separately, as if each one is not connected to other issues. David Bohm, a theoretical physicist, warned that the widespread distinctions among people that prevent people from working together for survival are largely caused by the kind of thought that treats things as inherently disconnected.

Peter Senge, a thought leader in Systems Dynamics who is director of the Center of Organizational Learning at MIT, stated that mastering Systems Thinking demands that you give up the practice of blaming other people or agents for your problems: "Everyone shares responsibility for problems generated by a system. That doesn't necessarily imply that everyone involved can exert equal leverage in changing the system." The observer and the actor are both part of the process— not apart from it. He asserted that Systems Thinking "is the antidote to [the] sense of helplessness" that comes when you are faced with increasing complexity.

The first step in Systems Thinking is seeing the whole as well as the parts that are interacting to give the system its characteristics and generate its outcomes. The next step is to recall or create a vision for the system that can provide context for imagining and testing possible interventions, anticipating both short-term effects and long-term unintended consequences. The next step is summoning the courage to convene a group of stakeholders to join in the transformation that you envision (Box 12-1).

Box 12-1:   **A Clinical Example of Systems Thinking**

In our county, we always tried to fill unmet needs of the residents as best we could within budget constraints. Our lead physician, a woman, noticed that in our family planning clinic we were serving, almost exclusively, young women of childbearing age. Where were the women beyond childbearing age having their gynecological care if they didn't have health insurance?

We tried to gather data from the community, but this was difficult because physicians were reluctant to reveal information on their patients for fear of being accused of discrimination. Officials at local hospitals did not know where these women were getting care.

A few of us met in a conference room and created a vision of healthy women over age 50. We advertised our "Mature Women's Clinic" through the Adult Medical Clinic in our building to determine if there was a demand for its services.

Fortunately, we were at the right place at the right time. Federal funding for our vision became available. In addition, our medical director contributed to the funding of our clinic. We offered mammograms, Pap smears, and physical exams 2 days a week to women in the target population. Visiting nurses promoted the clinic to women in the community who qualified.

Two physicians from the state medical school taught nurses how to perform physical assessments and enabled them to practice their skills, under close supervision, in the new clinic. Two of the nurses were initially assigned to the clinic, and others were available on busy days.

The clinic's schedule quickly filled. In 90-minute appointments, nurses assessed patients, provided education, and taught patients about age-related changes that were occurring. They detected breast masses, cervical dysplasia, malignancies, sexually transmitted infections, hypertension, diabetes, and other health problems. The ultimate goal of the clinic was to enable women, as they aged, to recognize their responsibility for their own health and well-being. Physicians who received referrals for further diagnostic studies and treatment were very supportive of the program.

When the clinic was expanded to be open 4 days a week, its schedule was filled for several weeks in advance. Patients were very complimentary of the care they received and the information they obtained.

When Medicare began covering mammograms and Pap smears, the clinic no longer accepted women age 65 and older. These women were quite upset, feeling that the care they had been receiving was superior to that they would receive from other clinics. Even though we appreciated their acknowledgment, limiting the population served to women between the ages of 50 and 65 enabled the clinic to see women in a more timely manner.

Community members got involved in the clinic. For example, the town's women's club donated small gift bags for each patient, and a garden shop contributed flowering plants. Today, the clinic continues its mission of addressing the health needs of uninsured women in this age group.

Conclusion

Systems Thinking is a lifelong study and practice. Using it, you are a thinker, teacher, learner, speaker, facilitator, ambassador, creator, and actor—and you increase the likelihood of leaving a positive legacy.

RESOURCES

Books and a Report

de Savigny D, Taghreed A (eds.). *Systems Thinking for Health Systems Strengthening*. Geneva: World Health Organization, 2009.

> *This report demonstrates how we can better capture the wisdom of diverse health system stakeholders in designing solutions to health system problems.*

Meadows DH. *Thinking in Systems: A Primer*. White River Junction, VT: Chelsea Green Publishing, 2007.

> *This book describes why systems fail and how to help them succeed. It includes a section on Causal Loops.*

Meadows DH, Randers J, Meadows D. *Limits to Growth: The 30-Year Update*. White River Junction, VT: Chelsea Green Publishing, 2004.

> *This book describes the dynamic forces of the global ecological challenge, provides alternative scenarios, and suggests general guidelines toward sustainability.*

Oshry B. *Seeing Systems: Unlocking the Mysteries of Organizational Life*. San Francisco: Berrett-Koehler Publishers, 2007.

> *An easy-to-read book on the power of hierarchy in human social interactions.*

Wheatley M. *Leadership and the New Science: Learning about Organization from an Orderly Universe*. San Francisco: Berrett-Koehler Publishers, 1994.

> *An understandable description of living systems principles as they apply to our organizations.*

"The Fifth Discipline" Series

Senge P. *The Fifth Discipline: The Art and Practice of the Learning Organization*. New York: Doubleday Publishers, 1990.

> *Systems Thinking is the fifth of five disciplines needed for leading a learning organization.*

Senge P, Roberts C, Kleiner A, et al. *The Fifth Discipline Fieldbook: Strategies and Tools for Building a Learning Organization*. New York: Doubleday Publishers, 1994.

> *This book provides practical tools and techniques for becoming a Systems Thinking practitioner.*

Senge P, Roberts C, Kleiner A, et al. *The Dance of Change: The Challenges to Sustaining Momentum in Learning Organizations*. New York: Doubleday Publishers. 1999.
> *Organization leaders offer their experience in transforming their organizations based on the human dynamics of change.*

Newsletter

The Systems Thinker. Available at: http://www.thesystemsthinker.com.
> *Published by Pegasus Communications, this newsletter is an easy way to understand current issues from a systemic perspective. Back issues are available.*

Commentary 12-1: Lessons Learned in Transforming the Veterans Health System

Kenneth W. Kizer

In 1994, I was asked to re-engineer the Veterans Health System (VHS). At the time, few people gave this effort any chance of succeeding. They said the VHS was too large, its bureaucracy was too sclerotic, the special interests were too entrenched, and the politics were too complicated. A few years later, however, the VHS had become a case study in radical organizational transformation and was being hailed as the largest and most successful health-care turnaround in U.S. history and a model for health-care reform.

The VHS is the largest health-care system in the United States. Administered by the Veterans Health Administration (VHA), a sub-cabinet agency in the Department of Veterans Affairs (VA), the VHS is the nation's only health-care organization having patients and facilities in all 50 states and almost every major metropolitan area of the country, as well as Puerto Rico, the Virgin Islands, Guam, and American Samoa. In federal fiscal year (FY) 2010, it had an operating budget of $45 billion, and its 8.3 million beneficiaries were served by 153 hospitals, 901 ambulatory care clinics, 135 nursing homes, 299 readjustment counseling centers, and 43 residential care facilities—and more than 222,000 full-time-equivalent employees (FTEEs), including some 14,000 physicians and 40,000 registered nurses. In addition to the care provided with VA assets, the VHS also paid $4.4 billion for out-of-network care and co-funded 133 state-operated veterans nursing homes.

The VHS operates the largest health professional training program in the United States, funding almost 10,000 graduate medical education positions for physicians and offering training in more than 40 other health professions. Of all VA medical centers, 85% are teaching hospitals. About 110,000 trainees receive clinical instruction at VA facilities each year through affiliations with more than 1,100 educational institutions.

The VHS is also a large research organization, having an intramural research program with dedicated funding of $575 million and a total annual research budget of almost $2 billion. It is an especially good setting to conduct research on medical care, health services delivery, and quality improvement (QI) because of its large and stable population of beneficiaries having chronic conditions. VA investigators publish about 10,000 articles annually in peer-reviewed journals.

Ironically, most of the 24 million U.S. veterans are not eligible for VA health care. The VHS was established to provide care for persons who suffered disabling injuries or illnesses while serving in the armed forces. In 1924, hospital care for indigent veterans without service-connected disabilities was authorized by Congress, establishing the VA's role as a provider of safety-net services. The VA is the nation's largest provider of psychiatric and behavioral health services, as well as the largest direct provider of services for homeless persons.

The Evolution of the VA's Dysfunction

Government-funded health-care benefits for veterans began in colonial days, but were originally limited to infirmary care provided by contract civilian providers or the equivalent then of the U.S. Public Health Service (USPHS). Limited inpatient services for veterans of the Union Army were authorized by President Abraham Lincoln after the Civil War in the newly established National Home for Disabled Volunteer Soldiers. However, the VHS did not really come into being until after World War I, when the population of veterans increased to 4 million and Congress transferred 57 USPHS hospitals to the Veterans Bureau. The Veterans Administration was established in 1930 as an independent federal agency to consolidate and streamline the multiple disparate veterans benefits programs. (The Veterans Administration was supplanted by the cabinet-level Department of Veterans Affairs in 1989.)

At the end of World War II, 12 million new veterans overwhelmed the VA, prompting the creation of a new VA Department of Medicine and Surgery. The VHS grew rapidly after this. More than 70 new VA hospitals were constructed over the next decade. Consistent with what was then viewed as the best medical care and its close affiliation with academic health centers, VA health care was patterned on a model that emphasized hospital inpatient care provided by medical specialists. It provided little primary care.

As the VHS grew, it became increasingly cumbersome and bureaucratic. Organizational leadership frequently changed and was often selected on the basis of one's political or military background. The VHS management style became centralized and hierarchical, similar to the military—even though such autocratic and rigid management practices were known not to work well in civilian, academic health-care organizations similar to the VHS. Untoward outlier occurrences often led to reactionary and ill-founded system-wide policies and micro-management from VA headquarters and the Congress. Excessive oversight, conflicted governance, inadequate funding, confusing or conflicting policies, and its "command-and-control" management approach created a punitive, fault-finding, risk-averse, "fishbowl-like" organizational culture that stifled innovation, diffused accountability, discouraged individual initiative, and eroded trust—internally and externally with stakeholders.

When I went to the VA at the end of 1994, care was fragmented, disjointed, hospital-centric, of unpredictable and irregular quality, expensive, and often difficult to access. Availability and predictability of services markedly varied among facilities. Construction and other capital-investment decisions were highly politicized and sometimes correlated poorly with need. Patients and families were dissatisfied.

VA personnel were dispirited and demoralized. Elected officials were angry, and many felt the VHS should be privatized.

Challenges to Change

When I was offered by President Bill Clinton the position of Undersecretary for Health—the chief executive officer (CEO) of the VHA and head of the VA health-care system—most of my colleagues advised me not to accept. They questioned how anyone could hope to address so many systemic problems while continuing to provide uninterrupted care to millions of patients. However, after years of varying success in changing Medi-Cal (California's Medicaid program) and other public health programs as Director of the California Department of Health Services, I thought the strong sense of mission of the VHS and its broad array of assets offered a novel opportunity to engineer more effective and more efficient delivery of health care. So I accepted President Clinton's offer.

Being an outsider to the VHS was both an advantage and a problem. As its first CEO to come from outside the organization in more than three decades, I did not have any relationships with its personnel or programs. This allowed me to be more dispassionate in making decisions, but it also meant that I did not know its unwritten history and did not have the internal or external interpersonal connections that were sometimes helpful in solving problems. To address this vulnerability, I selected a well-known and respected physician leader in the organization to be my deputy. I also cast a wide net to find new leaders for the organization.

Competing with or complicating efforts to address the care delivery issues were an array of other challenges, including:

- A new set of highly visible and contentious health concerns stemming from the 1990–1991 Persian Gulf War
- The variable understanding of health-care issues among some of the politically powerful veteran service organizations—who, in some cases, had vested interests in maintaining the status quo
- Often highly parochial issues of affiliated academic health centers
- The need to educate and train a large and diverse workforce in competencies needed to support the "new VA"—especially in Systems Thinking, QI, financial management, and population health
- The political risks associated with addressing problems such as medical errors or closing facilities
- A history of labor–management distrust and conflict
- Opposition to many of the needed changes by powerful special-interest groups, such as opposition by pharmaceutical manufacturers to establishing a national formulary or opposition by academic medical centers to our decreasing the number of specialist residency positions in order to create primary care slots

- Well-intentioned—but often naïve or misguided—intrusions and interference by White House or Congressional staff members
- The absence of any dedicated funds for the transformation—and, in fact, overall decreased funding in absolute dollars
- The short time that I would likely have to make major changes
- The complexities of engaging and enlisting the support of Congress, which had to approve or enact legislation to authorize critical elements of the transformation

Working with the Congress—essentially the VA's governing board—sometimes presented particular challenges. All members of Congress have veterans—and many have VHS facilities—in their districts, but their perceptions of the VA and their understanding of its mission vary greatly. In addition, the needs of the system sometimes conflict with the political needs of members of Congress. Other problems relating to Congress included:

- Its variable understanding of health care and veterans' problems
- Its sometimes lack of long-term vision or Systems Thinking
- Its tendency to place undue weight on anecdotes and individual stories
- Its highly charged partisan environment
- Its intolerance for errors and the dampening effect this has on innovation and implementing change
- The propensity of some members of Congress to publicly denigrate civil servants and use government agencies and "the bureaucracy" for political gain

The Transformation

In broad terms, the re-engineering of the VHS sought to improve quality, increase accountability, and provide better value. I designed the effort around a values-based vision for change: The VHS should provide a seamless continuum of consistent and predictable high-quality, patient-centered care of superior value. I sought to create a "high reliability organization" that could clearly demonstrate that it provided equal or better value than the private sector.

The re-engineering was based on an integrated strategy consisting of five primary objectives:

1. To increase accountability by creating an accountable management structure and management control system
2. To integrate and coordinate services across the continuum of care
3. To improve the quality of care and systematize quality improvement
4. To use funding to drive value-based performance
5. To modernize information management

Many interrelated and overlapping tactics were used to achieve these strategic objectives. Importantly, reducing cost was not a strategic goal *per se*, although I expected to achieve large savings by better coordinating services, improving quality, and aligning finances with desired outcomes.

To create an accountable management structure and management control system, we:

- Established a new operational structure based on regional accountable care organizations—the 22 Veterans Integrated Service Networks (VISNs)
- Implemented a new performance management system
- Decentralized much of the operational decision-making

Key tactics used to integrate and coordinate care included:

- Implementing universal primary care
- Getting Congress to rewrite the laws governing eligibility for care so that a person's total health needs could be addressed, not just his or her service-connected condition
- Establishing hundreds of new community-based outpatient clinics (CBOCs)
- Using a comprehensive care management approach
- Merging facilities
- Encouraging use of standardized care pathways and clinical guidelines
- Creating multidisciplinary "Strategic Healthcare Groups" and multi-institutional "service lines"
- Implementing a system-wide electronic health record

Performance measurement and public reporting of performance were cornerstones in improving quality of care. In addition, we sought to improve quality by:

- Promoting the use of evidence-based clinical guidelines
- Establishing clinical programs of excellence
- Instituting an evidence-based national formulary
- Pursuing population-based health promotion strategies
- Partnering with external organizations to enhance organizational capabilities
- Launching structured QI initiatives for specific clinical conditions and operational problems, such as care for cancer, HIV/AIDS, pressure ulcers, acute myocardial infarction, and hepatitis C—as well as pain management, end-of-life care, and performing postmortem examinations
- Building organizational competence in clinical QI by establishing the VA National Quality Scholars Fellowship Program and the VA Faculty Fellows Program for Improved Care for Patients at the End of Life
- Promoting rapid translation of research findings to clinical care by founding the Quality Enhancement Research Initiative (QUERI)

- Harvesting the lessons learned from hundreds of grassroots innovations through new knowledge management tools, such as the VA Lessons Learned Project

As a public health-care system, I felt that the VHS should take a lead role in the emerging national patient safety movement. We therefore worked closely with key national organizations on patient safety issues, established the National Patient Safety Partnership, helped fund the Harvard Executive Session on Medical Errors, and supported the National Patient Safety Foundation. In 1997, I launched a multi-pronged VHS patient safety initiative composed of five strategies:

- Building an organizational infrastructure to support patient safety, including establishing the VA National Center for Patient Safety and supporting dedicated patient safety personnel in VA facilities
- Creating an organizational culture of safety
- Implementing known safe practices
- Producing new knowledge about patient safety through research at new Patient Safety Centers of Inquiry that especially focused on learning from other high-risk industries
- Partnering with other organizations to facilitate rapid development of solutions to patient safety problems

We used funding to drive value-based performance by designing a capitation-based global payment resource allocation system—the Veterans Equitable Resource Allocation (VERA) methodology—and secured a Congressional mandate to use it. Because VERA was also designed to achieve equity in funding across the system, shifting hundreds of millions of dollars among the VISNs, this was an especially controversial change in the Congress. We also sought to diversify the funding base by improving collection of third-party payments.

We improved information-management capability by upgrading the system's information technology (IT) infrastructure to ensure a minimum level of system-wide connectivity and responsiveness to provide a communications platform to support the VISNs and a system-wide electronic health record. This enabled us to quickly implement the Computerized Patient Record System (CPRS) in 1997, which was combined with a new graphical user interface to create the Veterans Health Information Systems and Technology Architecture (VistA). Implementation of VistA at all of the VHS's then 172 hospitals occurred in six successive phases in less than 3 years—which, as of mid 2011, was still the largest and most rapid deployment of an electronic health record anywhere.

We also enhanced IT by such measures as implementing an automated cost-accounting system, an internally developed barcode medication administration system, and a "semi-smart" registration and access card.

Evidence of Change

By the end of 5 years, the VHS had markedly changed. It was treating 24% more patients and had:

- Implemented universal primary care
- Improved access with 302 new community-based outpatient clinics
- Markedly reduced waiting times
- Closed 29,000 acute-care hospital beds
- Reduced bed-days of care per 1,000 patients by 68%
- Reduced annual hospital admissions by 350,000
- Merged 52 hospitals into 25 locally integrated multi-campus facilities
- Eliminated 72% (2,793) of all forms and automated the remainder
- Secured passage of the Veterans Eligibility Reform Act of 1996, which eliminated most of the anachronistic restrictions on what care VHS could provide for individual patients
- Decreased staffing by 12% (25,867 FTEE positions) while concomitantly increasing the number of caregivers
- Substantially decreased annual operating costs
- Decreased annual expenditures per patient by more than 25% in constant dollars
- Improved patient satisfaction and achieved higher aggregate patient satisfaction ratings than in the private sector (In 1998, 80% of patients thought that care was definitely better than 2 years before.)
- Markedly improved quality of care according to standardized performance measures for a wide array of conditions.

Perhaps an especially telling composite measure of how veterans felt about the changes was that the number of veterans seeking care from the VHS increased from 4.5 million in 1999 to nearly 8 million in 2003, when the George W. Bush administration essentially closed the system to new non-indigent persons without service-connected disabilities.

Almost no new funds were appropriated for these changes. They were funded through redirecting savings achieved by redesigning processes of care and improving business processes.

Lessons Learned

Many lessons can be found in the transformation of the VHS, including the following:

- The government can provide high-quality and efficient patient-centered care.
- Rapid and dramatic change is possible in health care, even in large, politically sensitive, financially stressed, public-sector health-care systems.

- Improved quality, better service, and reduced cost can all be achieved simultaneously.
- Measuring and publicly reporting performance data is a powerful lever for change, but the data must be fed back to those who can make improvements.
- To improve performance, leaders must make clear that this is an organizational priority, ensure that everyone in the organization knows that it is a priority, and have a plan that includes clear goals, defined responsibilities, and measures of performance to assess progress.
- Decentralization of authority must be accompanied by broad understanding of mission-critical activities, clear delineation of responsibilities, unambiguous accountability, and performance monitoring.
- Focusing on changing organizational performance and processes is more productive than focusing on poor-performing individuals.
- To succeed, front-line clinicians must be continuously part of the planning for and implementation of changes in clinical processes.
- When undertaking major change, there can never be too much communication.
- If you wish to get different results, workforce education and training are essential and they must be supported with dedicated funding and time for training—especially difficult in public-sector agencies because training is an administrative cost and, therefore, prone to be cut.
- An integrated system of health care can be achieved with vertical and/or virtual integration as long as necessary information-management systems and clear contractual or partnership arrangements are present to support virtual integration.
- Most of a supporting infrastructure for change needs to be present before launching any major change process.
- Health-care systems operate as complex adaptive systems. Therefore, unintended consequences are inevitable and their occurrence—and the need to make mid-course corrections—needs to be anticipated.

Critical Success Factors

Many factors contributed to the success of the VHS transformation, but most prominent among these were:

- A particularly strong sense of mission among VA staff members
- A clear, values-based, actionable vision of a new future
- An integrated, multi-faceted change strategy, employing overlapping and mutually reinforcing tactics
- Alignment of funding with desired outcomes
- Use of automated information-management tools
- Strong and committed leadership that maintained an unwavering focus on the end goal

RESOURCES

Edmondson AC, Golden BR, Young GJ. *Turnaround at the Veterans Health Administration.* Boston: Harvard Business School, 2006.

> *This case study prepared by the Harvard Business School (HBS) is one of the few HBS case studies about health care and one of the very few about public-sector organizations.*

Kizer KW, Dudley RA. Extreme makeover—Transformation of the Veterans Health Care System. *Ann Rev Public Health* 2009; 30:18.1–18.27.

> *This overview of the transformation provides much objective detail and an extensive bibliography.*

Longman P. *Best Care Anywhere—Why VA Health Care Is Better Than Yours* (2nd ed.). Sausalito, CA: PoliPoint, 2010.

> *This book by an investigative journalist focuses on the role of the VA's electronic health record in facilitating the transformation of VA health care.*

Thibodeau N, Evans JH, Nagarajan NJ, Whittle J. Value creation in public enterprises: An empirical analysis of coordinated organizational changes in the Veterans Health Administration. *Accounting Review* 2007; 82:483–520.

> *Based on data from the initial years of the transformation, this report focuses on the improved economic performance of the system.*

Trevelyan EW. *The Performance Management System of the Veterans Health Administration.* Boston: Harvard School of Public Health, 2002.

> *This report evaluates the new performance management system implemented as part of the transformation.*

Young GJ. Managing organizational transformations: Lessons from the Veterans Health Administration. *California Management Review* 2000; 43:66–82.

> *This critique focuses on the role of leadership in effecting organizational change.*

13

Creating and Sustaining Change

Magda G. Peck

Think back over the major events of the past year or two that had an impact on you as a public health worker. How many major changes occurred?

Did colleagues come or go? Were your duties reassigned? Is a new boss shaking up your world? Within your organization, were there major budget cuts? Were key programs eliminated? Did fresh funding opportunities foster unexpected partnerships? Did you launch a new initiative to promote healthy behaviors and healthier communities?

How about larger forces at work in your community? Did economic hard times push fragile health-related nongovernmental organizations over the edge? Did a new community health center expand access to primary care? Did you experience a major victory on a public policy issue?

Change—for the better and worse—is always occurring. Much of the time it may seem that things are happening *to* you—by forces beyond your control. This does not change the fact that you have an obligation to shape the changes you believe are necessary to promote and protect the public's health. The leader within you needs to seize opportunities and respond effectively. (See Chapter 12.)

You are in the best position to determine what needs to be changed in your world—in response both to threats and opportunities. Tools abound for helping you make that happen. Personality-based assessments, such as the Myers-Briggs, FIRO-B, the Kirton Adaptation Index, and a host of 360-degree profile tools, offer data that describe and help us understand our preferences and styles. Used appropriately and thoughtfully, they can be powerful aids for making changes in ourselves. (See Chapter 10.)

This chapter focuses on working with others to change the influencing factors in your work and in your surroundings. Armed with knowledge, skills, and strategy, you and other public health workers have the collective power to create significant positive change for the greater good. Business leaders consider the missions and values of their businesses, understand surrounding market forces, and then work to increase profit. Your public health mission is about shaping change that yields healthier lives in healthier communities. Your bottom line is striving for the greatest good for the most people. To lead change to protect and promote the health and well-being of populations and communities, you must insist on evidence over opinion and champion social justice for all. To accomplish all this requires major changes.

Making Change Happen for the Public's Health

Your job is difficult because of the inherent complexity of most public health problems. For example, consider the challenge of reducing infant mortality. There are many factors that account for infant mortality, including the preconception health of women, access to quality health care before and during pregnancy as well as during labor and delivery, violence, poverty, and racism. If you want to create and sustain change to reduce infant mortality, you must face all of these challenges— and more. This is the case with most of the complex problems that we tackle: There is no single cause or single solution.

To make change, you cannot act alone. With other public health workers, you must rely on sound practices of communication, cooperation, coordination, and collaboration to align assets and build on shared strengths. You must master the practice of collaborative leadership, creating and fostering mutually beneficial relationships among individuals and organizations to achieve results that would not have occurred as well—or not at all—if you had not worked together. (See Chapter 15.)

For example, assuring the health and well-being of older adults requires strategic cooperation with people in multiple sectors, such as health and human services, housing, transportation, safety, and recreation. Only through effective collaboration can you promote healthy aging and the social inclusion and civic participation of older adults.

In addition to the challenges of complexity and collaboration, creating and sustaining change for the public's health calls for an understanding of the context of change. To be successful, you need to identify and engage diverse *stakeholders*— people and organizations that perceive they have a stake in, or are affected by, the proposed change.[1] There are both internal stakeholders within, and external stakeholders outside of, the organization undergoing change.

As a leader of change, you need to know the perspectives of internal and external stakeholders, and how much they understand and trust what is happening. You need to know how they feel about the change that is proposed or being imposed, and to what extent they are fearful, resistant, or supportive, given potential gains or losses from the change. So, if you are planning to develop school-based health centers in your community, perform a stakeholder analysis to identify, understand, and engage essential supporters as well as potential opponents—a range of people including principals, teachers, parents, clergy, and the media. Ask yourself if inside your organization there is sufficient support for expanding the scope of work, especially if this expansion is not accompanied by adequate new resources. (See Chapter 7.)

As a leader of change, you need to assess the external environment to identify potential opportunities and problem areas that can help or hinder change. Environmental scanning helps identify emerging issues, situations, and potential pitfalls that may affect the situation.[2] You may need to determine (a) anticipated support from the policymakers and the public, (b) current policies and regulations that may affect the situation, or (c) the public reputation and public image of your organization. In the above example on a school-based health center, do state laws or regulations allow such a health center to dispense prescription drugs? How well do public and private insurance plans cover the cost of school-based health care?

Learning from Business Models

Anticipating and managing change well is essential for businesses to increase their bottom-line profits. While public health has an additional "bottom line"— optimal health for everyone, every day, everywhere—we can learn from the business sector about creating and sustaining change successfully. Let's consider a business model for leading change that is timeless to understand why most proactive changes fail—and what you can do to get them to succeed.

John Kotter suggests the following eight stages for leading organizational change:

1. *Create a sense of urgency* based on a compelling reason for changing the way things are at present.
2. *Form a powerful guiding coalition* of people with power and influence who are invested in major change and initiate it.
3. *Create a vision* of what can be possible that does not seem possible at present.
4. To translate this possible vision into reality, *communicate the vision* in terms that inform and inspire everyone. (See Chapter 11.)
5. *Empower everyone to act on the vision* by providing sufficient resources, dedicated time, or relaxed rules.
6. *Plan for and create short-term successes.*
7. Since change initiatives must move beyond projects to have broader systems impact, *consolidate improvements and produce still more change.*
8. To sustain change over time, *institutionalize new approaches.* Your sustaining change requires changing the way work gets done throughout the organization or community.[3]

Kotter's sequential model can be challenging for leading change in public health. When public health works, it is invisible, providing, for example, safe food to eat, clean water to drink, and universal childhood immunization. The public therefore takes public health for granted. Feeling a sense of urgency—as required in Step 1—requires a visible problem or strongly perceived threat. After a century of public health successes, the U.S. public has become complacent. For example, although childhood immunizations were once presumed to be a universal good, immunizing all children for vaccine-preventable illnesses is not universally applied. Parents and physicians who have never seen measles or polio may minimize the importance of having children immunized. Others who doubt the safety of vaccines or erroneously state that their risks outweigh their benefits oppose childhood immunizations. Leaders for change may have a difficult time overcoming these attitudes and beliefs. Ironically, renewed outbreaks of vaccine-preventable childhood diseases, thought to have almost disappeared, are likely to fuel a fresh sense of urgency.

Chronic disease prevention represents additional challenges for leaders of change in public health, in part because adverse effects of unhealthy behaviors or environmental exposures may not manifest for many years into the future.

In Step 2, a guiding coalition must come together to make a compelling case for the need for change. However, public health priorities compete with other societal needs, such as affordable housing and public education. Generating a common vision (Step 3) and speaking as one voice for change (Step 4) may face similar challenges.

Practical frameworks and tools can help bring about sustainable changes for healthier communities by (a) identifying and aligning the right people and perspectives needed to create and support change, (b) assuring organizational and community readiness for enacting change, and (c) understanding the forces required to overcome resistance to change. Let's consider how to apply such frameworks and tools to improve public health.

TOOLS FOR ALIGNING PEOPLE AND PERSPECTIVES

Public health practice is collaborative—people working together for positive change. To be an effective leader for change, you need to know how to bring the right people together with diverse, complementary views to generate evidence and ideas, shape smart strategies, and translate plans into action. One approach for leading change in public health policy[4] defines three interactive components: (a) building a firm knowledge base among partners to design change, (b) formulating a clear social strategy to implement change, and (c) mustering the political will for making durable change—which is often overlooked or underestimated (Fig. 13-1). In other words, align (a) what we all must know with (b) what we must then do together based on what we know, and then (c) get others to do what must be done to get the desired results.

This framework is useful for understanding why things go right and how they can go terribly wrong. Consider the story of a local health department wanting to

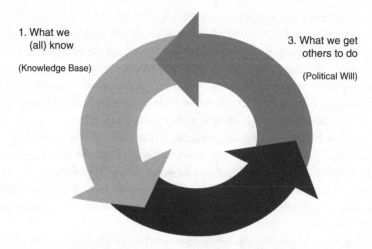

1. What we
   (all) know

(Knowledge Base)

3. What we get
   others to do

(Political Will)

2. What we do, together (Social Strategy)

Figure 13-1 Three essential elements for leading and sustaining change. (Adapted from: Richmond JB, Kotelchuck M. Political influences: Rethinking national health policy. In: McGuire CH, Foley RP, Gorr A, Richards RW, and Associates [Eds.]. *Handbook of Health Professions Education.* San Francisco: Jossey-Bass Publishers, 1983, pp. 386–404.)

work with others to reduce the rate of unintended pregnancy in its community. At that time, about half of all pregnancies had not been planned, timed, or wanted. Rates of unplanned pregnancy were highest among teenagers. Published evidence demonstrated that an effective strategy was increasing access to condoms and other forms of contraception in or near middle schools and high schools, together with programs to build self-esteem among students through after-school community service. The health department received a grant for a comprehensive school-based program to reduce teen pregnancy. However, it had not obtained sufficient support from key individuals and organizations in the community, including some socially conservative groups and some school board members. The headline in the local newspaper was: "Got Pencils? Got Condoms!" This was how some community leaders learned of the program. After contentious public hearings, the boards of several public schools suspended their schools' participation and the program was discontinued. In retrospect, program leaders recognized that having a great knowledge base and a strong social strategy, although necessary, were insufficient to overcome the lack of political will.

Consider another example: a state health department's program to send health tips to parents of newborns. A letter from "Pierre the Pelican" described the importance of breastfeeding and childhood immunizations. Generations of young parents pasted this letter into their children's scrapbooks. But when the program was eventually evaluated, it was found that it did not make a significant difference in parents' knowledge or practices about breastfeeding or immunizations.

Ultimately, the program was discontinued. Tradition (political will) was overridden by a lack of evidence (knowledge base) that it produced the desired results.

In contrast, consider application of the model proactively to design and implement a local ban on smoking in public places. First, local advocates, working in partnership, accumulated local data about knowledge, attitudes, and practices about smoking. They studied the medical and public health literature for evidence-based solutions, and they visited other communities where this policy change was successful. Second, they implemented a social marketing campaign concerning secondhand smoke, working with physicians and hospitals and offering free smoking-cessation services. Third, they built the political will to support a city ordinance by working with owners of theaters, bars, restaurants, and other businesses. Each of these three elements—convincing knowledge, workable programs, and political will—was necessary for transformative change.

Another tool that can help you engage and align the right people to make change happen is the Data To Action (DaTA) Triangle (Fig. 13-2).[5] You can use it to develop team-based work for the public's health.

The three corners of the DaTA Triangle—data, programs, and policy—correspond to three strengths you need for effective change teams. Some public health workers are strong in data and analysis, relying on data and evidence to shape change initiatives. Others, strong in "on-the-ground" field experience, know much about program planning and service delivery. Still others with much policy experience and political savvy have a broad perspective and often are strong in Systems Thinking (see Chapter 12). Each perspective is valid and needed. Yet too often people from each corner of the DaTA Triangle do not understand or appreciate the perspectives of people from the other corners, who are also essential for success. Service providers believe that demands for data and reports are impediments to caring for clients. Data analysts are frustrated by policymakers who misuse their data and service providers who resist collecting it. And policymakers sometimes demand data to prove that their ideas are right.

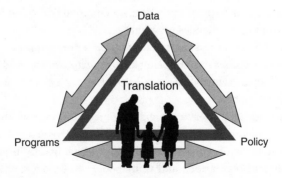

Figure 13-2 The Data To Action (DaTA) Triangle is a tool for aligning people to translate data into action. (Source: CityMatCH [www.citymatch.org])

You can use the DaTA Triangle to strengthen or reconstitute a change team. When you create a team using the DaTA Triangle, the team will have diversity, balance, and interdependence—all of which are keys to successful translation of ideas into action. There is a good probability for achieving desired organizational and systems change when leaders who have expertise in research and data analysis join forces with those who have experience in planning and providing programs and services and those who are policy-oriented and skilled in navigating political situations. Conversely, if one or more of the DaTA Triangle corners is weak or missing, the change process is less likely to succeed.

Another tool-based approach aims to align people to bring about change. Using evidence-based assessment instruments can give you and others information about your own preferences in creating and sustaining change. When diverse people come together to make change happen, by choice or by circumstance, they bring their preferred ways of working that are often well established by personality or habit. Think about the team of people with whom you now work, or when you have been assigned to work on a team to perform work. Have you noticed that some people always seem to want to keep things the ways they are, while others who are dissatisfied with the status quo challenge it? Still others can be relied on to ensure that everyone's perspective is presented. Conflict may arise between people on the team who prefer gradual, incremental change and others who prefer systemic change—between people who relish taking risky steps and others who resist even small changes. When different styles of dealing with change are managed well, the team can be more creative and find greater productivity.

The Change Style Indicator (CSI), a self-assessment instrument designed to capture individual preferences in approaching change, can be used in situations dealing with change.[6] The CSI calibrates *change style*, which can help you increase your flexibility in responding to change and better understand the preferences of others. When you use it in the context of teamwork and collaboration, it can help individuals and the groups in which they participate to better understand dynamics that happen when people with diverse change styles work together. This can be especially useful in public health practice, which requires inclusion and diversity in addressing complex challenges together.

The results of a CSI assessment place you on a continuum of change styles, ranging from being a *Conserver* to being an *Originator*. In the middle of the continuum between these two styles is the *Pragmatist*. Each change style has a set of associated characteristics.

Conservers work to preserve the existing structure of how things are. They prefer gradual, incremental, and continuous change. If you are a conserver, you generally appear to be organized, disciplined, and deliberate in your work. You know the rules and regulations and want people to follow them. For you, the details and facts matter. When faced with change, you strive for efficiency and prefer tested solutions.

Pragmatists tackle problems by practical, reasonable means to get a workable result. They tend to take the middle-of-the-road approach and are open to both sides of an argument. If the existing structure lends itself to getting the work done, fine; if not, they may support greater changes. If you are a pragmatist, you are likely to appear flexible, agreeable, and team-oriented. When working with a team, your broad perspectives may make it harder to commit to a course of action when you are faced with multiple options. Pragmatists can serve as mediators and bridgers between Conservers and Originators, who may be at odds with each other on how to get work done.

Originators can be relied upon to challenge existing assumptions, rules, and structures. They may be viewed as visionary and as promoters of innovation. If you are an Originator, you likely are an eager agent of change willing to set aside the status quo and welcome risk and uncertainty.

Each change style can have strong perceptions of the other styles, which can lead to conflict and dysfunction within teams and organizations. Conservers may seem to others to be cautious, bureaucratic, or traditional, or to hold the group back by sticking to the rules—no matter what. To others, Originators may seem spontaneous, undisciplined, or unorganized, although they know just where to find specific files in their cluttered offices. In their thirst for new ideas, they may seem irreverent toward how things have been done, or advocate change for the sake of change. Conservers may see Originators as being impulsive, starting things they don't finish, or lacking an appreciation of already proven ways. Originators may view Conservers as having their heads in the sand, lacking new ideas, or being stuck in the status quo. While Conservers want to keep things running smoothly and build on what works, Originators are pushing the envelope to pursue new possibilities others have not imagined. And both Conservers and Originators may view Pragmatists as indecisive or noncommittal. Through use of the CSI approach, you can reframe conflict from a position of "right or wrong" to one of differences in perspective and style.[6]

Awareness and understanding of differences in preferences and styles also can translate into better collaboration and more creative solutions. A combination of styles can translate a bold idea into a workable solution with measurable results. A void in any one of these three styles in a team can leave a team stuck. Full of ideas and possibilities, Originators provide inspiration for new initiatives. Full of practicality and energy, Pragmatists are great at turning that new concept into a concrete reality. With their attention to detail and reliable follow-through, Conservers can be relied on to refine the solution and make sure the final product is on time and on target. When the strengths of the each style are appreciated and aligned strategically, major positive change is more likely to be sustained.

The CSI tool can help you better understand your individual and collective contribution to your organization and community. CSI findings, based on individual assessment, can help you identify a preferred work environment in which you can be an effective and valued agent of change.

All three styles have strengths—none is better than another. CSI is not about competence or effectiveness, but about "hard-wired" preferences. Knowing and using your style and the styles of others can help you anticipate common pitfalls and improve change outcomes.

TOOLS FOR ASSESSING READINESS FOR CHANGE

In response to a persistent problem in community health, public health workers and their organizations may choose to adopt practices or policies that have been shown to work. However, all too often they neglect to ask a fundamental question: "How ready are we to seize this opportunity?" In other words, they miss the opportunity to assess their combined readiness for change.

Another practical tool can help you and others assess your combined readiness for change. Readiness Tenting is based on five elements:

1. Partners planning to use new approaches to address a shared public health challenge must articulate, in understandable terms, clear *reasons* for using a specific approach with a specific population at a specific time. Together they must make a unified, compelling case for pursuing the strategy for the desired change.
2. They must describe intended, measurable *results* of changing practices and/or policies.
3. Everyone must agree on the primary *roles and responsibilities* of the people and organizations that will implement the desired programmatic or policy changes.
4. All key people in the change initiative must recognize and accept individual and institutional *risks and rewards* in the proposed activities.
5. There must be adequate human and financial resources, sufficient time, and political will to complete the initiative.[7]

Using a structured tool for community engagement, Readiness Tenting invites self-assessment and collective discussion for each of these five elements. It uses the metaphor of raising a tent. Change team participants first calibrate their individual scores on the strength of each of the elements (1 is very weak; 5 is very strong). After comparing perspectives and interacting among themselves, members of the group agree on a single consensus score for each of the five elements. The tent's shape—revealed by connecting the plotted scores across the tent's five "poles"—describes the readiness status of the group to change. Figure 13-3 shows the ideal readiness tent shape, called "Palladian Power," resulting from the highest possible consensus scores across all five tent poles.

Public health workers sometimes participate in change initiatives in which participants are driven by a common passion for change and willing to take whatever risks are necessary—but little progress is made because there is no clear plan or

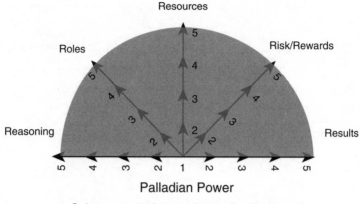

Figure 13-3 Palladian Power.

no expectations. If no additional resources are obtained to fuel the work, the "tent" cannot rise or may have a dysfunctional configuration called a "Balanced Heart" (Fig. 13-4). In this configuration, the change process is inadequately supported by a clear rationale, planning, measurable results, or adequate resources.

Let's examine an alternate scenario. A few talented grant writers or a small group of colleagues submit a well-written proposal for a project to bring about change. If the project gets funded, a variety of busy people have each agreed to work on it for a small percentage of time—but the project is not a priority for any of these people and it does not have a clear leader. The "tent" here is likely to have a "Witch's Hat" configuration (Fig. 13-5): While the grant proposal may seem

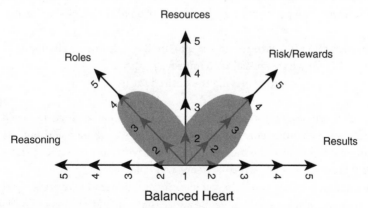

Figure 13-4 Balanced Heart.

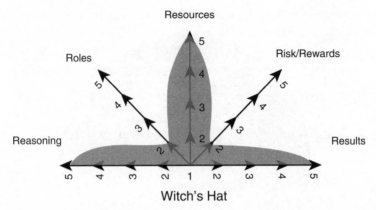

Witch's Hat

Great plan and resources, but who will do the work?

Figure 13-5 Witch's Hat.

impressive, there is inadequate human capital and insufficient institutional buy-in to translate the proposal into action for sustainable change.

TOOLS FOR OVERCOMING RESISTANCE TO CHANGE

As you start any change process, expect that there will be resistance. Some people are satisfied with the current state of affairs. Others believe that change will not improve the situation—or will make it worse. Still others believe that change is not feasible or will cost too much.

To counter resistance, you may want to consider the Change Formula[8]:

$$D \times V \times F > R$$

R stands for Resistance to significant change in policies or programs affecting public health. R can be overcome by a combination of three counterforces:

1. Dissatisfaction (D) with the status quo, fueling a desire for change
2. Vision (V) for what is possible to improve health
3. First steps (F) toward achieving the desired future

Each of these counterforces is necessary to bring about change, but each counterforce alone is insufficient to overcome resistance to change without the other two forces. And because the model is multiplicative, if any one of the three counterforces is absent (equal to zero), change will fail to occur.

The Change Formula can help you identify and understand counterforces that can overcome resistance to change. Be aware that small First Steps (F) are important but are unlikely to grow to scale for larger systems change without fueling sustained Dissatisfaction (D) with how things are. A sufficient number of people have to want to change the status quo. Disseminating compelling reports on a problem or writing an "op-ed" piece for the local newspaper may raise awareness and Dissatisfaction. Accompanying a growing desire for change, there must be a compelling Vision (V) for what can be possible.

Conclusion

Change is difficult. Assessing your organization's readiness and capacity for sustainable and effective change is necessary for success. Measuring progress helps to ensure that partners and others feel that they are on the right path. Change leaders must understand and practice effective strategies and they must also have strong personal resilience to sustain themselves through the journey from the present state to a new future.

References

1. Kee JE, Newcomer K. *Transforming Public and Nonprofit Organizations: Stewardship for Leading Change*. Vienna, VA: Management Concepts, Inc., 2008.
2. Albright KS. Environmental scanning: Radar for success. *Information Management Journal* 2004; 38:38.
3. Kotter J. The eight stage process. In: *Leading Change*. Boston: Harvard Business School Press, 1996, p. 33.
4. Richmond JB, Kotelchuck M. Political influences: Rethinking national health policy. In: McGuire CH, Foley RP, Gorr A, Richards RW, and Associates (Eds.). *Handbook of Health Professions Education*. San Francisco: Jossey-Bass Publishers, 1983, pp. 386–404.
5. CityMatCH. *Data To Action (DaTA) Triangle*. Available at: http://webmedia.unmc.edu/community/ citymatch/CityLights/CLs p00. pdf. Accessed on October 18, 2010.
6. Musselwhite WC, Ingram RP. *Change Style Indicator Facilitator Guide*. Greensboro, NC: Discovery Learning Press, 1995.
7. Peck M (CityMatCH). *Readiness Tenting for Change*. Available at: http://www.citymatch.org/ ppor_how.php. Accessed on October 19, 2010.
8. *Change Equation–Beckhard*. Available at: http://www.valuebasedmanagement.net/methods_ beckhard_change _model.html. Accessed on October 18, 2010.

RESOURCES

Books

Heath C, Heath D. *Switch: How to Change Things When Change Is Hard*. New York: Broadway Books, 2010.

> *Using great stories of people and organizations wanting to make large and small changes happen, this accessible book lays out a three-part framework for making the "switch."*

Kee JE, Newcomer KE. *Transforming Public and Nonprofit Organizations: Stewardship for Leading Change*. Vienna, VA: Management Concepts, 2008.

> *This practical public administration text is designed to assist workers in the public and nonprofit sectors lead change processes for the greater good.*

Kotter J. *Leading Change*. Boston: Harvard Business School Publishing, 1996.

> *This accessible, timeless textbook on the change process is written for the business sector but is applicable to public health practice. It is a primer on why most transformative changes fail, and what leaders can do to increase the odds of success.*

Kotter J, Cohen D. *The Heart of Change*. Boston: Harvard Business School Publishing, 2002.
> *This follow-up book to Leading Change tells the stories of people and companies undergoing transformational changes in the context of Kotter's eight-step approach to change.*

Kotter J. *A Sense of Urgency*. Boston: Harvard Business School Publishing, 2008.
> *This book adds to Kotter's eight-step approach by focusing on the first step: creating a sense of urgency.*

Musselwhite C, with Jones R. *Dangerous Opportunities: Making Change Work*. Bloomington, IN: Xlibris Corporation, 2004.
> *This book, from the founder of Discovery Learning and creator of the Change Style Indicator, shows the reader how to use this tool effectively.*

Assessment Tool

The Change Style Indicator (CSI). A product of Discovery Learning, Greensboro, NC. Available at: http://www.discoverylearning.com. Accessed on July 15, 2011.
> *The Change Style Indicator is administered by a certified trainer. It is used to help individuals assess their Change Styles and use their profiles for being strategic agents for change.*

Tool Kit

The Readiness Tenting Toolkit, www.citymatch.org
> *Developed by CityMatCH founding chief executive officer Magda Peck in 1997, this tool kit for public health action learning collaboratives has helped public health teams navigate the change process.*

Commentary 13-1: Fluoridation: Bringing About and Maintaining Change

Myron Allukian, Jr.

Less pain, less infection, and lower dental bills. About 4 million people on 141 public water systems in Massachusetts are receiving these health and economic benefits of fluoridation. But it wasn't always this way.

In 1967, Massachusetts ranked 48th among the states in percentage of people living in fluoridated communities—only about 8% of its population—compared with 53% for the United States as a whole.[1] The state health commissioner had stated that by, age 13, 99% of children in the state had bad teeth and that 10% of them had never seen a dentist. The average 16-year-old in the state had 15 teeth affected by tooth decay. Only a few communities were fluoridated because fluoridation had been a controversial and political issue in Massachusetts for many years.

The Problem Personified

"TAKE THEM OUT. TAKE THEM ALL OUT!"

These were the cries of a 10-year-old boy with a dental abscess at a community health center. Both of his parents and his 18-year-old brother had no teeth at all. For this family and for this community, dental care was having your infected teeth removed. There had to be a better way.

My colleagues and I performed a needs assessment of adults in this Boston neighborhood and found that half of adults had no upper teeth and one third had no teeth at all. There had to be a better way.

What could we do? There weren't enough dentists in the city or state to treat—or willing to treat—everyone who needed dental care. We needed to focus on prevention. Fluoridation of public water supplies was clearly the answer to prevent future tragedies. Fluoridation is the foundation to better oral health.

From 1957 to 1967, the law in Massachusetts required that people in a given city or town needed to vote, in a public referendum, in favor of fluoridating its water supply before its board of health could order fluoridation. In 1967, a state legislative commission on dental health recommended that this law be changed.

In 1968, we worked with the Massachusetts Citizens' Committee for Dental Health (MCCDH), a group of citizens interested in better dental health, to change the state law so that, on recommendation of the state health commissioner, the board of health of any town could order fluoridation.[2] This order could be halted only if 10% or more of the registered voters of that town signed a petition, within

90 days, requesting a public referendum to determine whether the water supply in that town would be fluoridated. If the public vote was subsequently against fluoridation, it could not be implemented at that time.

THE PLAN

Changing the law took vision, passion, persistence, a well-organized and informed constituency, and much difficult work. Ultimately, we were successful. Once we changed the state fluoridation law, we aimed to get Boston fluoridated. Since its water supply was part of a larger water system of 31 other cities and towns, we realized that a regional approach would be much more cost-effective. We had to develop a plan.[3]

First, we needed to find out whether there was sufficient interest in fluoridation among the 32 communities served by the Metropolitan Water District (MWD) in the Boston area. In early 1969, the MCCDH asked the mayor of Boston to write a letter to the 31 other communities in the MWD to determine their interest in regional fluoridation. When most of the communities demonstrated interest, a joint committee for regional fluoridation was formed. This committee had 16 members, reflecting a wide range of disciplines, including administration, community organization, dentistry, water supply engineering, health education, law, medicine, and public health. We then formed a small working committee to draft a strategy and plans for consideration by the joint committee, which were then implemented. Over a 6-year period, an operational program was developed.

Critical Steps

COMMUNITY PROFILES

For each community in the MWD, we collected information on the child population, current status of fluoridation, and attitudes toward regional action. We identified key people and collected information on the organization of local government. In about half of the communities, there was a favorable attitude toward fluoridation; the response was mixed among the others.

SURVEY

We performed an informal survey based on community questionnaires. We interviewed members of boards of health of all the communities. On fluoridation, 25 of the 31 boards had a favorable position, one was unfavorable, and five had no position. We determined the attitudes of key individuals in these communities.

REGIONAL MEETING

We convened a regional meeting for local health officials and representatives of all 32 communities. Almost all participated. Commissioners of the city and state health departments, representatives of the MWD, the presidents of the Massachusetts Dental Society and the Massachusetts Health Officers Association, and representatives of the MCCDH, the Massachusetts Medical Society, the New England Water Works Association, and the regional office of the then U.S. Department of Health, Education, and Welfare attended—as well as student representatives from each of the three dental schools in Boston. We presented information that demonstrated that half of the many new cavities among children in the area could be prevented through fluoridation—at a savings of approximately $7 million over a 20-year period.

Members of our working committee then encouraged the communities to order fluoridation. In some communities, grassroots support was needed before and after the board of health ordered fluoridation. We undertook an intensive educational and supportive process. Within 4 months after the regional meeting, 27 of the 32 boards of health—representing 91% of the 2 million people in these communities—had ordered fluoridation. In two communities that later held referenda on fluoridation, the fluoridation order was upheld by a ratio of 4 to 1. The orders of the boards of health were uncontested in the other communities. Five communities did not order fluoridation and remained neutral.

Once a majority of the 32 communities had ordered fluoridation, the state health department ordered it for the entire MWD. However, the MWD commissioner did not comply with the order immediately and requested a legal opinion from the state's attorney general. A year later, after a legislative hearing on a bill to require fluoridation for these communities, the attorney general issued a decision that the MWD had to fluoridate the water supply of the 32 towns in the district.

Financing and Legislation

Initially, the MWD commissioner succeeded in getting the state legislature to appropriate $25,000 to finance an engineering feasibility study. Subsequently, a legislative appropriation of $100,000 was made for the design of fluoridation facilities. Later, an appropriation of $1.15 million for construction was authorized by the state legislature. For each of these legislative appropriations, our coalition stimulated strong continuous community support.

Construction and installation of equipment was completed in early 1978. However, under the threat of a preliminary restraining order, the MWD commission voluntarily stopped progress on fluoridation. But, a month later, the county superior court denied the restraining order. Fluoridation was implemented the next day. Within the next 15 days, a dozen anti-fluoridation bills were filed with the state legislature, but all of them were defeated.

Success

As a result of the Greater Boston Area becoming fluoridated, Massachusetts increased its ranking to 24th in the nation in fluoridation status—as half of its population resided in fluoridated communities.

Our work demonstrated that a well-organized interagency program can succeed in eliciting official community support for a regional approach to fluoridation. During the 8-year period of this initiative, at least 70 bills were submitted to the state legislature to block or weaken our fluoridation efforts. All were defeated. And we demonstrated that a regional approach to fluoridation for several municipalities on the same central water supply can be more practical and economical.

The key to the success of our efforts was the collective action and support of a number of public agencies and nonprofit organizations, working together toward a common goal. The support of many dentists and physicians who had provided care for individual legislators and had discussed fluoridation with them was also helpful. We found that there was a significant correlation between (a) a dentist or physician being in favor of fluoridation and having discussed fluoridation with a legislator, and (b) the legislator's support of fluoridation. First-term legislators who lived in fluoridated communities were also more likely to support fluoridation. We concluded that practicing dentists and physicians have a responsibility to educate all of their patients about the benefits of fluoridation, especially patients who are legislators or community decision-makers.[4]

By 2010, almost 4 million residents living in 141 communities in Massachusetts were receiving the health and economic benefits of community water fluoridation. Massachusetts is now 65% fluoridated, compared to 73% for the nation as a whole, and it is ranked 32nd among the states.[5]

Critical to our success was our transformation of the City of Boston's Bureau of Community Dental Programs, beginning in 1970.[6] It provided key leadership in fluoridation and other oral health initiatives. Its basic goal was to improve dental health for the Boston community. It went from a crisis-oriented dental treatment program for children only to a population-based family and neighborhood dental program. Its primary objectives were:

- To provide stimulation, consultation, and expertise for private, voluntary, and public agencies, organizations, and institutions to respond to the dental needs of the Boston community
- To stimulate, develop, implement, support, and evaluate preventive and dental care programs to improve dental health

This dental program became a great resource for Boston and the state by bringing many non-dental organizations and agencies together for a common goal: better oral health.

We found that a well-planned city dental program can have a meaningful impact on the dental health of inner-city communities, as well as improving the accessibility, quality, and scope of dental services provided in these communities. We also found that the program served as a beacon for better oral health for the rest of the state, with a focus on prevention and fluoridation.

The Future

Fluoridation of community water supplies is the foundation to improve the oral health of a community, state, or nation. Additional initiatives and programs must be designed and implemented to build on the benefits of fluoridation in order to:

- Strengthen the dental public health infrastructure
- Improve access to dental care for underserved populations
- Make oral health a much higher priority on the local, state, and national levels to reduce and eliminate disparities in oral health
- Include oral health as a key component of all federally funded health programs
- Promote and use individual and population-based preventive programs and services, such as by providing oral health education in all schools and school-based dental prevention programs in high-risk communities
- Improve the oral health component of Medicaid and Medicare
- Modify and augment the oral health workforce, including training more dentists from minority backgrounds in dentistry and dental public health
- Make dental practice acts less restrictive and more responsive to the needs of the public in such areas as national reciprocity of licensees and expanded duties for dental hygienists and assistants
- Explore new and less-expensive primary dental care models, such as by using dental therapists and advanced dental hygiene practitioners
- Support fluoridation of additional communities—27% of U.S. communities with public water supplies still do not have fluoridation[7]

In conclusion, the key elements in our ability to bring about and sustain change were:

- Assessing community needs and resources
- Defining the problem and developing a cost-effective solution
- Agreeing to a common goal
- Executing an action plan with a well-informed and organized constituency
- Providing guidance
- Being patient, persuasive, and persistent

References

1. Allukian M. Fluoridation—A continual struggle in Massachusetts. *Harvard Dental Alumni Bulletin* 1968; 28:77–80.
2. Hendricks JR, Allukian M. Water fluoridation in Massachusetts: A thirty-year review. *J Mass Dental Soc* 1998; 42:8–17.
3. Allukian M, Steinhurst J, Dunning JM. Community organization and a regional approach to fluoridation of the Greater Boston area. *J Am Dental Assoc* 1981; 104:491–493.
4. Allukian M, Ackerman J, Steinhurst J. Factors that influence the attitudes of first-term Massachusetts legislators toward fluoridation. *J Am Dental Assoc* 1981; 104:494–496.
5. Centers for Disease Control and Prevention. *2008 Water Fluoridation Statistics.* October 22, 2010. Available at: http://www.cdc.gov/fluoridation/statistics/2008stats.htm. Accessed on December 13, 2010.
6. Allukian M. The role of a city dental program in improving the dental health of inner-city communities. *J Public Health Dentistry* 1981; 41:98–102.
7. Allukian M Jr. The neglected epidemic and the Surgeon General's report: A call to action for better oral health. *Am J Public Health* 2008; 98(Suppl 9): S82–S85.

Commentary 13-2: Build the Stomach for the Journey*

Ronald Heifetz, Alexander Grashow, and Martin Linsky

Adaptive work generates what can feel like maddening digressions, detours, and pettiness. People often lose sight of what is truly at stake or resort to creative tactics to maintain equilibrium in the short run. All of this can leave you deeply discouraged or burn you out. You may start questioning whether the whole thing is worth it and be tempted to downgrade your aspiration. You may numb yourself to these frustrations. Or you may decide to throw in the towel. It is hard to stay in the game in the face of hopelessness or despair. But to lead change, you need the ability to operate in despair and keep going. And that calls for building the stomach for the journey.

Building resilience is similar to training for a marathon. You need to start somewhere (for example, running a mile or two each day for a few weeks and then gradually working up to the longer distances). In an organizational context, this kind of training can take the form of staying in a tough conversation longer than you normally would, naming an undiscussable problem facing your team, and not changing the subject at the first sarcastic joke designed to move off the uncomfortable topic.

Marathoners in training use benchmarks. You can track your progress if you have clearly defined short-term goals along the way. Targeting a monthly or quarterly goal that feels realistic may help you build stamina for the long haul. Or bringing warring factions together in the same room for even just a few minutes may be good practice for conducting a longer meeting later.

To further build your stomach for the adaptive leadership journey, keep reminding yourself of your purposes. Runners look forward, not down. Staying focused on the goal ahead will help keep you from becoming preoccupied or overwhelmed by the number of steps necessary to get there.

Early in his career, Alexander and a colleague worked with the New York City Department of Health, assessing the patient-care capacity in all forty-seven of the city's public hospitals and health-care centers. They met with resistance at the first few centers they visited. Uncooperative managers refused to supply the necessary data because they were anxious that they would not come out looking good. After these visits, Alexander and his colleague were exhausted. To stay in the game, the two of them made a decision: after each subsequent visit, they would

* Excerpted from Heifetz R, Grashow A, Linsky M. *The Practice of Adaptive Leadership: Tools and Tactics for Changing Your Organization and the World*. Boston: Harvard Business Press, 2009, pp. 260–262.

spend time together reminding themselves of their long-term goals and eating a healthy lunch rather than comfort food to keep their spirits up.

Building a strong stomach requires relentlessness. You probably have a limit to how hard you are willing to push an initiative forward. If opponents of your intervention sense that limit, they will know exactly how hard they have to resist. One of the best practitioners of leadership we know used to say at the beginning of tough meetings when everyone knew this was going to be a difficult conversation, "I am willing to stay in this meeting as long as necessary." As soon as he indicated that he was there for however long it would take, people for whom the issue was not such a high priority would begin to back away rather than stall or sabotage the discussion. He would then be that much closer to getting the needed work done.

Leading adaptive change will almost certainly test the limits of your patience. Even after you have accomplished a lot—for example, increased market share, built more low-income housing, or put your issue on the top team's agenda for the first time—you might well find yourself having trouble celebrating that progress because you know how much more work remains to be done.

Impatience can hurt you in numerous ways. You raise a tough question at a meeting and do not get an immediate response. So you jump right back in and keep pounding on the question. Each time you pound, you send the message that you are the only person responsible for that question. You own it. And the more you pound away, the less willing people are to share ownership of the question themselves. And if they do not feel any ownership of the question, they will have less investment in whatever the resolution turns out to be.

Where are you supposed to find the patience when there is such a long way to go on the issues for which you feel so strongly? You can find patience by tapping into your ability to feel compassion for others involved in the change effort. Compassion comes from understanding other people's dilemma, being aware of how much you are asking of them. Your awareness of their potential losses will calm you down and give you patience as they travel a journey that may be more difficult for them than it is for you.

14

Facilitating Negotiation and Mediation

Giorgio A. Piccagli

This chapter focuses on basic principles of negotiation and mediation and their application. *Negotiation* is a process of working with others to reach an agreement. *Mediation* is facilitated negotiation. Negotiation and mediation may involve conflict resolution, deal-making, or complex problem-solving among parties with differing viewpoints, positions, or interests.

The first part of this chapter focuses on two-party negotiation, although the principles can be applied to multi-party negotiations. The second part focuses on multi-party mediation, although the principles can be applied to mediation between two parties.

Negotiation, mediation, arbitration,* and litigation** fall on a continuum of self-determination and cost. As you move from negotiation to litigation, costs generally increase, and self-determination and the ability to tailor solutions to specific problems without affecting other issues decline.

Negotiation

Consider the following situation:

> You and your boss are in a tug-of-war with a rope, and you are bigger and stronger. The winner will get 10 points for every 6 inches that the rope's center marker is on that person's side after 3 minutes. The loser will lose an equal number of points. Everyone in your office is looking on. What do you do?

---

* Arbitration is defined as "the process by which parties to a dispute submit their differences to the judgment of an impartial person or group." (www.thefreedictionary.com)

** Litigation is "the act or process of bringing or contesting a legal action in court." (www.thefreedictionary.com)

Many people see negotiation as a tug-of-war—not comfortable. It is positional—it proceeds by taking and abandoning a series of positions before settling. It is a "zero–sum" game: What you win, the other person loses. Even worse, it pits results against relationship. If you win, you may harm your relationship with your boss; if you lose on purpose, you may harm your reputation with your co-workers—and your boss. Seeing negotiation as a tug-of-war may link your self-concept to the outcome.

There is an alternative form of negotiation—one that builds relationships, models cooperative behavior, and produces custom solutions. In some cases, it provides unexpected value for both sides—a "win–win" solution. It is especially suited to evidence-based public health practice in a complex environment.

This alternative is *interest-based negotiation*—also called *integrative negotiation*. It proceeds very differently than positional negotiation proceeds; it aims to jointly satisfy the interests of multiple parties and works by examining issues from the perspectives of all involved parties.

Interest-based negotiation differs not only from positional negotiation, but also from distributive negotiation, whose purpose is to distribute a fixed value: How shall we split this $100? Interest-based negotiation can generate more value for the involved parties than simply splitting the money.

Interest-based negotiation also differs from two other ways to resolve differences and conflicts: the use of power and the assertion of rights, the law.

Interest-based negotiation does not guarantee success. Like any tool, it is more suited to certain types of problems than others. Used properly and skillfully, however, interest-based negotiation holds the promise of creating more value for more parties, in less time, and less expensively, than many alternatives.

Interest-based negotiation is built around three core concepts:

1. Establishing a collaborative frame
2. Focusing on interests—not positions
3. Communicating effectively

Three additional factors enhance the likelihood of successful outcomes: goals, relationships, and leverage.

CORE CONCEPT #1: ESTABLISHING A COLLABORATIVE FRAME

In our interdependent world, with incompletely specified problems, missing information, and ambiguous situations, adopting and communicating a collaborative frame is extremely valuable. Are you and others competitors or collaborators? Are your interests aligned or opposed? Very often, the answer to these two questions is: "Both." Focusing on the collaborative elements helps address even the competitive elements of a situation.

Regulatory agencies may be mandated to protect a population, but also to facilitate the success of those who are regulated. Similarly, those who are regulated ideally have an interest in the safety of customers, employees, or neighbors. Both groups may have an interest in a healthy, educated, and employed population. When you recognize both common and divergent interests, you are more likely to open avenues for collaboration.

Adopting a collaborative frame does not mean surrendering your responsibilities or interests to the other party. It means finding and communicating a way to work together in addressing what is likely a jointly owned problem. It is an active choice—not simply the passive recognition of the nature of the situation.

Approaching negotiation with a collaborative orientation can help to:

- Communicate that collaborative frame, possibly transforming a "zero–sum" game to a "win-win" situation
- Find joint interests, possibly leading to generation of unexpected value
- Find ways to work together during difficult times
- Generate a more complete understanding of the multiple aspects of issues
- Generate a fuller set of corrective options

Your abilities to perceive the interdependence of the involved parties and to effectively signal a willingness to collaborate are major determinants of the conduct of a negotiation and its outcomes. You can do this best by focusing on interests—not positions—and by listening in order to understand.

Collaboration, Agreement, and Shared Values

Do not operate from the assumption that you can collaborate only with people who hold the same values as you do. Similar values are neither necessary nor sufficient for agreement or collaboration. In fact, sometimes shared values lead to conflict, as when multiple parties value the same thing and compete to control it. And having different values—or different valuation of the same object—is sometimes essential to agreement and collaboration (Box 14-1).

Another useful approach is to contextualize a limited disagreement within a larger scope of agreements. Listing the areas on which the disagreeing parties agree can moderate a disagreement, thereby (a) reducing the likelihood of seeing the other party as an enemy, and (b) increasing the possibility that each party will come to see the other as an essential partner in solving a shared problem.

People who disagree about a position often have the same goals, but different ways of achieving them. In the debate on gun control, both sides are concerned with freedom and physical security, but each side sees threats to freedom and security differently. Transforming these two sides from seeing the other as the problem to seeing themselves as collaborators in solving a jointly owned problem is very helpful in achieving resolution. This transformation in relationship should

---

Box 14-1: **The Orange**

Two parties each need a whole orange. Neither one has use for half of it. Only one orange is available. Who will have it?

Splitting the orange will satisfy no one's needs. The two parties could compete for the orange (power), or they could explore who has a stronger claim to it (rights).

Alternatively, they could discuss the situation, finding out in the process that one needs the flesh of the orange to make a glass of juice, and the other needs its rind to make a cake. By indicating their needs and specifying the parts of the contested orange necessary to meet these needs, both parties can be satisfied.

This resolution depends on the two parties having different needs (interests) and different valuations (the peel is of no value to one, the flesh to the other)—and on the exchange of information. Counter to our tendency to simplify, this negotiation and others depends on "complexification" of the orange—a recognition that the whole has different parts and that each may be valued differently. Recognition of such differences can occur with many objects of a negotiation and can help lead to agreement.

---

precede a search for solutions to identified problems. Proposed solutions will less likely be rejected by the other party after the transformation, making agreement more likely to be reached and implemented.

Building the Habit of Agreement

Often, negotiating parties will be negotiating not only the primary issue, but also the negotiating procedures. If the parties cannot reach agreement on the primary issue, they should try to find something—anything—on which they agree, such as the shape of the negotiating table, the schedule of negotiation sessions, or simply that the issue is of concern to both parties. That agreement—however trivial—can become the starting point for other agreements, including an agreement on the primary issue.

CORE CONCEPT #2: FOCUSING ON INTERESTS—NOT POSITIONS

Two people are in a library; one is seated at a table in front of a closed window. The second person approaches and says, "Excuse me. I'd like the window open." The first person replies, "I want it closed." The second replies, "Open." Back and forth they go: "Closed . . . Open . . . Closed . . . Open . . . ."

How will they get beyond this impasse? By a battle of wills? By checking the library regulations? They can do so by finding out how both of them can be satisfied. That is easier to accomplish when information on interests is exchanged—"I want fresh air." "I want to avoid a draft."—then checking for options that satisfy the interests of both of them. Looking around, they see two possible solutions: (a) They can leave the window closed, but open a door that does not create a draft. Or, (b) the first person can move to another seat—out of the draft created by opening the window—and the second person can sit in front of the window. Notice, however, each person must be willing to collaborate with the other to reach this resolution.

Wanting the window open or closed is a position—a desire to achieve a certain end. Focusing the disagreement on these positions frames it as "win–lose" situation and creates an impasse. A desire to have fresh air and a desire to avoid a draft are interests, narrowly defined. A desire to be physically comfortable is a broader definition of the same interest—a framing that can lead to an agreement. In this framing, the similarity between the parties is highlighted: "We are alike, we want the same thing." The previous framing "fresh air" or "no draft" defines what the larger interest means to each person—specifying needs to be satisfied for them to agree.

Once the two people jointly owned the problem and identified a shared desire for physical comfort, they recognized possible solutions that could satisfy them both.

We often analyze a situation based on our outlook—influenced by many factors, such as experiences, values, inclinations, and roles. We then decide what we think must be done and try to convince others to do it. In contrast, interest-based negotiation is based on the parties *jointly* defining, analyzing, and solving a problem. Many institutions and systems are based on both positional and adversarial processes. Positional processes, whether initially adversary or not, tend to inject or exacerbate adversary elements and yield suboptimal results. A position is often the means to accomplish an end. And the end is often the satisfaction of an unstated need or interest.

Interest-based negotiation is designed to minimize or eliminate the following four characteristics of positional negotiation:

- It is adversarial and polarizing.
- It obscures information or supports misinformation.
- It generates suboptimal solutions.
- It obscures the agreement underlying the disagreement.

Interest-based negotiation functions by highlighting underlying common interests and using them as a pathway to agreement. Discussion to understand the issues of both parties, in the context of a collaborative frame, increases the likelihood of actions that satisfy these interests. As in the library example, parties to a dispute may share the same interest, but define it in different ways or focus on different aspects of it.

Disputes are often presented in a positional form: "We should undertake Action X." "No, we should undertake Action Y." Disputes are difficult to resolve in this form. So, how do you get parties in a dispute to retreat from their positions to their needs?

Here are a few ways for you to accomplish this:

- *Ask, "Why?"*: When presented with a demand for action, ask for the reason behind it. But beware: This can be interpreted as a demand for justification and can exacerbate the dispute.
- *Ask for the consequences*: "What would that allow you do?" By asking for the consequence—rather than the cause—of a request, you may discover a party's interest in a less threatening way.
- *Disclose your interest and ask the other party or parties to disclose their interests*: Disclose and then count on reciprocity. "I'll show you mine, if you show me yours."

Don't limit your discovery work to what can be done at the negotiating table. If an issue has media or industry attention, review media reports or industry "in-house" reports to better understand the concerns of the negotiating parties and others, and how organizational and financial factors may be affecting these concerns. If you know one of the parties or know others who do, speak with them away from the negotiation table—where they may be more open to discussing their concerns and interests.

Types of Interests

There are three types of interests:

- Psychological, related to the people who are negotiating
- Substantive, related to the issue at hand
- Procedural, related to how things are done.

Look beyond the issue being negotiated. One party may have interests that arise from the individual negotiator's concerns or that are related to how he or she will negotiate. For example, a wage dispute between union and management—in addition to addressing financial issues—may involve the need of the union negotiators or the management negotiators to appear strong to their members or superiors. These interests are not extraneous distractions to be pushed aside. As a negotiator or a facilitator of a negotiation, explore ways of satisfying the psychological as well as the substantive needs of each side. These needs might include the need for both sides to show themselves to be able leaders, tough negotiators undeterred by the other side, or champions for their members or shareholders.

Psychological and procedural interests provide opportunities for negotiators to (a) demonstrate an understanding of the interests of the other party and a willingness to collaborate, and (b) provide a first agreement in the negotiation, as the following real-world example illustrates.

> During the 1982 disarmament talks between the United States and the Soviet Union on weapons to destroy and procedures for verification—a positional discussion—the two sides were stalemated. Then the chief negotiators went for a walk in the woods. They ended up talking about their hopes and fears for their grandchildren and their countries, and what the world would be like with an agreement and without it. When they returned to the negotiating table, they created a draft agreement based on this shared vision of the future. (Unfortunately, this agreement was not subsequently ratified by their governments.)

Like the library example, this negotiation started off positionally. The discussion about grandchildren, while personal and "off topic," enabled the negotiators to get out of their roles as representatives of opposing countries and identify shared psychological interests. The conversation transformed their relationship to one of grandparents with similar concerns. And it allowed them to discover, highlight, and adopt a collaborative frame. After this transformation and adoption of a collaborative frame, they developed an agreement.

Note another important shift that happened during the walk. Rather than debating how they would reduce stockpiles or production from the present situation, they discovered a jointly desired future and generated options in that context. Rather than competing with changes from the present, they collaborated in building a future—a jointly desired future. Their physical activity, their side-by-side position, and their distancing themselves from the negotiating table helped them to reach agreement. Personal relationship, established either before or during a negotiation, increases the likelihood of reaching agreement.

The failure of the U.S. and Soviet governments to ratify the draft agreement, however, highlights the importance of having decision-making authority at the negotiating table or taking steps to bring decision-makers to support a draft agreement—especially when they have not directly experienced the transformative dynamic of a negotiation.

The range and scope of public health practice disciplines and settings make it hard to identify interests in a particular negotiation in advance. It is not unusual, however, to be able to predict that interests will involve scientific evidence, health and safety, and social justice. Issues in negotiation often point to interests relating to finance, independence and freedom, security, reputation, and respect; these are interests of both individuals and organizations.

CORE CONCEPT #3: COMMUNICATE EFFECTIVELY

Communicating effectively means communicating your interests and a collaborative frame, avoiding unnecessary conflict, and understanding the interests of the other party or parties.

State Your Interests

Successful negotiation depends on the free flow of information. Each side should provide and elicit information—and avoid erecting barriers to the flow of information. This does not mean that negotiators should immediately "show all their cards." But negotiations often fail to generate results because one or both parties have withheld important information.

If distrust exists among negotiators, disclosure should occur cautiously, with each side gauging the trustworthiness of the other by how they treat disclosures—whether they reciprocate with their own disclosures or try to use the initial disclosure against the disclosing party. Negotiators should determine what information they need to give, to get, and to guard. Each should seek out and recognize relevant information, disclose it, and avoid unnecessary barriers to the flow of information. It is difficult for parties to participate in meeting the other's needs if they do not know what these needs are or do not understand them.

Avoid Unnecessary Conflict

Since parties need to feel comfortable with providing information, avoid unnecessary conflict and its chilling effect. Careful choice of language can help avoid unnecessary conflict. Appropriate framing of a situation can facilitate the flow of information. Following are some useful ways to do this.

- _Separate people from the problem, and intent from effects. Use contributory language—not responsibility language_. Just as medicines have side effects, policies have unintended consequences. In facilitating negotiation, separate effects from intents—do not infer intents from effects. Do not use responsibility language, such as, "You are responsible for these consequences." Use contributory language instead: "These actions contribute to these consequences." Contributory language is generally more reflective of a multi-causal reality and less likely to put the other party on the defensive, opening the conversation to the search for other contributions. Some contributions may lie in the parties' actions and some in external factors. Parties who realize the multiple contributions—including their own—to an undesired situation may transform from adversaries to collaborators.
- _Use depersonalizing language_. Reframing a situation into depersonalizing language is helpful—such as from "The situation your actions support. . ." to "The situation we both face. . . ." This reframing does not attribute intent or blame the other party. However, it acknowledges that the situation needs to be altered.

- *"Help me understand."* When feeling the urge to ask, "How can you possibly think X?" consider saying instead, "Help me understand your view on that."

All of these features—not inferring intent, not attributing responsibility, and not identifying the other party with the situation—make it easier for both parties to look at the situation without defensiveness, guilt, or loss of face. These steps are easier when practiced without pressure. Some good advice: Adopting some of these reframing practices in everyday activities will make it easier for you to use them under pressure of negotiations.

Actively Listen for Understanding

Recognizing information when it is provided is a challenge, especially under stress. You should explicitly confirm your understanding. The following example illustrates this point.

> A Jesuit seminarian was taking a 4-hour oral exam in theology, administered by an elderly priest. As the seminarian answered the priest's questions, he was encouraged by the priest frequently nodding his head affirmatively. At the end of the exam, the priest informed the seminarian that he had failed the exam.
> "How could that be, father?" asked the seminarian. "Throughout the exam, you were nodding up and down."
> The priest responded, "I wanted to let you know that I could hear you."

There can be great differences between what you *think* you say and what you *actually* say—and among what speakers want to say, think they said, actually said, and what you heard. To bridge these differences, you need to employ *active listening*, also known as empathic listening or assertive listening. You can use the following four techniques to ensure that all parties have heard and have understand the same thing:

1. *Listen for understanding.* Think back to when another person was talking. Were you listening to understand his or her points or were you thinking of how you could respond to them? Psychological noise consists of our internal conversations that impede our ability to hear and understand what another person is saying. If you do not understand the concerns of the other party, you cannot address or satisfy them.
2. *Manage the noise.* You cannot eliminate your concerns about your performance or your judgments about other parties—your noise—but you can learn to manage them. Know they are there. Acknowledge them. Do not let them build up. And return to listening.
3. *Reflect facts, feelings, and concerns.* In negotiation, reflection is critical to success. Reflect—repeat what you have heard—about the other party's interests and

concerns and the strength of these interests and concerns. Restate what the other person has said without any processing—without judgment, agreement, or argument. Said one negotiator, "When I heard the other party repeat our points, I knew we could deal." Understanding the other party or restating the other party's position does not mean you are agreeing with that person.

4. *Seek verification or clarification*. This avoids what happened in the example of the oral exam in theology—a misunderstanding. If you simply ask, "Do I have that right?" after a reflection, the other party's response will provide verification or clarification. A clarification may deepen everyone's understanding. Your attempt to understand will be appreciated and will likely lead to a reciprocal attempt to understand and clarify your interests, concerns, and feelings.

A former prosecutor, who now teaches negotiation to law students, found that his best interrogators were not the meanest or cruelest or the best questioners—but rather the best listeners. They heard hesitations or other clues that led them to new revelations. Similarly, the U.S. military has found that the most effective interrogators are those who are most perceptive, who can read subtle signs in the answers and behaviors of those being questioned—not the harshest or most cruel.

Significant meaning is communicated not only through words, but also through tone and expression, especially when emotional subjects are being discussed and there is conflict between what one is saying and what one is feeling. Do not limit your active listening to spoken words. Enlarge it to include perception more generally. Do not focus only on what someone is saying. Look for other cues, especially in emotional situations. As Yogi Berra said, "You can observe a lot just by watching."

A PROCESS FOR APPLYING THE CORE CONCEPTS

You can use a simple, flexible four-phase process for negotiation, conflict resolution, and multidimensional problem-solving. It can be used in two-party and multi-party negotiations—both formal and informal negotiations. The basic process has the following four phases.

Phase 1: Identify Interests and Generate an Agenda for the Negotiation Structured Around These Interests

State your interests. Identify the other party's interests. Listen and reflect, verify and clarify. Model a collaborative frame by avoiding unnecessary conflict, using depersonalized language, and separating people from the problem. Create two lists of interests, your own and the other party's. Based on these lists, identify common and disparate interests. These two lists of interests will form the agenda for the rest of the negotiation. While there is no limit to the number of interests involved, it is often useful to identify the top three or four interests for the parties and to proceed on these interests.

Phase 2: Generate New Understanding — Discuss These Interests

Choose a common interest and explore it. This choice needs to be strategic. Sometimes it is best to choose an interest that appears simplest and sometimes one that appears most important. Understand what this interest means to the other party, and help the other party understand what it means to you. Listen actively. During this exchange, parties are likely to experience "Aha!" moments—new discoveries, different understandings. When you are done with one interest, move on to another one—ultimately discussing all interests to the satisfaction of each party. Avoid jumping to "solutions" during this process, as the "solutions" may be suboptimal—satisfying one party more than another, or satisfying one set of interests more than others. If a suggestion arises, say, "Thank you, I've made a note of that so we can revisit it when we are ready to look at solutions."

Phase 3: Generate Options — Brainstorm How to Address Interests, Not Positions

Generate ideas. Do not evaluate. Build on suggestions made by the other party to make them more useful. Do not self-censor—"off-the-wall" ideas may open up new possibilities. Suggest ideas to satisfy your interests as well as those of the other party. Making suggestions that satisfy the other party's interests is a powerful way of opening up new possibilities.

Phase 4: Select Options That Best Satisfy Interests and Record Agreements

Develop objective criteria for selecting the best options generated in the previous phase. And then apply them. Discuss remaining options and identify needs for research. Model a collaborative frame through active listening.

Flexibility of Process

This process does not proceed in a rigid lockstep order. Especially in negotiations you do not control, you may choose to do one of the following:

- Enter negotiation in a positional manner, as in the library example. Move to discover the interests behind those positions.
- Begin the negotiation with an extensive discussion of a specific interest. Return later to identify the other interests.
- Find any previously unrecognized interest as it emerges and add it to the agenda.

You may find yourself in an unstructured negotiation—one that does not proceed naturally or by design according to the above phases. Especially if you do not control the negotiation, consider using "organizing moves," such as (a) regularly indicating your sense of where the discussion stands, (b) pointing out how the issue being discussed relates to the larger task, (c) summarizing parts of the conversation, (d) clarifying points that may be unclear, and (e) modifying the list of interests.

Timing the Discussion of Potential Solutions

Timing of suggested solutions is critical. Too early is likely to lead to a positional negotiation, contrary to the goal of interest-based negotiation. Before establishing a working relationship, one party's suggestion of a potential solution is likely to be rejected—in a process called "reactive devaluation." Delaying the search for potential solutions to better understand the full nature of the problem enhances the likelihood of an agreement and its value.

Modifying the Process of Negotiation for Conflict Resolution

The process of negotiating for conflict resolution is not different from negotiating for making a deal, but the point of entry into the process is different.

In the absence of conflict, negotiation begins with identification and discussion of concerns, desires, objectives, and interests. In the presence of conflict, negotiation likely begins with identification and discussion of grievances. While the grievances may be in the past, their resolution—especially when the parties have an ongoing relationship—lies in building a jointly desired future, as in the walk in the woods by the U.S. and Soviet negotiators. Listen to the grievances and identify underlying interests by reframing the grievance and using other techniques discussed earlier.

Multiple Parties

Collaborative arrangements (see Chapter 15) and community-based planning are public health activities likely to bring together more than two parties. In these situations, a facilitator is likely to be especially useful. The first phase is likely to be longer, with each party stating its interests or concerns before additional work is done. The second and subsequent phases become more challenging, given the need to reach agreement among multiple parties. (Multi-party approaches are discussed in greater detail in the section on mediation that follows.)

OTHER SUCCESS FACTORS

Three additional factors can improve your success in negotiation: clear goals, relationships, and leverage.

Clear Goals

Identify clear goals before a negotiation begins because they profoundly affect the entire negotiation. Clear goals define what you want, such as guidelines, joint action, risk reduction, a partnership, or a contract. They provide a beacon to guide your negotiation. Clear goals also form the basis for determining if the negotiation has been successful. An agreement that does not address the issues is not helpful. The purpose of a negotiation is not to come to agreement or to gain concessions from the other party, but rather to satisfy the interests of both parties. Ambitious goals can energize, motivate, and sharpen one's imagination—making both parties analyze and negotiate more effectively.

Relationships

The nature of a relationship not only affects the response to a request or result of a negotiation, but also determines whether you will accept the request or participate in negotiation. Relations can change the frame from competitive to collaborative. Imagine your reaction when a person—someone you do not know, find irritating, or expect never to deal with again—asks you to do something you do not want to do. Now imagine your reaction to the same request from a valued colleague, friend, or someone with whom you have a continuing relationship. You will likely dismiss the first request and comply with the second— or work to modify it into a request that satisfies the other party and is acceptable to you.

Working relationships are also important at the negotiation table to continue the discussion, to get past challenging phases, and to generate results. Whether or not you have a prior relationship, you can generate and strengthen a working relationship at the negotiation table with small steps, such as favors, disclosures, or concessions. Active listening helps identify opportunities to take these strengthening steps.

Leverage

A lever is a simple machine used to multiply power. *Leverage* is a way of achieving an objective, such as moving a party, by augmenting the resources you have. There are three kinds of leverage:

> *Positive leverage* is the power to give the other party something it wants: "Eat your spinach and you can have some ice cream."
> *Negative leverage* is the power to withhold something the other party wants: "If you don't eat your spinach, no ice cream for you."
> *Normative leverage* is justifying the action you want taken on the basis of either societal or group norms or the other party's goals or interests: "You said you wanted to be strong; eat your spinach and you will be."

Of these three, normative leverage is the strongest in getting parties to move. Normative leverage is giving the other party reason to do what you want by showing that it is in line with his or her stated interests and values.

THE BEST ALTERNATIVE TO A NEGOTIATED AGREEMENT (BATNA) AND ITS USES

Getting Parties to the Negotiating Table and Keeping Them There

Interest-based negotiation is not the only way to deal with a difference between parties. A party could go to the legislature and lobby for a law limiting your activity in a certain area, or conduct a media campaign against your activity. These avenues are also available to you and can be powerful adjuncts to your work at the negotiation table. What would lead the other party to negotiate with you instead of following other options?

One way to answer this question is to look at the *Best Alternative to a Negotiated Agreement (BATNA)*. In a simple system, no party would accept a negotiated agreement worse than the BATNA. Why would a vendor accept a 50-cent unit price at the negotiation table when she can get $1 with certainty elsewhere? But public health issues are usually complex and incompletely defined, and have multiple possible outcomes—not a single, certain one.

If the negotiators from the other party indicate they have no incentive to negotiate because they have better payoffs elsewhere (a higher BATNA), engage them in a discussion of the probability of achieving their BATNA: "In what proportion of cases was that BATNA reached? What were the circumstances that led to it? Do these circumstances apply in the current situation? What were the costs involved?"

The discussion arising from answers to the questions should lead to an estimate of the *Most Likely Alternative to a Negotiated Agreement (MLATNA)*, which is the appropriate comparison to a negotiated agreement—not the BATNA, with its low probability.

The other party's estimate of its BATNA may be too high, and a discussion may help the negotiators realize it. Or its BATNA may be correct, and you may wish to take steps to worsen it. Legislative action, a media information campaign, and other enforcement actions may worsen the other party's BATNA and lead it to find negotiation advantageous. Sometimes if you give a credible indication of your likely action to lower the other party's BATNA, it is sufficient to get them to the negotiating table.

Mediation

Mediation is facilitated negotiation. In addition to the parties, there is a facilitator—a mediator who assists the parties in exploring the issues and in coming to an agreement. This section pertains to mediation among more than two parties, which can become complex. However, the principles are the same if there are only two parties.

Given the increasingly interdisciplinary nature of work in public health, you may be called upon to participate in or even lead a mediation or group problem-solving process. As a party to mediation, you can use the processes, core concepts, and additional success factors for negotiation that were discussed earlier. Experienced mediators often follow a process similar to the four-phase process described for negotiation. You can assist the mediator by engaging in *organizing moves* during the mediation (described earlier), even if the mediator does not.

FACILITATING THE MEDIATION

Professional mediators are bound to neutrality, not favoring one side or the other, and are often also bound to avoid substantive contributions—focusing instead on creating and managing the process to elicit the parties' concerns and ideas. Your neutrality is especially important in conflict resolution. As a public health worker involved in multi-party mediation, you might not be in a position to give up substantive contributions. In fact, you may find that one of the most useful roles you can play is to focus the discussions on health effects—and even provide your technical expertise to the discussions of the possible effects of various courses of action. Whatever approach you take, a discussion of your role early on is helpful in avoiding later misunderstandings.

However you deal with neutrality, two approaches will be helpful. First, raise a topic by asking a question of the group rather than making an assertion: "Do we have a clear idea of the effect of action X?" or "Is anyone concerned that action X will lead to Y?," rather than "But that is going to result in Z." Second, make the group responsible for the answers, rather than assuming that responsibility yourself. For example, the group may discuss options whose consequences are not well known or are controversial. Rather than taking on the responsibility for researching these consequences, you can assist the group in determining these consequences by drawing on the expertise and work of group members. This process involves your organizing, facilitating, and managing a common effort.

Good organization of the mediation is critical because the parties often do not know each other, operate in different fields, represent different organizations, and have different priorities, professional associations, and directives. In multi-party mediation, you should check in periodically with all parties to find out what each party's concerns are and to get a sense of how and where the process is going.

In your role as facilitator, you do not have command and control and often have to act by suggestion or influence. With major responsibilities for communication among parties, your role makes you "Listener-in-Chief."

MEDIATION PHASES: USEFUL ACTIONS

The following are actions that can be especially useful to you in your role as mediator. The basic principles of negotiation also apply.

Before the Start

If time allows, talk to all participants individually, clarifying the purpose of the meeting, answering questions, and soliciting their concerns about substance and process.

Opening Statement

After parties introduce themselves, make a statement about the purpose of the mediation, summarizing the concerns you have heard (if appropriate) and indicating your role. Involve the group in creating or approving ground rules for the mediation, rather than your imposing them.

Work groups are often formed to plan *how* to proceed (implementation planning)—not *what* to do. Clarify any constraints on the mediation. For example, certain courses of action may not be possible, perhaps for financial or legal reasons, or because prior decisions cannot be altered.

As facilitator, you can help the group understand that the time spent in setting up the process for mediation is probably more productive than the time spent trying to resolve a stalled mediation.

Phase 1: Solicit Concerns

Invite all participants to state their concerns, such as achieving specific results or avoiding particular adverse effects—going in order of how people are seated. Give each participant the option to defer speaking until later. Enable all participants—each with a different perspective and style—to participate, not just the dominant ones.

Record, verify, and clarify. As participants speak, record their main points. Listen for underlying interests, common themes, and significant differences. Clarify and accurately summarize what has been said. Solicit their verification or clarification of your summaries. Using flip charts or other tools can enable all participants to clearly review the evolution of the discussion and actively participate. In many situations, it may be best for you to ask someone else to be the recorder.

The preliminary discussion may trigger additional thoughts from the participants. Solicit them.

Remind participants that you are now only collecting concerns, not discussing them yet.

Next, consolidate the participants' comments, linking comments to concerns, which will serve as an agenda for later discussion. This will allow participants to see that they have been included and where their comments fit in the bigger picture. It also begins to demonstrate shared concerns. Invite verification and clarification.

Phase 2: Facilitate the Information-Gathering and Information-Sharing

Lead the group in discussing each item.

Phase 3: Facilitate the Brainstorming

When all topics have been discussed, ask the group to brainstorm approaches to resolving each issue. Keep the discussion wide open. Do not allow participants to make analyses of others' statements.

Phase 4: Lead the Selection of Criteria and Their Application

Lead the group in addressing how participants will choose from among the many options suggested. Ask which approaches are consistent with the objectives and concerns that formed the agenda. Determine if there is (a) information from evaluation of similar approaches, (b) professional standards, and/or (c) relevant scientific findings. Consider the cost and effectiveness of various options.

Record the agreement, including next steps, dates, and parties responsible.

Do not be surprised if this stage reveals differences among participants' preferences for different approaches, and even among participants' perceptions of facts about various approaches. Discuss these differences. And test participants' perceptions and beliefs against objective standards, which will likely increase the commitment of group members to the eventual decision.

In any multi-party mediation, expect differences at every step: (a) in the definition of the problem, (b) in the selection of information to examine, (c) in the interpretation of data, (d) in the selection of appropriate actions, and (e) in assessing the results of the action chosen. Each difference provides an opportunity for more complete understanding of the situation and a negotiated consensus.

USEFUL FACILITATION PRACTICES

During the second and subsequent phases, you can help the group significantly by engaging in the following activities:

- *Organizing and mapping ("You are here")*: A complex conversation among multiple parties may lose its focus as it develops. This makes your use of the organizing moves mentioned in the section on negotiation even more important: summarizing statements or periods of conversation, catching points and clarifying their meaning in the discussion, returning the focus to the point.
- *Leading active listening*: It is not unusual for participants to fail to hear important points, especially from individuals with whom they disagree. As "Listener-in-Chief," catch possible breakthrough comments, check whether they have registered, and ask for clarification and verification. This may enable participants to hear something for the first time. Reflect facts and feelings back to speakers. When appropriate, ask whether a concern is shared by others.
- *Asking open-ended questions*: The success of interest-based mediation depends on the free exchange of information. As mediator, your job is to make people comfortable to speak the facts as they know them and to provide their

interpretations of situations: "Can you tell us more about this issue?" "Can you help us understand your view on this?"

- *Being a cheerleader*: People generate more options and more settlements when optimistic. So praise work done so far, thank participants for being forthcoming, and express optimism that the group will succeed.

- *Going quickly by going slowly*: Groups are often disappointed by the sluggishness of their own decision-making. But the quality of "solutions" improves if discussion of them is delayed until the group has completely described the problem, especially in complex situations. Do not jump immediately from the statement of the problem to a search for solutions. Take breaks, either during a session or when the group has reached an impasse. But if there is an impasse, state the nature of the difficulty so participants can think about it during the break. Use breaks to speak to participants individually about what they see, how they feel, and what they would suggest. Let people know that you will be speaking to members of the group and why. Be transparent in your actions. If the group is divided, avoid impressions of favoritism.

- *Providing a choice, not a demand*: If the group does not want to consider X, even though it must, ask the group a question with a choice: "Would you like to do X now or later?" "Would you rather do X by listening to each other's views or by collecting relevant facts?"

TWO OVERRIDING CAUTIONS

Be prepared for the following two developments, especially if multiple public health disciplines or sectors are involved.

The Tower of Babel

Help the group understand that every profession has its own "dialect," requiring everyone to learn a new language and to "translate" their terms into terms commonly understood by members of the group.

Divergent and Convergent Phases

All group work, especially among diverse participants who do not frequently work together, involves a divergent phase and a convergent phase. In the divergent phase, participants examine their situation from multiple perspectives—not necessarily clearly linked to a decision or agreement. Before the conversation starts to converge, participants may be overwhelmed by complexity and unsure about how to proceed—dissatisfied, discouraged, or pessimistic about progress.

Your success in facilitating mediation depends as much on managing expectations, normalizing reactions, perceiving the mood and energy of the group, and naming the issue and inviting the group to participate in determining how to address it as it does on your technical expertise or your ability to convene and chair a meeting.

Conclusion

If you keep a collaborative approach, a focus on interests, and active listening in mind and practice them outside of negotiation and mediation, you will find success where previously you found resistance. If you use those core principles in the basic four-phase process—state concerns leading to an interest-based agenda, gather information about those interests, generate options to satisfy these interests, and select an option using "objective" criteria—you will find that acknowledged disagreement can improve decisions.

You will find it easier to get participants to the table, keep them there, and achieve a useful resolution if you define your goals, build relationships, and use the leverage you have from understanding the interests and BATNAs of the parties.

The prime danger is not ignorance, but inaction. When people first confront a new technique, the danger is that they will freeze because they feel they lack perfect skills. There is nothing magic in negotiation and mediation. Many of the tools involved are familiar with from other problem-solving work. People have remarkably good instincts about what is happening and what should be done, even though they sometimes lack the vocabulary to put it into words or implement it. Remember that sincerity trumps technique. If you bring your "self" to the negotiation or mediation, your sincerity will be perceived—and often reciprocated. Perfection comes later.

RESOURCES

Books

Fisher R, Ertel D. *Getting Ready to Negotiate: The Getting to Yes Workbook*. New York: Penguin Books, 1995.
> *A valuable step-by-step guide to the application of the principles in this chapter, especially useful in preparing for negotiation.*

Fisher R, Shapiro D. *Beyond Reason, Using Emotions as You Negotiate*. New York: Penguin Books, 2006.
> *This book can help you to understand, use, and control your emotions during negotiation.*

Fisher R, Ury L, Patton B. *Getting To Yes: Negotiating Agreement Without Giving In*. New York: Penguin Books, 1991.
> *This book is filled with insights and retains its value as your experience grows. It has a useful summary for quick review of key points.*

Kritek PB. *Negotiating at an Uneven Table: Developing Moral Courage in Resolving Our Conflicts*. Hoboken, NJ: Jossey-Bass, 2002.

Marcus LJ, Dorn BC, Kritek PB, et al. *Renegotiating Health Care: Resolving Conflict to Build Collaboration*. Hoboken, NJ: Jossey-Bass, 1995.
> *These two books are valuable for negotiations related to public health and medical care.*

Shell R. *Bargaining for Advantage: Negotiation Strategies for Reasonable People* (2nd ed.). New York: Penguin Books, 2006.
> *This book is especially helpful for negotiations in business or professional situations with adversarial elements. It highlights the role of relationships and leverage.*

Stone D, Patton B, Heen S, Fisher R. *Difficult Conversations: How to Discuss What Matters Most.* New York: Penguin Books, 2010.

> *This book is especially useful for situations likely to "push your buttons." It addresses the complex interplay of fact, emotion, and self-concept and provides a practical way to deal with that complexity.*

Web Sites

www.iaf-methods.org

> *This Web site of the International Association of Facilitators provides free access to many methods related to multi-party decision processes and building consensus.*

www.mediate.com

> *A comprehensive source of articles, blogs, videos, and other information for negotiation and mediation.*

www.nafcm.org

> *This Web site of the National Association for Community Mediation can help locate your nearest community mediation association. Community mediation associations frequently provide both training and practice opportunities in conflict resolution and mediation.*

Commentary 14-1: Lessons Learned About Negotiation from a Career in Public Health

David J. Sencer

Although I don't consider myself primarily a negotiator, I recognize that some basic skills in negotiation that I learned over many years are helpful in being an effective public health leader. Here are a few of the lessons that I've learned, with examples from the time I was Director of the Centers of the Disease Control (CDC).

In positions of leadership, negotiation is for the most part negotiating with a higher unit in the hierarchy, whereas mediation is usually working to bring equals into agreement. The same principles hold for both.

1. Establish Yourself as Being Completely Honest and Admit There are Times You Don't Know an Answer

In 1965, a woman from Ghana was seen with a rash, which the CDC laboratory diagnosed as smallpox. Epidemiologically and clinically, this was chickenpox, but we made the decision to manage it as smallpox. Subsequently, it was proven to be chickenpox. Shortly thereafter, I testified for the first time before Congress. Although the subject was measles vaccine, I was suddenly asked, "Why, with all your experts, can't you tell the difference between smallpox and chickenpox?" My answer—"We made a mistake"—set the stage for 12 years of trust between Congress and CDC.

CDC's communication strategy during the 2009–2010 influenza pandemic was exemplary because CDC representatives were not afraid to admit that they didn't know all the answers—and that what is stated today may change by tomorrow.

2. Establish Your Position by Having the Best Science on Your Side When Creating Public Policy

For example, in 1962, the Surgeon General wanted the U.S. Public Health Service to buy all of the oral polio vaccine (OPV) and distribute it to state health departments. This strategy had been used in 1956 with the administration of Salk vaccine, which protected school-age children but did not reach those at greatest risk—disadvantaged preschool children. Also, this strategy focused public awareness on one preventable disease but neglected others. The alternative that we proposed—and that was adopted—provided vaccines (diphtheria-pertussis-tetanus [DPT] as well as OPV) for children under age 5 and funded states so they could organize their own programs to immunize children. Our alternative was less appealing to the public, but represented sounder public health science.

Another example of this lesson learned was when we at CDC insisted that the Food and Drug Administration and an intravenous (IV) fluid manufacturer recall large batches of contaminated IV fluids, based on our strong epidemiologic evidence—even in the absence of laboratory confirmation of the contamination. Once again, we established our position by having the best science on our side.

3. When Negotiating, Know When To "Fold"

For example, CDC proposed a program to improve clinical laboratory services that would have been based on giving grants to states to establish quality-control programs and to train laboratory workers—a traditional public health approach. However, the Secretary of the Department of Health, Education and Welfare (HEW, the predecessor to the Department of Health and Human Services) insisted on accomplishing lab improvement through a licensure program. The Secretary of HEW insisted that if we were going to improve the quality of clinical laboratories, there must be "teeth" (enforcement capabilities in the program), which states did not have. So we gave up our position—the traditional public health approach—knowing that ultimately the HEW Secretary's position would ensure improvement of clinical laboratories.

4. Be Willing To Take Risks When You Are Convinced Your Side is Right

In 1976, a new and potentially virulent strain of influenza virus appeared and although it did not seem to be spreading, we at CDC decided to immunize the susceptible population—most U.S. residents. To prepare for a possible epidemic, we were, in effect, stockpiling antibodies in people, rather than stockpiling antigen (vaccine) in warehouses. Although this decision was endorsed by the scientific and public health communities to protect the U.S. population against a serious pathogen, it involved some scientific and political risks, given that we were using a new vaccine. When problems arose with this vaccine, the program was terminated and it became a political issue. Ultimately, I lost my job as CDC Director because of this decision.

15

Collaborating with Others

Darrin K. Hicks and Carl E. Larson

Collaboration is the preferred way for public health organizations to operate. Collaboration can lead to increased accountability, more community and family engagement, consistent implementation of programs and delivery of services, improved cost-effectiveness, less unnecessary duplication and fragmentation of services, and, most importantly, significant improvements in the public's health.

Successful collaboration depends on a process through which stakeholders can communicate needs, weigh options, allocate resources and responsibilities, and make decisions. It depends on a climate of communication that fosters trust, shared commitment, mutual accountability, and a willingness to share risk.

Collaboration, Commitment, and Health Outcomes

Collaboration is a process through which people or organizations with diverse interests, backgrounds, and types of expertise work together to create new ways of understanding the causes of public problems and to consider novel solutions to these problems. Collaboration is also a means for forging new partnerships to implement programs that improve public health—partnerships designed to increase the scope of services, to eliminate waste and duplication, and to ensure that necessary resources are used to deliver these programs.

Collaboration has structural and process dimensions that are interrelated. In its *structural* dimension, collaboration is a means of organizing and managing the delivery of services, typically through the creation of new partnerships and other systems-level reform. In its *process* dimension, collaboration refers to the methods that groups use to identify needs, to share perspectives on important issues, to talk through any differences in perspectives, and to make consensual decisions that result in policy changes. The quality of a collaborative process directly affects the character of its partnerships and the quality of its outcomes.

Collaboration is a communicative process. All of its work is accomplished in and through communication. Therefore, it is necessary to clearly identify the various communicative processes present in various stages of collaboration and to measure their presence and, especially, their quality. It is important to measure the levels of stakeholder participation and the diversity and strength of network ties, and to focus on the ways in which communication creates, maintains, and transforms the identities of participants and thereby the responsibilities they will accept in relation to each other. This entails measuring the inclusiveness of the process, the standing of stakeholders, and the authenticity of the collaboration.

Collaborative structures are dynamic relationships that have been institutionalized. Collaborative relationships are built on the mutual commitment of two or more agents acting as a single body to accomplish a common goal. It takes much mutual commitment to collaborate—including commitments from all parties to work, if necessary, in unfamiliar areas and towards accomplishing collaborative goals, even if they do not necessarily further their own interests. The outcome of collaboration depends on the forms, functions, and quality of these relationships.

Parties create mutual commitment jointly, by communicating to each other that they are committed to accomplishing some goal together. When this occurs, possibilities for joint intention and mutual commitment emerge. Collaboratives can intend to do something together as a single body and be accountable to the general public or a government for accomplishing the goal.[1] This profound shift from "I" to "we" is at the heart of collaboration.[2] (See Chapter 13.)

The manner in which you communicate with others establishes the nature of your relationship with them. You experience this relationship in terms of the commitment that you have to it—a commitment that, in turn, motivates how much time and effort you will expend in accomplishing shared goals. The intensity of your commitment is interpreted from your language, your behavior, and the tone it establishes—a tone that is a way of communicating your orientation to the relationship. The process is circular and mutually constitutive; a change in one dimension of this process will result in permutations in the other two.

This process of generating and sustaining mutual commitment pervades every aspect of a collaborative initiative, from the initial meeting of interested stakeholders though the delivery of services. For example, in a collaborative initiative, stakeholders have commitments to:

1. Direct their work towards addressing serious problems that require collaboration for their solution
2. Establish and work within a *high-quality collaborative process*—one that is judged by stakeholders to be fair, open, and credible, and that can motivate stakeholders to engage other stakeholders in committing to the collaborative
3. Work with trust and respect for each other
4. Develop a new group identity and prioritize this identity and its interests when addressing the problem
5. Make resources available for the group to succeed

6. Select an implementing agency that has the requisite resources to implement the program and the cooperation of other agencies to ensure efficiency and effectiveness

Commitments #1 through #4 are considered *process* commitments; #5 and #6, *implementation* commitments. In addition, team leaders have a commitment to the integrity and fidelity (strict faithfulness to obligations) of the programs they implement. Also, front-line providers (those who work with targeted populations, such as physicians, nurses, and educators) have a commitment to deliver programs to those whom they serve. Both of these commitments are considered *program* commitments. Process commitments can drive implementation commitments, which, in turn, can drive program commitments.

The success and sustainability of a collaborative initiative is correlated with the level of the initial stakeholders' commitment and their ability to generate additional commitments from those who oversee and implement public health programs. The initial commitment to address problems by a collaborative process forms the basis for all of the other forms of commitment.

Two Features of a High-Quality Collaborative Process

Two features characterizing highly successful collaboration are strong process leadership and an open and credible process.[2] The presence of an open and credible process is what drives collaborative commitment. A collaborative process is open and credible when (a) stakeholders perceive that everyone has an equal opportunity to directly influence the decisions to be made, and (b) it is clear to all participants that decisions were not made in advance — with the process simply serving as legitimatization for these decisions. Stakeholders must be confident that the process is free from behind-the-scenes manipulation, that safeguards are present to check the disproportionate influence of powerful individuals, and that decisions are likely to affect the problem that the participants are addressing. People will perceive processes as fairer if they have an opportunity to influence these processes before decisions are made.[3,4]

Participants' judgments that a process is fair reflect interpersonal trust and determine whether people will cooperate.[5] Within a group, people continually "read" processes for cues to ascertain their personal status. When people perceive that they are being treated fairly—understood in terms of positive attributions of trust, neutrality, and standing—they will, in turn, feel valued, respected, and cared for by the group. As a result, they will see their individual identities in terms of their group membership—an identification which, in turn, results in an increased commitment to the group's projects and goals. In addition, they will see the integrity of the process as an expression of the group's integrity.

A high-quality collaborative process has the following five features:[6]

IT IS INCLUSIVE

Ideally, everyone affected by a problem is invited to participate in reflecting on the nature of the problem and designing plans to address it. An inclusive process moves beyond proportional representation towards reflecting the perspectives, experiences, and concerns of the broader community. Inclusion is a means for ensuring the presence of "unusual voices"—offering minority or different perspectives—in the process as well as those with command of resources. A diversity of views may help compensate for a non-diverse group of stakeholders because stakeholders may perceive the presence of "unusual voices" as a sign of genuine inclusiveness.

IT TREATS ALL STAKEHOLDERS EQUALLY

All stakeholders have an equal opportunity to influence the final decision. This opportunity is often experienced, ironically, as all participants feeling that they have a disproportionate chance to affect the final decision—that what they say could command the attention of the entire group and that their arguments could be persuasive. The process is free of favoritism. Each group needs to justify its position; nothing is taken for granted. (See Chapter 14.)

IT IS AUTHENTIC

Each participant believes that there is a good chance that what the group decides will actually be implemented. Stakeholders must believe that there are not powerful forces pulling the strings. A good process does not begin with the solution, but builds a transformative dialogue in which a novel solution can be created.

IT FOCUSES ON THE PROBLEM

Stakeholders trust each other enough to focus on the problem they collectively face, rather than trying to garner resources for their home organizations. The process must consider the real needs of the entire community, how each stakeholder contributes to the problem, and how each might contribute to its solution. The most important criterion for determining the merits of a proposal should be its focus on the problem.

IT IS REVISABLE

The process is open to revision if it has been unfair. There are sufficient opportunities to challenge decisions. And stakeholders feel they can contest decisions without fear of retribution.

High-quality collaborative processes are instrumental in keeping stakeholders engaged, fostering strong interagency partnerships, enrolling and retaining clients in programs, increasing the level of community involvement, ensuring that caregivers build strong relationships with those they serve, and implementing programs with fidelity.

The quality of the collaborative process should be understood and measured in the beginning stages of program implementation. The care taken to improve the quality of the process early in the development of the program or initiative will pay dividends later.

Successful programs share an important characteristic: Their success depends on the quality of the relationship between, for example, caregivers and clients, or among members of a community health organization. The stronger the relationship, the better programs perform. High-quality collaborative processes promote high-quality relationships that build off each other—and have a positive impact on critical interactions between, for example, caregivers and clients.

Strong process leadership differs considerably from traditional, hierarchical models of leadership that generally involve strong advocacy of a specific opinion. Process leadership involves bringing the appropriate people into the decision-making process and keeping them there through difficult periods, facilitating expression of divergent points of view while respecting differences and fostering convergence. It ensures that all stakeholders feel competent, trusted, and valued throughout the process. Strong process leaders promote high-quality collaborative processes.

Establishing a High-Quality Collaborative Process

Many factors determine the success of a collaborative process, but the most important is the quality of communication. Communication concerning goals facilitates teamwork, collaboration, and other forms of collective effort. It also generates the following types of energy:

- *Mental energy*: Creating strategies, thinking of options, developing plans, playing out scenarios, solving problems—all of the many mental operations involved in answering the question, "How are we going to get there?"
- *Physical energy*: Doing the work, gathering resources, building and testing a collaborative process—all of the many physical tasks necessary to reach a goal
- *Emotional energy*: Confidence, belief in one's self and one's partners, and a willingness to try, to persevere, to overcome obstacles, to remain optimistic, to never believe that you're helpless

Relative to other kinds of collaborative work, public health leaders enjoy distinctive advantages. Most collaborators in public health are people who are attracted to the goals of public health, rather than motivated by extrinsic rewards. So, public health leaders have an initial reservoir of energy on which to build.

They can build on this energy by articulating goals so as to inspire broader commitment to them, and by demonstrating their own commitment to these goals. Sustaining the energies of group members and keeping them focused on the goals represents the essence of leadership.

In the process, beware of factors that can drain energy, such as the following:

- _Competing goals_: For example, when the "managed" goal in "managed care" competes with the "care" goal
- _Relationship issues_: When dysfunctional relationships have an adverse impact on the performance of the group
- _Control issues_: When the question "Who's in charge?" becomes more important than "What should we do?"
- _Differing values_: When contention over team values or identity distracts team members from the goal
- _Helplessness_: When a team seriously doubts its ability to have an impact or when it goes through the motions without actually expecting any change

The kinds of energy present in a group and its focus determine the outcomes of the group's work. Effective leadership creates and sustains a communication climate that keeps constructive energy focused on the goals of the group.

The Communication Climate

As a leader, you should create a climate for communication that keeps constructive energy focused on the goals. The primary factor in accomplishing this is your behavior. Your behavior is contagious and is likely to be reflected in the behavior of those around you.

Behave the way you want others to behave. If you are trying to create an open and supportive climate, then your behavior should be open and supportive. And you should explain why you are open and supportive so others will not have to guess at your intent or your motives, and will be in a better position to help you.

Each member of your team is likely to perform better if you can establish supportive norms, such as the following:

- "It's okay to ask for help. Jump in and help each other out."
- "Don't wait until it's a crisis. Don't hide your problem until it gets to be a problem for everybody."
- "Keep performance and personality issues separate. Don't complain about somebody just because you don't like them."
- "Whenever you see something that's adversely affecting performance, let's talk about it. Performance is everyone's responsibility."

Open and supportive communication is best served by warm, personal energy. In contrast, cold energy is associated with low levels of safety and trust. A cold communication climate may be efficient, but it is distant, impersonal, and business-like.

To summarize, a group is likely to succeed if:

- Members occasionally get "jolts" of commitment from their leader.
- Their collective mental, physical, and emotional energy remains focused on the goals.
- With guidance from you as their leader, they construct a communication climate that is open and supportive.
- They recognize and manage energy drains.

Plugging the Energy Drains

Great leaders create a communication climate in which it is safe for any member of the group to report and discuss anything that is likely to adversely affect the group's work. As a result, the group can recognize "the elephant in the room" and address critical issues early.

As a leader, you must recognize and address any issue that is having an adverse impact on the performance of the group. The true test of your leadership is the extent to which you can encourage the group to commit all of its mental, physical, and emotional energy to the group's goals.

As a leader, your behavior is the primary mechanism for instilling a norm in the group to plug its energy drains. Your visible commitment—"walking the talk"—models behavior for all members of the group. As a result, everyone becomes responsible for the performance of the group. Everyone wants the group to succeed. Each group member learns that there are consequences associated with success—or failure.

Adopting a common methodology and a common language are ways to reinforce the group's norm. One methodology to accomplish this is *tagging*, which is raising an issue that needs to be discussed and resolved because it is affecting the performance of a group. You can "tag" an issue when you raise it to a more conscious level, point to it, or call it to the attention of others (Box 15-1).

If you decide to use tagging, you should do the following:

- *Prepare and plan tags*: Plan each tag carefully. Get feedback from one or two people before using each tag.
- *Avoid blaming anyone for the situation you are describing in the tag*: It does not matter how it got to be the way it is or who is responsible for it. Concentrate on what the group needs to do to improve the situation.

Box 15-1: **An Example of a "Tag" from a Team Member to the Entire Team**

"There's something that has been bothering me, and I'd like to know if anyone else is concerned about it. It's about our team. What we're doing—reducing deaths and disease from tobacco—is important and something we're all committed to. Most of the time, we work very well at it.

"But it's that time of the year again. Budget requests. So we'll probably see morale dropping, competition increasing, a lot of the same old backbiting and arguing about whose work is more important. And our work as a team will suffer.

"Does this bother anyone else, or is it just me?"

(Pause, Listen, and Discuss)

"I don't think it does much good to talk about who is guilty or past grievances. Can we talk about ideas? Who can think of something we can try—something we can do differently this year that might help?"

A good tag will usually have the following four parts:

Goal: What we're doing and why it's important

Observation: What I see happening that is affecting our performance

Pause and Listen for Feedback: For example, "Anyone else see what I'm talking about?"

Suggestion: Something we might try. Suggestions might come from yourself or others.

Give it a try. Think of a situation that should be tagged. Plan the tag by writing a sentence or two for each of these four parts.

- *Pause and listen*: Spend a minimal amount of time talking about the way you see the situation. Allow most of the time for other people to discuss how they see the situation.
- *Try something*: Enable the group to try something—anything. As long as you can help group members to remain in an experimental mode, they ultimately will find a solution to a problem.

Conclusion

Collaboration can create the conditions for more effective public health practice and improve program outcomes. Many factors contribute to the success of a collaborative achieving its goal and determine a leader's success. Nothing is more important than the communication climate created and sustained by the leader together with the group. An open and supportive communication climate is necessary for designing and sustaining a high-quality collaborative process.

The quality of the collaborative process and the communication climate ultimately determine the focus of the group's mental, physical, and emotional energy for attaining the goal. That energy is contagious. It can spread from the initial working group to an entire agency or organization. It can support the energy of frontline providers to build strong and successful relationships with those in need.

References

1. Gilbert M. Obligation and joint commitment. *Utilitas* 1999; 11:143–163.
2. Chrislip DD, Larson C. *Collaborative Leadership: How Citizens and Civic Leaders Can Make a Difference.* San Francisco: Jossey-Bass, 1994.
3. Lind EA, Kaufer R, Earley PC. Voice, control and procedural justice: Instrumental and non-instrumental concerns in fairness judgments. *J Personality Social Psychology* 1990; 59:952–959.
4. Tyler TR, Boeckmann R, Smith H, Huo Y. *Social Justice in a Diverse Society.* Boulder, CO: Westview, 1997: 88–90.
5. Lind EA. Fairness heuristic theory: Justice judgments are pivotal cognitions in organizational relations. In Greenberg J, Cropanzano R, eds. *Advances in Organizational Justice.* Stanford, CA: Stanford University Press, 2001: 56–88.
6. Hicks D. The promises of deliberative democracy. *Rhetoric and Public Affairs* 2002; 5:223–260.

RESOURCES

Books

Brown J, Isaacs D. *The World Café: Shaping Our Futures Through Conversations That Matter.* San Francisco: Berrett-Koehler Publishers, 2005.

This book describes how to create a "world café," a method for strategic collaboration that can engage members of a community or a group to talk about the future and about changes that they desire.

Chrislip DD. *The Collaborative Leadership Fieldbook.* San Francisco: Jossey-Bass, 2002.

This book is one of the most comprehensive and practical guides for how to establish and implement a truly collaborative process, including how to include stakeholders, set goals for your collaborative process, and create conditions for genuine dialogue.

Chrislip DD, Larson C. *Collaborative Leadership: How Citizens and Civic Leaders Can Make a Difference.* San Francisco: Jossey-Bass, 1994.

This book presents the two essential features of any successful civic collaboration: an open and credible process and strong process leadership. It uses case studies of 52 highly successful collaborations to explain how to implement these features in your own collaborations.

LaFasto F, Larson C. *When Teams Work Best: 6,000 Team Members and Leaders Tell What It Takes to Succeed.* Thousand Oaks, CA: Sage, 2001.

This book offers theoretically sound and practical advice for creating an open and positive team climate, with emphasis on how to identify and remedy the most common communication problems that can arise in collaborations.

Tyler T, Blader S. *Cooperation in Groups: Procedural Justice, Social Identity, and Behavioral Engagement.* Philadelphia: Psychology Press, 2000.

This book explains how people judge the quality of collaborative processes and how these judgments motivate the behavior of stakeholders. It helps one to understand why group members react as they do in collaborations.

Article

Ansell C, Gash A. Collaborative governance in theory and practice. *J Public Administration Research Theory* 2008; 18:543–571.

This meta-analysis of 137 collaborative initiatives identifies the essential components of successful public–private partnerships, with an especially fine account of how to deal with power differences.

Learning Modules on Collaborative Leadership

Turning Point Leadership National Excellence Collaborative, Robert Wood Johnson Foundation. Collaborative Leadership Learning Modules: A Comprehensive Series. Available at: http://www. turningpointprogram.org/toolkit/content/cllearncomp.htm. Also available from the National Public Health Leadership Development Network, St. Louis, MO, telephone: (314) 977–8145.

This series provides skill-building instruction for developing the capacity for collaborative leadership.

Commentary 15-1: Lessons Learned from Establishing a Collaborative Graduate Program That Evolved into a Collaborative School of Public Health

Audrey Gotsch and Michael R. Greenberg

In the early 1980s, New Jersey was the most populous state (population then: 7.4 million) without formal graduate education in public health. Yet the state had significant levels of many public health problems, including high rates of cancer, ambient air pollution, hazardous waste, substance abuse, and lead poisoning as well as other health problems related to substandard housing. Consequently, there was an enormous pent-up demand for academic education in public health.

Together we helped to create the first collaborative graduate program in public health (New Jersey Graduate Program in Public Health) to be accredited by the Council on Education for Public Health (in 1986), and also contributed to the subsequent establishment of the first collaborative school of public health to be accredited (in 2001)—the University of Medicine and Dentistry of New Jersey (UMDNJ)-School of Public Health. Today the School has 208 faculty members and 380 students.[1]

The two institutions that formed the New Jersey Graduate Program in Public Health and ultimately the School of Public Health were UMDNJ and Rutgers University. When the School was formed, the New Jersey Institute of Technology and the Public Health Research Institute also joined the collaboration, although the Public Health Research Institute is not currently included as an independent collaborator with the School due to a merger with UMDNJ. Based at UMDNJ, the School of Public Health is one of eight independent schools within UMDNJ— along with two medical schools, a school of osteopathic medicine, a dental school, a school of nursing, a graduate school of biomedical sciences, and a school of health related professions. The School of Public Health has worked closely with the other UMDNJ and Rutgers schools to develop dual-degree programs as well as research and service projects and, to a lesser extent, with the New Jersey Institute of Technology. The Rutgers primary partner has been the Edward J. Bloustein School of Planning and Public Policy, which also has an undergraduate public health program.

We have discovered that there are many advantages in a collaborative school, including shared resources for administration, less competition among faculty in the collaborating institutions, and development of collaborative research projects and community service programs. These projects and programs, which build on the strengths of each participating institution, are more effective than if they had been undertaken by one institution.

In the process of establishing and nurturing the growth of the collaborative program and the subsequent collaborative School of Public Health, we have learned several important lessons about collaboration that may be useful to you as you design and implement collaborative activities—be they projects, programs, departments, or schools of public health.

Think Big, but Start Small

When collaborating, start with a small group of committed, highly motivated people who know each other and share common goals. The initial collaborative New Jersey Graduate Program in Public Health and the subsequent collaborative UMDNJ-School of Public Health grew out of strong working relationships among participants who, over several years of working together on various projects, had come to know and respect one other. This was critical for the development of a sound foundation for the collaborative School of Public Health.

Develop a Shared Vision and Mission

When the School was founded, we invited all stakeholders to participate in developing a vision and mission statement. We agreed that our shared vision was: "The UMDNJ-School of Public Health is a nationally recognized, statewide partnership of educators, researchers, and practitioners working to improve the health and well-being of communities and populations." Our stakeholders also developed a mission statement that the School of Public Health is a "statewide, multi-institutional, multi-campus scholarly community dedicated to improving the health of diverse populations in New Jersey and elsewhere through collaborative research, teaching, and service." Not only did we develop these shared vision and mission statements after many hours of discussion and vetting by our stakeholders, but we widely disseminated the School's vision and mission to all faculty members and other stakeholders and regularly referred to them in annual reports, grant proposals, and other documents.

Obtain and Maintain Institutional Commitment

Institutional commitment is vital. We developed and have maintained a strong commitment for the School of Public Health from the senior leadership of the institutional partners. We initially presented information to our institutions' senior leadership on the need for the school and its projected value to research, education, and service. Support was secured from the president of UMDNJ to serve as the lead institution—a critical element to meet accreditation requirements.

We have helped to sustain support through successive senior leaders at our institutions by emphasizing the quality of the work of our faculty, students, and alumni; regular face-to-face meetings; and written communications that demonstrate the value of the School of Public Health to the universities and the State of New Jersey—and to public health education, research, and service.

Build from Existing Strengths

In developing collaboration, it is wise to build from existing strengths, and not try to take on too much at once. The School of Public Health evolved from a strong collaborative graduate public health program that was initially established by a department of environmental and community medicine within a medical school at UMDNJ and a school of planning and public policy at Rutgers. The program initially built on strengths in environmental health science and environmental health policy and then on capabilities in epidemiology, health education and behavioral science, health systems and policy, and biostatistics. Development of these strengths attracted faculty members and students and enabled the Program and later the School to develop research and education that focused on environmental health and other public health problems of concern in New Jersey. Additional academic concentrations were added to the degree programs as the disciplines of the faculty expanded with the growth of the School.

Develop and Implement a Strategic Plan

Strategic planning is vital. Initially and at regular intervals, we helped to develop a strategic plan for the School to meet the School's mission. The strategic plan was developed and supported by faculty from each of the institutions, as well as representatives of the alumni, students, staff, state departments, and community agencies. We have promoted adherence to the strategic plan and achievement of outcome measures that are used for annual planning and budgeting.

Ensure Equity Among Collaborators

When collaborating, make sure that all collaborators are treated equitably. Extensive negotiations enabled the establishment and application of equitable policies among the collaborating institutions on such issues as faculty appointments, governance, and tuition reimbursement. For example, when a faculty member who is based in a collaborating institution teaches a course in the School of Public Health or when a School of Public Health student takes a course in a collaborating institution, the faculty member's home institution receives financial credit for that tuition. In addition, faculty members in collaborating institutions hold positions on standing committees that are designated by the School's bylaws and are awarded equal faculty status within the School based on their faculty appointment at their home institution rather than serving as adjunct faculty members. While the School does award adjunct faculty appointments, these appointments are reserved for practicing professionals who share their expertise with our students.

Communicate Frequently and Widely

In collaborative work, frequent and widely disseminated communication is critical. We have promoted ongoing collaboration through regular communication channels such as newsletters and annual reports in print and online, and more frequent communication among administrators, faculty members, students, and staff members on all campuses and in all units of the School. Electronic media have greatly enhanced our communication channels.

Sustain Collaboration

Sustainability is a major challenge in any endeavor. Perhaps our greatest set of challenges has been in sustaining collaboration as time has passed and many of the people who were most directly involved in establishing the School of Public Health have moved on to different roles or have retired. We have attempted to achieve sustainability by creating a culture in the School that promotes and rewards collaboration among faculty members and students and among all collaborating institutions. In addition, the School's bylaws and policies have been embedded with practices that ensure that collaboration is maintained by the participants.

Collaboration is not easy. Our experience in helping to establish and develop the UMDNJ-School of Public Health has been challenging. It has been a very gratifying experience, however, to enable New Jersey's only school of public health to achieve its vision and fulfill its mission by preparing the next generation of public health professionals to improve the health of communities and populations through collaborative research, teaching, and service.

Reference

1. Greenberg M, Gotsch A, Rhoads G, Schneider D. Building and sustaining a multiuniversity and multicampus program or school of public health. *Am J Public Health* 2008; 98:1556–1558.

Commentary 15-2: A Funder's Work to Facilitate and Nurture Collaboration

Martin D. Cohen

In many jurisdictions, public health and human services are provided by multiple organizations—state, county, and municipal governmental agencies, nongovernmental organizations, community coalitions, individual practitioners, and private businesses. Often, these organizations have multiple funding sources that dictate how, and to which populations, services will be provided. At the community level, this pattern of service delivery and funding often results in fragmented systems of care, duplication of effort, and missed opportunities for service improvement. To address these issues, many providers have joined together through formal or informal collaborations that address specific public health issues, or address the needs of a particular geographic area or special population. Such collaborations have often resulted in significant improvement in health outcomes at the community level.

As successful as collaborations can be for improving public health services, getting organizations to work together is not an easy task. There are often organizational issues, such as competing agendas, inflexible processes, and time constraints. And there are the human elements: ego, pride, and dismissal of any idea that is not one's own. Therefore, collaborations also require a fair amount of facilitating and nurturing to take hold and be successful.

As a regional philanthropy addressing community health needs, the MetroWest Community Health Care Foundation has, since its inception in 1999, sought to improve how local services are planned and delivered in 25 communities west of Boston. The Foundation, formed from the sale of two local community hospitals, has as its mission "to improve the health status of the community, its individuals, and families through informed and innovative leadership." The Foundation's work is primarily that of a grantmaker, providing funds to support local public health and community services, but it has used its grantmaking as a platform to seek improvements in how community organizations work together to benefit those living in its target communities.

In 2000, a community needs assessment sponsored by MetroWest Medical Center found that there was a need to improve psychiatric and substance abuse services in the region.[1] At the same time, the Foundation observed that there were at least 15 community organizations concerned with provision of mental health and/or substance abuse services. Many of these organizations directly competed for limited state and local funds, including those from the Foundation. And, while there was a clear community focus on providing treatment services, there were no formal community initiatives that focused on prevention of, or early intervention for, behavioral health problems.

In 2001, the Foundation convened mental health and substance abuse agencies in the area to establish the MetroWest Task Force on Mental Health and Substance Abuse to examine mental health and substance abuse services in the region and make recommendations as to how these services could be better organized, financed, and delivered for the benefit of consumers and their families.[2] While there were other community coalitions in the region then, this was the first totally devoted to behavioral health.

The 34-member Task Force met over a 6-month period. The Foundation hosted the meetings and its president served as its chair. Other Foundation staff members also provided support. The group reviewed key indicators of service delivery, surveyed community needs, developed an understanding of the programs and services available in the region, and identified gaps in service delivery. The Task Force also became a forum for discussing common problems or issues in the delivery of care, such as inadequate reimbursement rates, difficulty in attracting qualified staff, and problems in engaging the region's growing immigrant population. These discussions came to be viewed by Task Force members as important as the work to develop recommendations.

In July 2001, the Task Force issued its final report, which contained recommendations for improving behavioral health care in the region. The Foundation encouraged Task Force members to continue to meet regularly to discuss how to implement the recommendations. It also challenged the group to develop collaborative approaches that could address the needs identified in the group's final report, and sought joint funding proposals from Task Force members that would support these approaches.

One need that generated significant cross-agency interest was the lack of mental health and substance abuse resources for young adults between the ages of 16 and 24, especially those who were making the transition out of state custody (such as foster care, juvenile justice, and children's mental health services). The Task Force asked the Foundation for help to better understand what kinds of programs and evidence-based services were available for this population. The Foundation responded by providing a small planning grant, which the Task Force used to engage a consultant to review the literature and develop plans for a pilot program that could be launched in the region.

The Task Force presented a plan to the Foundation for the creation of a young adult resources center, which would address the physical and behavioral health needs of young adults and assist them with education, employment, housing, and legal assistance. At the core of this model was a unique collaborative approach to service delivery, in which agencies providing these services would all commit to providing their expertise "under one roof." In all, five community agencies agreed to partner in establishing the young adult resource center.

For its part, the Foundation agreed to match this level of provider collaboration by creating a funders' collaborative that would pool funds to "seed" the project.

The Foundation also nominated the project for support under the Local Funding Partners Program of the Robert Wood Johnson Foundation. In 2007, the project was approved and received $496,000, which was matched by the Foundation and three other local funders.

The Tempo Young Adult Resource Center has now been operating for 4 years. It serves over 300 annually and has produced positive outcomes for most participants—67% improved their educational attainment level, 87% found appropriate housing, 92% remained drug-free and sober, and 99% of those on probation met their probation requirements.[3] In addition, the five participating provider organizations have changed the way they work together. Staff members from these agencies who previously did not know about the work of their counterparts or had considered them competitors now saw each other as extensions of themselves. The positive collaboration among these agencies has extended to other projects in the region, including work to improve the access of minorities to services.

For the Foundation, the work of the Task Force, the creation of the Center, and the positive outcomes for those served by the program demonstrate the importance of joining forces. But what does it mean to facilitate and nurture collaboration?

For the Foundation, fostering collaboration means creating the opportunity for community organizations to act as a team—in this case, the work of the Task Force. It also means creating incentives for organizations to *want* to collaborate. The Foundation used its grant funds both as a carrot—to prod organizations to develop collaborative models—and as a tool—to facilitate the planning and development needed for the collaborative to further develop its goals and to plan their implementation.

Fostering collaboration means *leading* when it is appropriate to do so, and *following* when the participants are firmly in control of the process. It also means modeling the desired behavior. For example, an important role the Foundation played in creating the Center was establishing a funders' collaborative to financially support its development—clearly demonstrating to the participants that the Foundation and other local funders valued a collaborative model enough for them to put aside *their* operating differences to fund the Center.

Developing a successful collaboration cannot be rushed. It takes time. The development of the Center took 3 years of planning and development before it was funded. This time span allowed the participating agencies to develop the working relationships needed for the project to succeed. Building relationships takes time—and there are often elements of a process that cannot be predicted beforehand. These include understanding each other's strengths and weaknesses, adjusting to differences in personalities and organizational cultures, and developing protocols needed for ongoing communication. While it might have been faster for one organization to try to develop the array of services provided by the Center, the collaborative allowed the project to capitalize on the expertise and knowledge of the participating agencies.

Collaborations succeed when there are clearly stated shared goals or purposes among the partners. The work of the Task Force helped to frame a common set of needs and actions that the group could focus on. Targeting a specific age group helped to further refine the goals of the partner agencies. Collaborations also succeed when participating organizations recognize and adjust to potentially competing agendas, which have the potential to undermine the collaboration process.

In a successful collaboration, there must be some form of mutual benefit that accrues to all partners. In other words, each partner needs to get something out of the collaboration. Sometimes, it may be new resources, such as a grant. But often there are other benefits that come from being part of the collaboration—publicity or recognition; access to new technology and business practices; education, training, and research opportunities; or just the added status of being connected to the project. Defining the benefits to be derived from the establishment of the Center helped to attract partners to the collaboration and to keep them involved.

Transparency is also vital to success. The more partners see, the more they will be invested. Transparency means having access to all important information, developments, and plans for the collaborative. In our collaborative process, partners shared critical documents throughout the process of developing a grant proposal, including agency budgets. They also developed written agreements that clarified the expectations, roles, and responsibilities of the partners once the program was established.

Finally, collaboration does not mean equality. In any collaboration, partners will have differing levels of participation, work, decision-making, and responsibility. There must be in the group a designated leader who can make decisions on behalf of all of the partners. Initially developing an understanding on this principle and clarifying how the group will make decisions throughout the partnership will help ensure its survival. For our collaborative project, a local agency, the Wayside Youth & Family Support Network, was vested with ultimate fiduciary responsibility, thus giving it decision-making authority for important financial decisions.

Funders, especially community-based foundations, are well suited to foster collaboration. Very often, their stature in the community and the promise of funding make them natural conveners who can bring disparate groups together to address complex issues. Their grantmaking can catalyze the work of community partners, helping to translate good ideas into innovative projects and programs. And their ability to form funder collaboratives can both model the desired behavior they seek to promote among community partners and create a more dynamic funding environment to support positive change for improved personal and community health.

References

1. *Final Report: Health & Human Service Needs Assessment of the MetroWest Community*. Framingham, MA: MetroWest Medical Center, Tenet Health Systems, Inc., 2000, p. 44.

2. MetroWest Mental Health & Substance Abuse Task Force. *Final Report & Recommendations*. Framingham, MA: MetroWest Community Health Care Foundation, 2001.

3. Saulnier B, Goodman G, Planchta-Elliott S. Young adults value participation, meaningful employment, and unconditional caring. *Focal Point: Transitions to Adulthood* 2010; 24:23.

Index

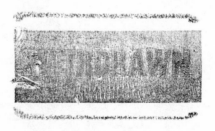